Herbal
Emissaries

Herbal Emissaries

BRINGING CHINESE HERBS TO THE WEST

A guide to gardening,
herbal wisdom, and well-being

STEVEN FOSTER and YUE CHONGXI

Healing Arts Press
Rochester, Vermont

Healing Arts Press
One Park Street
Rochester, Vermont 05767

LIBRARY OF CONGRESS CATALOGING-IN-PUBLICATION DATA

Foster, Steven, 1957–
     Herbal emissaries : bringing Chinese herbs to the West : a guide to gardening, herbal wisdom, and well-being / Steven Foster and Yue Chongxi.
          p.   cm.
     Includes bibliographical references and index.
     ISBN 0-89281-349-0 (pbk.)
     1. Herbs—Therapeutic use.   2. Medicinal plants—China.   3. Herb gardening. I. Yue, Chongxi. II. Title.
RM666.H33F67 1992
615'.321'0951—dc20   92-1054
                                                                                        CIP

Printed and bound in the United States

10 9 8 7 6 5 4 3 2 1

Photographs by Steven Foster.
Text design by Virginia Scott.

Healing Arts Press is a division of Inner Traditions International, Ltd.

Distributed to the book trade in the United States by American International Distribution Corporation (AIDC)

Distributed to the book trade in Canada by Book Center, Inc., Montreal, Quebec

Contents

Preface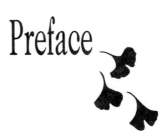

On May 14, 1987, I received a phone call that changed my life. The deep, heavily-accented voice stated, "This is Yue Chongxi from Beijing. I am in San Francisco. Can you pick me up at Little Rock Airport in three days?"

I could only answer yes.

Not knowing what to expect, my family and I—then in our remote Ozark location in Izard County, Arkansas—prepared for a Chinese visitor, Professor Yue Chongxi. He planned to be with us for at least eight weeks, which as it turned out stretched to eight months.

On the two-and-a-half hour drive to the airport, the chronology of events leading to Professor Yue's arrival flooded my mind. Through my long association with Dr. Shiu Ying Hu, a Chinese-born botanist who has spent her career at Harvard University's Arnold Arboretum, I had developed an interest in documenting Chinese medicinal plants found in American gardens. She had met Professor Yue in 1984 and suggested that he write me.

I began to correspond with Professor Yue in December 1984. A researcher with the Institute of Chinese Materia Medica of the Academy of Traditional Chinese Medicine, Beijing, he had indicated his desire to travel to America in his very first letter to me. I extended an invitation to him, thinking that the possibility of his visit was remote at best.

In 1986 through the Ozarks Resource Center, a nonprofit organization in Missouri, I was able to raise money for his trip. At the time I was director of their Ozark Beneficial Plant Project. We were charged with documenting beneficial plants of the Ozark Plateau, as well as plants with medicinal, fiber, and food uses from other regions that might be cultivated in our area.

By the end of 1986, Professor Yue had been denied a visa twice by the American Embassy in Beijing. Since before his call I had not heard from him for several months, with three days' notice of his arrival, I was less than well prepared for a foreign visitor whose diet, habits, needs, and ability to speak English (I knew no Chinese) were a complete mystery to me. Let alone the fact that he was coming from one of the world's most populated cities to "No Town, U.S.A.," deep in the Ozark foothills.

My American stereotypes of the Chinese began to crumble when the six-foot two Professor Yue emerged from the terminal. I soon learned that he was completely adaptable to any situation at hand. He made himself comfortable in an Ozark cabin and prepared gourmet Chinese meals from a limited selection of fresh foods. We quickly developed our own short-hand, bridging differences in botanical and medical terms. We became fast friends. Shortly after his arrival, our family no longer called him "Professor Yue." We knew him as "Lao Yue," a respectful nickname meaning "old Yue."

Lao has been a researcher with the Academy of Traditional Chinese Medicine since 1956, a year before I was born. The academy is China's main institution for researching traditional medicine, including the use of herbs and acupuncture. In his work, Lao has traveled to every province of China except Tibet and Taiwan, surveying folk medicine, collecting drug plants, and following leads on possible new drug plants. He has collaborated on more than ten books, including the 1977 edition of the *Pharmacopeia of the People's Republic of China*, the nation's official drug compendium, which includes over 700 plant drugs.

Dr. Hu had once mentioned that Lao was from a well-known medical family. Beyond that I knew little about him. Soon after his arrival I learned the depth of her statement. The Yue family has been known as traditional pharmacists and physicians in Beijing for over 400 years. Until a few years after liberation, the family operated Tong-Ren-Tang, Beijing's oldest pharmacy, in the same location since 1669. From the end of the Ming dynasty to the present day, Tong-Ren-Tang has served the pharmacy needs of the people of China.

During our eight months together, Lao shared his rich personal experience in the course of endless detailed discussions, interviews, and conversations on various aspects of the source plants used in traditional

Chinese medicine. Many of these plants are known in America as herbal products, flower garden subjects, ornamental trees and shrubs, or weeds. We visited several botanical gardens together, attended herb conferences, visited herb businesses, and collected specimens of American medicinal plants for the Institute of Chinese Materia Medica's herbarium. One result of these experiences and my subsequent trip to Beijing in 1988 to visit Lao Yue is this book.

Many people helped in the process of bringing Lao and myself together. Foremost among them is Dr. Shiu Ying Hu, botanist (retired) at Arnold Arboretum, Harvard University. Not only did she initiate our first contact, but she also assisted at various stages, among other ways by hosting Lao Yue's research at Harvard for five months in 1988. Without her help this collaboration and project would not have been possible.

The following persons also helped at various stages in arranging Professor Yue's travel to and stay in America: Howard Harrison of the American College of Traditional Chinese Medicine; Ken Murdock of Murdock Healthcare; Loren Israelsen, attorney at law; Lavinia McKinney and Sally Goodwin of Elixir Farm Botanicals; Ron Hughes and Denise Henderson of the Ozark Resources Center; Allen Yue; and Lisa O'Maley of the Shen Foundation.

Assistance and support that made the collaboration possible was generously provided by Ella Alford, Yolande Jurzykowski, the Threshold Foundation, and the Ozark Beneficial Plant Project of the Ozark Resources Center. Our heartfelt thanks to all of you.

We gratefully acknowledge the support of Dr. Hu Shilin of the Institute of Chinese Materia Medica, Academy of Traditional Chinese Medicine, in helping make Lao Yue's trip to America—as well as my trip to Beijing—possible. Huang Yiping, Zheng Meiyi, and Zhao Zhongzhen of the Institute provided useful English interpretations for Chinese concepts. Zhao Yan of the Institute of Medicinal Plant Development, Dr. Wang Kaimin of the National Institute for the Control of Pharmaceutical and Biological Products, Liu Tamu of the Beijing Botanical Garden, and officials of Tong-Ren-Tang Pharmaceutical Factory offered hospitality beyond the call of duty and thoughtful answers to the questions of a naive American. My deep gratitude goes to Jia Shu Ping, Le Yang, Yue Dong Ping, Song Hong Shu, and Yue Su Jun for offering warm friendship to a foreigner.

A number of people supplied useful information on Chinese medicinal plants throughout the research process. Thanks go to Mark Blumenthal,

American Botanical Council; Rebecca Perry, Lloyd Library and Museum; Dr. James A. Duke, Germplasm Resources Laboratory, USDA; Dr. Al Leung, AYSL Corporation, and Dr. Clifford M. Foust, Department of History, University of Maryland who provided critical comments on the Rhubarb (*Rheum*) chapter.

I would also like to acknowledge the support and patience of the staff of Inner Traditions, including Leslie Colket and Ehud Sperling. A special thanks to Cornelia Bland Wright for making a difficult editing task look easy. Thanks are also due to Mary Pat Boian for helping to keep me on track at the final stages of review.

Finally, due to circumstances beyond our reach, it was not possible for Lao Yue to review my changes once the final manuscript was completed. Therefore, any errors are not those of the above-named friends and colleagues or my coauthor, but are mine alone.

Steven Foster
Eureka Springs, Arkansas
December 1991

Introduction

CHINESE HERBS IN THE WEST

The herbalist's appreciation of plants reaches to the beginnings of human memory. That appreciation has led to using plants to enhance flavor and preserve foods, to conjure precious fragrances to excite all the senses, and to heal the ills that befall the human form. Nowhere is this thread of human history so prevalent, lasting, and deep as in China.

The famous plant hunter, Ernest "Chinese" Wilson (1876–1930), is responsible for the introduction of over 1,500 Asian plants species to Western horticulture. He was a renowned collector for the famous English Veitch Brothers horticultural firm and for Harvard University's Arnold Arboretum. One of his many books is titled *China: The Mother of Plants*. This title is very fitting; with an estimated 30,000 flowering plant species, China possesses the most diversified and rich flora in the temperate zones.

At least 5,000 of those plant species can be documented as having been traditionally utilized as medicinal plants in China. Approximately 500 plants species serve as "drugs" in modern traditional Chinese medicine. Many of these plants are used as foods. The line between foods and drugs is often obscure. In China, plants used as "drugs" are distinguished from plants used as "herbs" or "folk medicines." The 1985 edition of the *Pharmacopeia of the People's Republic of China* includes about 500 official plant drugs. The 1977 edition of the *Pharmacopeia* listed approximately 700 species; this 30 percent reduction in official plant drugs from the 1977 to 1985 editions is due to the fact that many drug plants were dropped because they were not widely available.

Since Chinese-American relations began to warm in the early 1970s, a tremendous interest in Chinese herbal folk traditions and traditional Chinese medicine (TCM) has emerged. TCM has captured the fancy of the West perhaps more than any other single aspect of Chinese culture. Over the past twenty years, the West has experienced an ever-increasing interest in a wide variety of alternative medical practices. One form of treatment that has made greater legal inroads than any other single therapy is acupuncture. Just fifteen years ago, acupuncture in the West consisted of little more than fantastic reports of needles being used for anesthesia in surgery or for treating conditions ranging from arthritis to migraine headaches. Today, more than half of the states in America license non-physician acupuncturists.

American acceptance of herbal medicine may indeed, like acupuncture, sneak through the back door from China. Soon after the revolution that ended with "liberation" in 1949, Mao Zedong delivered a mandate to the Chinese people to validate the efficacy of traditional remedies. "Weed through the old and bring forth the new," he ordered—then combine the best of Western medicine and traditional remedies. The successful integration of TCM and Western medicine in the People's Republic of China is a model for the role of herbal medicine in the modern world. Increased worldwide interest in traditional herbal medicine among scientists, pharmaceutical companies, governments, and international organizations can be largely attributed to the remarkable success of herbal medicine in the People's Republic of China.

This interest has resulted in dozens of English-language books about TCM and the medicinal plants it uses. Some books are for popular consumption, while others are targeted at the hundreds of acupuncturists or other health care practitioners who now incorporate Chinese herbs in their practice. These books explain traditional uses, theory, prescriptions, and practice. However no book in English has focused on a broad coverage of source plants used in Chinese tradition, a number of which are also known as ornamentals, weeds, or herbs to Westerners. We hope that this book will fill that gap.

Herbal Emissaries

This is a book about human-plant interactions. It is about how some Chinese herbs came to be known in America—but not necessarily as medicinal plants! Most Chinese medicinal plants served over the centuries as emissaries of their culture based on their physical characteristics, their reflection of the curious beauty of the Far East. Now, thanks to the new interest in alternative medical practices, these plants are serving more and more as emissaries of the medical tradition they have been a part of for thousands of years.

Many Chinese medicinal plants are better known to the vast majority of Americans as ornamental garden perennials, among them day lilies, forsythia, chrysanthemums, and peonies. Others are known as shade or fruit-producing trees, such as white mulberry, ginkgos, or the silk tree. Some, like privet, are best known as hedge plants. We regard Japanese honeysuckle and kudzu as noxious weeds, but the Chinese view them as medicinal plants.

Some important Chinese herbs such as the Baikal scullcap (*Scutellaria baicalensis*) are best known in the West among rock gardening enthusiasts. Gardenias are best known as cut flowers grown by florists. Still other plants, like the hardy rubber tree (*Eucommia ulmoides*), are known as rare exotics, primarily found in the collections of botanical gardens and arboreta.

Through a joint exchange program with the Guangdong College of Traditional Chinese Medicine, the University of California at Berkeley Botanical Garden, and the American College of Traditional Chinese Medicine in San Francisco, a special garden of Chinese medicinal plants has been established at the University of California at Berkeley Botanical Gardens. Some Chinese medicinal plants that cannot be seen elsewhere in the United States are found at this garden. Whether they are considered garden ornamentals, weeds, rock garden specimens, or rare cultivated plants, they all have one thing in common. They are all important herbal medicines in Chinese tradition.

Since a time thousands of years ago when early humans made the transition from hunter-gatherer to agricultural societies, plants have traveled with humans. Hundreds of plant species were adopted from their wild haunts and cultivated for food, fiber, medicinal, or other uses. As humans moved from one location to settle in another, we have taken seeds or other propagules of these plants to cultivate for basic needs. These plants have included vegetables, culinary herbs, medicinal herbs, fruit-producing trees and shrubs, and other useful plants. Plants commonly referred to as "weeds" have tagged along, perhaps attaching their seeds to clothing or animal fur, establishing themselves in new locations without human's consciously intending to introduce them. Still other plants have been introduced to one region from another because of their beauty. These ornamentals include trees, shrubs, and garden flowers. All of these non native or alien plants, whether cultivated or naturalized (established without deliberate cultivation), are known as *exotics* in any given flora.

North America has about 18,000 species of native flowering plants. An equal or greater number of plants are exotics in America, either cultivated for food or ornamental use or established as weeds. Over 20,000 plant species, both exotics and natives, are found in American horticulture. It is estimated that between 14 to 18 percent of plant species growing in eastern North America are weeds. Two thirds are from Europe, and the other third is mostly from Asia, along with a few subtropical American representatives.

Starting with the explorations of Marco Polo in the thirteenth century and the landing in China by Portuguese sea traders in the sixteenth century, there has been a steady flow of plant introductions from East to West. Linnaeus's famous *Species Plantarum*, a botanical compendium published in 1753, described one hundred species of Chinese plants. By the late eighteenth century, Britain's Royal Botanical Gardens at Kew was actively introducing Chinese plants. When the first volume of William Aiton's *Hortus Kewensis*, or catalog of plants cultivated in the Royal Gardens at Kew, was published in 1789, Chinese plants in English gardens included the hollyhock (*Alcea rosea*), camellia (*Camellia japonica*), golden rain tree, (*Koelreuteria paniculata*), tree of heaven (*Ailanthus altissima*), crape myrtle (*Lagerstroemia indica*), matrimony vine (*Lycium chinense*), and gardenia (*Gardenia jasminoides*), to name a few.

The major objective of most Western botanists in China has been to discover useful plants, especially ornamental flowers, shrubs, and trees, that are hardy in northern climates. Of all parts of the world from which plants may be introduced to North America, temperate East Asia has held the most promise because of the similarity of climates and the great diversity of plants. Most plant introductions that were grown for curiosity or ornament were bought from East Asia by Jesuit, Swedish, Russian, Portuguese, English, or French collectors during the previous two centuries. Collectors like Ernest Wilson and the Dutch-born, turn-of-the-century U.S Department of Agriculture (USDA) collector, Frank N. Meyer (1875–1918) introduced more than 3000 types of economic and ornamental plants to the West. Although virtually all of Wilson's and Meyer's introductions were intended as ornamentals or food plants, many of them, coincidentally, are Chinese medicinal herbs. Indeed, American flower gardens, fields, forests, and parks are a rich source of Chinese medicinal plants.

Plants have not traveled in only one direction. Nearly one hundred of the species of exotic plants that have been introduced to China from other regions have, over the centuries, been adopted as medicinal herbs. Some exotic plants arrived in China from other regions in prehistoric times. Hemp (*Cannabis sativa*), once thought to be a Chinese native, is now believed to have been introduced as an exotic plant to China from southwest Asia by Neolithic man at least five thousand years ago. The African species *Sesame orientale*, the source of sesame seed, was recorded in Chinese herbals in the first century A.D. Mediterranean herbs, well-known in European and American herb gardens, such as rosemary (*Rosmarinus officinalis*), were known in China and adopted for medicinal use as early as 739 A.D. The tropical South American red pepper (*Capsicum frutescens*) was recorded to be adopted as a medicinal plant in China by 1621. People of the ancient world traveled extensively, and plants migrated with them (S. Y. Hu 1990).

Chinese immigrants who arrived in the Americas in the eighteenth and nineteenth centuries brought medicinal herb products from their homeland. They developed their own cultural centers, the Chinatowns of major American cities. Until about twenty years ago, Chinese herbs were available only as dried plant materials in exotic Chinatown pharmacies, or Chinese groceries.

When interest in herbs for health purposes began to reemerge in the early 1970s, with the help of warming relations between the United States and China, Chinese medicinal herb products began appearing on the shelves of American health and natural food stores. Now, many Chinese herbs are familiar to herb consumers in the United States. They include dang-gui (*Angelica sinensis*), schisandra or *wei-zi* (*Schisandra chinensis*), Chinese licorice root or *gan-cao* (*Glycyrrhiza uralensis*), Asian ginseng (*Panax ginseng*), and the traditional Chinese herbal product *ci-wu-jia* (*Eleutherococcus senticosus*), sold in the United States as Siberian ginseng or eleuthero. The system of healing that has produced these herb products is one of the oldest and most highly developed medical systems the world has ever known. By combining its vast wisdom and experience with scientific developments, it has emerged as an important modern health care system.

FROM ANCIENT MEDICAL SYSTEM TO MODERN HEALTH CARE

Traditional Chinese medicine is an integral part of the culture, not just of today, but of a continuous tradition going back at least five thousand years. From the beginnings of imperial rule over four thousand years ago to the end of the Qing dynasty, which ended in 1911, more than 10,000 books on traditional Chinese medicine, including four hundred herbals (or *ben cao*), were written. *Huang Ti Nei Ching Su Wen*, the *Internal Classic* or *The Yellow Emperor's Internal Classic*, one of the oldest and most comprehensive extant medical works in China, was written around 300 B.C. Its 18 volumes encompassed basic TCM theory, information on hygiene, clinical symptoms, acupuncture and moxibustion, and prescriptions and drugs. It also recorded the theories of the viscera and bowels, meridians, and yin and yang.

The oldest comprehensive herbal, the *Shen Nong Ben Cao Jing*, written about two thousand years ago and attributed to the "Divine Plowman Emperor" Shen Nong, contains 365 drugs, one for every day of the year, which are divided into three classes. The first class included "superior" herbs that were considered nonpoisonous, had rejuvenating properties, and could be taken for long periods of time without side effects. Medicines in the second or middle class were said to have a tonic effect, but could be toxic depending upon the dose and duration of administration. The third class included "inferior" medicines that were used for the cure of specific conditions, but could be considered potentially toxic and should only be used for acute conditions over a short period of time. The original text of this herbal was lost long ago; all that we have now is a list of the drug names with their simple functions and properties.

The next important herbal is *Xin Xia Ben Cao (Tang Ben Cao)*, written by Su-gong, Li-ji, and 20 other officers of the court. It was published by the government of the Tang dynasty in 659 A.D. and is thus the world's first official pharmacopeia. The most famous herbal is *Ben Cao Gang Mu*, which includes 1,892 drugs, published in 1596. Its author, Li Shi-zhen, compared closely related species and enumerated their similarities and differences. In his plant descriptions, he was the first to distinguish between true source plants and adulterants. The scientific arrangement of his text agrees closely with modern systems of botanical classification. His completed work consisted of 16 parts in 52 volumes. Its illustrations are rather crude, but the book is still considered one of the most important Chinese *materia medica* and has been translated into seven languages.

These works and many others mentioned in the text serve as the basis for modern TCM, a system of health care that incorporates hundreds of herbal medicines, acupuncture, and other modalities to provide primary health care for over one quarter of the world's population. TCM is a unique medical system with its own theories of disease, "energy," and ways of perceiving uses of plants. The system includes tongue and pulse diagnosis, acupuncture, and herbal prescriptions, which may consist of from three to over 100 medicinal plant ingredients. The Chinese distinguish between plants used as "drugs" in TCM and "herbs." Approximately 500 plant species produce TCM drugs. Root drugs are most important, seeds and fruits are second in importance, and leaf drugs are the least important.

It is remarkable during these days of the rapid technological development of modern western medicine that the wisdom of the ancient system of TCM has been preserved, enhanced, and crystallized for application to modern health care problems. The *Internal Classic* in addition to the ancient *ben cao* are still essential textbooks in schools of TCM, both in China and the West.

In 1929 the Koumintang government of the Republic of China attempted to eliminate TCM by banning traditional medicine in order to clear the way for the development of modern medicine. TCM was suppressed and declared illegal. The ensuing forty years were a time of great upheaval in China, marked by civil war and periods of occupation by the Japanese, but TCM continued to thrive.

Soon after the People's Republic of China was established in 1949, the government recognized that TCM could play a major role in national health care. A policy was formulated, based on the health care needs of the country, that strove to develop, systematize, and enhance the practice of TCM. An effort was made to bring together and train TCM doctors to optimize the initiative. Western-style medical institutions developed education programs to teach Western-trained physicians about TCM. Using modern scientific methods, the pharmacology, chemistry, and clinical applications of TCM were gradually modernized. Public health policy mandated that Chinese and Western medicine be integrated, developed, and researched in a planned and rational way. A concerted effort was made to protect, utilize, and develop Chinese medicinal plant resources. The results of these public health policies not only preserved and enhanced TCM in China, but brought it to the attention of the rest of the world as well (Wang Pei 1983).

Today China recognizes three systems of medicine—Western medicine, TCM, and a combination of the two systems. However, preventative medicine takes precedence over the three systems of treatment mentioned above. Up to 80 percent of the people in China's vast rural areas still rely upon TCM for their health care. In urban areas about 40 percent of the population choose to use TCM, especially the elderly who believe in and rely on this ancient system of health care.

In 1952, three years after the establishment of the People's Republic of China, five schools of TCM were established. Now there is an institute of advanced TCM training in each province and autonomous region of China. The development of extensive education programs is one of the major modern achievements of TCM.

Chinese scientists have instituted extensive and sophisticated screening and production programs for medicinal plants. In modern China, numerous institutions with hundreds of chemists, botanists, and medical researchers study traditional drugs. Western scientific methods are used to document herbal medicine source plants in all parts of China. Botanical, pharmacological, chemical, and clinical studies have been carried out, catapulting TCM into the modern world. Indeed, the dozens of technical botanical, chemical, pharmacological and clinical Chinese herbals produced over the past two decades make most American herb books look like the work of amateurs in comparison. The Chinese have also produced a number of excellent provincial illustrated field guides to medicinal plants. China has now emerged as a world leader in medicinal plant research.

The main institution for the modern advancement of TCM is the China Academy of Traditional Chinese Medicine in Beijing. Founded in 1955 as a national center for research, health care, and teaching about TCM, the academy has 16 institutes, including two hospitals, that employ more than 3,300 researchers and technicians.

The research of some of these institutes is worth mentioning here. The Institute of Chinese Materia Medica is a World Health Organization collaborating center for traditional medicine. Over the past 35 years, more than 300 researchers in the institute have carried out extensive investigations of Chinese medicinal plants. One of their major achievements was the isolation from sweet Annie, or *qing-hao* (*Artemisia annua*), of a substance to treat quinine-resistant malaria. This has been used in China with nearly 100 percent success in thousands of cases. This institute is just one of several medicinal plant research groups in Beijing alone.

Founded in 1983, the Institute for Medicinal Plant Development (IMPLAD), located on the outskirts of Beijing, employs more than 350 scientists in nine departments carrying out research on various aspects of Chinese medicinal plants. Its researchers include botanists, agronomists, organic and analytical chemists, and pharmacologists. IMPLAD's primary focus, alongside research on traditional drugs, is the development of new medicinal plant resources. Areas of research include production techniques, new processing and extraction methods, tissue culture experimentation, and chemical and pharmacological studies. Scientists at IMPLAD's Department of Medicinal Fungi have developed an injectable immunostimulant drug from the reishi mushroom (*Ganoderma lucidum*) that can be used as an adjunct therapy for cancer patients undergoing chemotherapy. Other IMPLAD researchers have successfully cultivated the rare Chinese orchid *Gastrodia elata*, used to promote male virility, for the first time. Previously, this expensive and rare orchid could only be harvested in the wild. IMPLAD also has the largest medicinal plant garden in north China, which covers at least three acres and contains over 1,300 species of medicinal plants. A large greenhouse contains specimens of important economic plants of the tropics. IMPLAD has two branch institutes located in tropical regions, one in Yunnan province in southwest China and another on Hainan Island in the South China Sea.

One of the greatest achievements of Chinese research programs is the systematic identification of the exact source plants used in TCM. China's version of the Food and Drug Administration (FDA), the National Institute for the Control of Pharmaceutical and Biological Products (NICPBP), produces China's official drug compendium, *The Pharmacopeia of the People's Republic of China*. A country's pharmacopeia is a listing and description of drugs officially recognized by the medical establishment or government. For example, the United States Pharmacopeia (USP) has been published and periodically updated since 1820. The NICPBP maintains 40 regional offices that monitor traditional drug production, collection, and identification. They set standards for the identity and use of "official" plant medicines used in TCM. The NICPBP employs over 800 staff members, including 400 scientists, 100 of whom are professors and associate professors. Thirty scientists in the TCM division are involved in teaching, research, and testing. Their outstanding collection of herbal medicine samples contains 80,000 specimens of drug plants from all over China, along with specimens of substitutes or adulterants. This collection is used for quality-control research.

The NICPBP has edited a new English-language work on Chinese medicinal plants, *Colour Atlas of Chinese Traditional Drugs*, vol. 1, (Beijing: Science Press, 1987). The first of three volumes, it lists 150 drugs, with botanical descriptions, descriptions of the dried herb, identification characteristics, and notes on the use and form of the herb.

Other medicinal plant research institutions in China include the Shanghai Institute of Materia Medica, world renowned for its studies on the chemistry of medicinal herbs. Researchers there have recently isolated huperzine A, a substance obtained from Chinese club moss, which shows promise in the treatment of Alzheimer's disease. The Institute of Chinese Materia Medica in Sichuan province is famous within China for the quality of its research. Sichuan produces more herbal medicines than any other province. In 1988 a new institution was established in Guangxi province to study "ethnic medicines" used by minority groups in China.

There are over 100 nationalities in China. The Han people comprise about 98 percent of the population. The remaining 2 percent of the population includes such groups as the Dai people of southwest China, the nomadic tribes of Inner Mongolia, and the Tibetan people to the west. Each of the minority population groups has its own distinct traditional medicine and medicinal plants.

The Chinese make a clear distinction between plants used as "drugs" in TCM and the "herbs," folk medicines or nationality medicines that are used by people in the countryside and are not recognized as drugs in TCM. While 500 plants are used as "official drugs" in TCM, about 4,500 folk medicines are documented in China. The distinction is as clear as the gap between herbal medicine and Western medicine in the United States. An herbalist in a remote village may take pride in being able to cure a disease that doctors of TCM may not have success in treating. Intensive research on nationality or folk plant uses has resulted in the addition of some of the nationality folk medicines to China's official drug compendiums.

Part of Prof. Yue's work has been to travel to remote regions to study such folk cures. He and several other researchers once traveled to Hainan Island in the South China Sea to follow up on a report of an herb that was reportedly successfully used as a contraceptive. What the researchers found, however, was that it was used primarily by women in their mid-forties and had only a 40 percent success rate!

These are just a few of the research institutions that have helped to modernize, systematize, and raise TCM to a new level of understanding and utilization. The scientific information they have developed has served as a bridge between traditional knowledge and the modern world. This research, coupled with several thousand years of traditional wisdom, has established TCM as a health care system that serves about one quarter of the world's population.

In *Herbal Emissaries* we draw on that knowledge to present new information on Chinese herbs to a Western audience. Most of the plants in the book are familiar to Westerners as exotic introductions to horticulture, as weeds, or as herb products that are available not only in Chinatown herb shops, but also in health and natural food stores all over North America. This book is meant to serve as a bridge between East and West—the American people and the Chinese people.

Using Plants as Drugs in Traditional Chinese Medicine

Yue Chongxi

What is the traditional Chinese *materia medica?* Some might answer, "Traditional Chinese *materia medica* is the roots of herbs and the barks of trees." This is only partly true. Another person might answer, "It is licorice roots, Chinese rhubarb and so on." That answer is not exact, either. Many nationalities in China use the herbs in their own way, just as other countries, including the United States, Russia, and others do: the way the herbs are used is as important as the ingredients themselves. Perhaps a correct answer to the question is that the traditional Chinese *materia medica* is a group of natural drugs and their preparations that are used according to the theories of TCM.

Some traditional Chinese drugs are based on animal and mineral ingredients, but plants are by far the most commonly used Chinese drugs. The major plant parts used are the root and the fruit (including seeds). *The Handbook of Traditional Drugs*, the first drug book published after the liberation of 1949, lists 517 different drugs, which can be broken down according to their ingredients:

Roots: 120	Fruits: 130	Herbs (leaf and stem): 50
Leaves: 15	Flowers: 40	Bark: 20
Stems: 25	Animal parts: 45	Minerals: 30

THE PRINCIPLES OF CHINESE *MATERIA MEDICA*

In order to use traditional Chinese medicine effectively in clinical situations, traditional doctors must have a firm grasp of its rules and characteristics. These include the four properties and five flavors, the "trend" of the functions or effects of the drug, the attributive channel through which the drug enters the body, compatible applications of the drug, and incompatibilities in prescriptions. In Western tradition, herbalists pay little attention to the four properties and five flavors of traditional Chinese drugs, and are primarily concerned with the effects. But the four properties and five tastes are the guiding principles behind using Chinese *materia medica.*

Properties

The four properties are cold, hot, warm, and cool. The general principle of treatment is to treat heat-syndrome diseases with cold-natured drugs, and cold-syndromes with warm-natured drugs. Patients with heat-syndrome diseases have heat-related symptoms, including fever, or a red face. They need cold-natured drugs. Patients with cold-syndrome diseases have a pale face, poor appetite, and a feeling of weakness in the limbs. They need warm-natured drugs. If the doctor makes a wrong judgment about the property of the disease it is like lighting charcoal in hot weather or adding frost to snow. The doctor will not only fail to cure the disease, he or she may make the condition worse.

Recently, many people in China have begun to pay attention to the properties of food. Drugs have long been recognized as having different properties, but foods do as well. For example, the bitter gourd has a cold nature; the mung bean is cool-natured, as is the soft-shelled turtle. Longan and litchi fruits are hot natured, mutton is warm natured, and pig meat is mild, or has a neutral nature.

Flavors

The five flavors of TCM are sour, bitter, sweet, hot (acrid), and salty. In ancient times, traditional doctors found that the different taste of drugs produced different clinical results. Acrid (pungent or hot) has the function of expelling cold. Sour has an astringent function. Sweet has the ability to mitigate or alleviate pain. Bitter drugs have the function of hardening or drying tissue. Salty drugs are able to soften hard lumps, such as tumors.

Bland flavors belong to the sweet category, while astringent drugs or foods belong to the sour category. Ginger is hot (acrid), so it can expel cold. Schisandra has five tastes, but the major one is sour, so it has the ability to stop sweating. Astringent nuts are sour, so they can stop diarrhea. Ginseng is slightly sweet and helps to invigorate vital energy. Licorice root has the ability to regulate and enhance the functions of other drugs and reduce poisonous qualities of somewhat toxic drugs. Salty drugs, such as oyster shell, can soften tumors and are used to treat the first stages of cancers. Some drugs have more than one flavor; the first , or primary, taste of the drug is used to determine its properties.

Trends of Drug Functions

There are four trends of drug functions: lifting, lowering, floating, and sinking. These four terms show the way in which the drug acts. Drug actions have different "directions." Diseases are also classified according to their direction. For example, a cough rises from the bottom to the top. Sweat moves from the interior to the exterior. Diarrhea moves from the middle part to the bottom. Menstrual dysfunctions travel downward. In TCM the rule is to use drugs that have an opposite direction to the direction of the disease. For treating coughs, traditional doctors use antitussive or antiasthmatic drugs whose effects are downward. Treating hernias calls for drugs with "lifting and floating" actions, such as citrus seeds.

While most drugs have only one direction, the action of some drugs moves in two directions. For example *Cimicifuga* (cohosh) has the ability to first rise, then move lower. The function of kudzu vine is lower at first, then rises. Ginseng can move in several directions. Therefore, it is not only good for patients with high blood pressure, but with low blood pressure as well. Methods of preparation or combining prescriptions can also change the direction of drugs.

Some drugs have another characteristic—the ability to lead other medicines to specific places in the body. The root of balloonflower (*Platycodon*), for example, can lead drugs to a higher area of the body, so it is used as an ingredient in prescriptions for colds, coughs, and head ailments. *Achyranthes bidentata* (*niu-xi*) can take other herbs to lower regions, so it is useful in prescriptions for diseases centered below the diaphragm.

Attributive Channels

The attributive channel indicates the particular meridian, organ, or group of organs in the body, on which a drug has a major effect. In the theory of TCM there are five viscera (the five *yin* orbs)—heart, liver, spleen, lung, and kidneys. There are six bowels (the six *yang* orbs)—gallbladder, stomach, large intestine, small intestine, bladder and the "triple burners" in the human body. The triple burner refers to three parts of the abdominal cavity. The upper burner is the part that includes the heart and lungs, and lies above the diaphragm. The middle burner is the part of the abdomen housing the spleen and stomach. It lies between the navel and diaphragm. The lower burner represents the abdominal cavity below the navel, housing the kidney, urinary bladder, intestines, but includes the liver as well because of its relationship to the kidney (Liu 1988, vol. 1, p. 23). Separately, the viscera and bowels belong to twelve channels (some scholars believe there are fourteen channels). Sometimes a traditional herbal drug enters more than one channel. Certain cold-natured herbs, for example, are specifically used for clearing away "liver-fire" or for clearing away "stomach fire." Some herbs are general tonics, while others may be specifically tonic for the kidneys, spleen, or other organs.

PROCESSING TRADITIONAL CHINESE DRUGS

The processing of traditional Chinese drugs, *pao-zhi*, is based on the theories of TCM, clinical uses by TCM doctors, and the production of Chinese drugs. While in Western herbalism most drugs are used in their crude form, in China almost all drugs are processed in a variety of ways before use. The main purpose is to increase the clinical effect, enhancing the quality and the safe use of the medicine. Processing can also fulfill other requirements.

Standards of cleanliness and purity of collected materials are maintained through careful processing. Since plants, animals, and minerals are natural substances, they are often collected with foreign matter or additional parts that are not considered medicinal. For example, Japanese honeysuckle flowers can be used, but the leaves that are attached to them must be removed. Fruits sometimes have stems attached. Tree bark often is covered with lichens and mosses. All of the foreign matter can affect the healing properties of the drug and should be removed during the sorting and cleaning process.

Certain prescriptions call for the drugs to be powdered, broken into particles of a specific size, or sliced. Soaking or moistening the drugs with water makes them easier to slice. Mineral drugs and shell drugs are very hard, so in order to powder them more easily they are forged (baked) under high heat to make them more fragile. The processes of cleaning, roasting, and frying drugs kills most of the insects and microorganisms, thus reducing mildew or insect infestations in storage.

Some plants are specially treated to remove or reduce the toxicity or side effects. For example, the chemical constituents of crude *fu-zi* (*Aconitum*, or monkshood root) is very poisonous. After intricate washing, soaking, steaming, or boiling, the toxic chemical components of *fu-zi* are dramatically reduced, so it can be used safely. We know that the *Croton tiglium* seed can cause severe diarrhea; after the oil is removed from the seed, this reaction is less severe.

By treating a drug with other substances, the original effect of the drug can be changed or increased in order to enhance its effects. The character and taste of crude *Rehmannia glutinosa* (rehmannia root) is slightly sweet and cold. It has the function of nourishing the yin and cooling the blood, but after steaming with yellow wine, its character and taste changes to slightly sweet with a warming effect, and it nourishes the yin while enriching the blood. Careful processing changes the original effects of the plant slightly. The root of *Arisaema* (jack-in-the-pulpit) has the function of expelling wind and dispersing phlegm. After processing with the bile of cows or sheep, the function is altered so that it removes heat and disperses phlegm, while relieving muscle spasms.

Processing can also increase the effect of the drug. After processing *Aristolochia* (dutchman's pipe) with honey, it has more power to strengthen the lungs and stop coughs. *Corydalis yanhusuo* (Chinese corydalis) stops pain much more effectively after it is processed with vinegar, which increases the solubility of the active alkaloid in the plant.

Processing Methods

Pao-zhi, processing, has two parts. One involves cleaning the drugs by hand or cutting them with knives or scissors, but does not include the use of water or fire. The other uses water, fire, or both. Recently, scholars have identified three divisions of drug processing according to traditional methods. The first step is cleaning and sorting. Foreign matter is sorted from the medicinal part of the plant through sifting, shaving, winnowing, grinding, powdering, etc. The second step is cutting or slicing the drug, using only water to moisten and soften it, so that it can be cut more easily.

The third division uses water, heat, or both to process drugs. Some drugs are processed with water, heat, and alcohol, including yellow (rice) wine; some with vinegar; and some with honey and salt. The common method of processing is steaming or stir-frying the drug. There are at least three methods of stir-frying including frying the crude drug only, frying the drug mixed with the burnt clay from brick cooking stoves, and frying the drug mixed with wheat bran.

The processing methods produce different "functions" or effects on the crude drug. After a drug is processed with alcohol, it can lead other drugs to "move up" in the body. Processing a drug with vinegar can have the effect of aiding its efficacy in expelling blood stasis (bruises), stopping pain, expelling wetness, and detoxification. After drugs are processed with salt they may have the effect of relaxing the bowels and promoting diuresis, curing red eyes and swelling, making tendons and bones strong, and softening hard lumps or dry feces. Processing drugs with ginger can enhance the function of heating the middle burner and can stop vomiting, eliminate phlegm, and relax the side effects of other drugs. After processing with honey, drugs can more effectively nourish the blood, invigorate vital energy, nourish the lungs and intestines, and relax the bowels.

PRESCRIPTIONS

One of the characteristics of TCM is that most herbs are used in prescriptions with 3 or more herbs, there are sometimes 10 and up to 50 or 100 herbs in a single prescription. Many subbordinate drugs cooperate with a major ingredient in a prescription to produce a better effect on one particular organ or condition. According to the theories of TCM, the prescriptions are separated into the monarch or main drug, minister drugs, assistant drugs, and guide drugs. The monarch drug "rules" the prescription and has the primary effect on the diseased condition. The minister drug helps to synergistically increase the effect of the monarch drug.

The assistant drug may have several functions. It can be used to help the monarch drug or sometimes to help to treat a disease complex. For example, if a patient's liver is diseased and has set off additional problems with the spleen, the monarch drug treats the liver's condition and the assistant drug helps with the diseased condition of the spleen. The assistant can also "supervise" the function of other drugs, increasing or decreasing their effects on certain organs. Lastly, the assistant can serve as an antagonist to the effects of other drugs in the prescription, altering their effects.

The guide drug is added to enhance the efficacy of medicines; for example, onion or ginger can be used to mediate the properties of other herbs. Using licorice root, ginger, and alum with the crude drug *Pinellia* (a member of the arum family), can substantially reduce the toxicity of

Pinellia. The guide drug can also improve the taste of the prescription; licorice root is often used for this purpose.

After hundreds of years of practice and experience in clinical situations, recipes for prescriptions have become very scientific and exact. More than 80,000 prescriptions are recorded, whose precise quantities and proportions are crucial to their efficacy. A person once asked a famous doctor of TCM who specialized in pediatrics for help. His child had been unsuccessfully treated by another physician. After seeing the original prescription, the doctor said that this was a suitable prescription for the child and that if he had been the child's first physician, he would have used the same prescription. Why did the child fail to respond to the treatment? The doctor decided to check the prescription again. He found that in fact, the first doctor had made a mistake in the prescription and had transposed the weights of two drugs, almond and licorice root. The doctor corrected the weights and gave the same prescription to the child. After only two or three doses, the child returned to health. From this story we can see that in TCM, the compatible proportions of the ingredients in a prescription are very important.

How to
Use This Book

Herbal Emissaries is divided into five main parts: Major Chinese Medicinal Herbs, Garden Flowers, Ornamental Shrubs, Ornamental Trees, and Familiar Weeds. In each part, plants are arranged alphabetically by their best-known English common name. All of the plants included are exotics in America that are used as important drug plants in TCM or are used as "herbs" or "folk medicine" in Chinese traditions. Forty-four plants are covered.

The Chinese use the term *drug* in a very different sense from the American one. They use it to refer to both the source plant and the specific end product used to treat disease. There is also, as mentioned earlier, a vast difference between a drug plant and an herb used in folk or ethnic medicines.

The chapters on individual plants include 16 to 18 headings. The first group of headings provides information on how the plant is described. First comes information on the "Botanical name," the name used by scientists the world over to distinguish one particular plant from others. Here we have chosen the botanical name by which the plant is most widely known. Botanical names are also known as Latin binomials. They are composed of two parts. The first word is the genus name, and the second word is the specific epithet, or species name. After the species name comes an abbreviation, such as "L." This is an abbreviation of the name of the botanist who created the botanical name, and indicates to the "botanical authority." For example, "L." refers to the "father" of modern botanical nomenclature, Linnaeus. This is a useful point of reference, especially if a plant is listed by more than one scientific name in modern or historical works. The next section in many chapters is a listing of "Botanical synonyms," obsolete or relatively little-known scientific names that are found in the historical literature or some modern books.

Under the "Chinese names" heading are listed the name or names of the traditional Chinese form of the plant used. These names are not necessarily the Chinese name of the source plant itself, but the name of the traditional herb product derived from the plant. If more than one plant part is treated in the chapter, several names are listed. The English name of the plant part is listed in parenthesis after the Chinese name.

Under "English names" you will find the most common names by which the source plant is known. Generally, the first name listed has been adopted as the primary chapter name. If the plant is little known to Americans by an English common name, the names in this section follow those proposed by Shiu Ying Hu in her *An Enumeration of Chinese Materia Medica* (1980).

"Pharmaceutical names" is the next heading. These represent Latinized names of the "drug" produced from the source plant. Pharmaceutical names listed follow those in *The Pharmacopeia of the People's Republic of China* (1985) or S.Y. Hu's *An Enumeration of Chinese Materia Medica* (1980). The "Family" is a simple two-part listing of the scientific plant family name, followed by the common name of the plant family. Sometimes more than one family name is listed, if the plant is placed in different plants families by modern botanists. Some plant families, like the mint family, are known by two names: the *Labiatae* or the *Lamiaceae*. The first name is the old way of writing the botanical family name. The second is a new way of expressing the family name, with the suffix "aceae," used for all plant families. In these cases, the new name is given in parentheses after the older family name.

The main text entries provide more in-depth information about the properties, characteristics, and handling of the source plant and the drug or drugs derived from it. The first of these deals with the plant's "History" and gives basic background information about the plant and the human relationship to the plant, both in the East and the West. Historical aspects of the plant's introduction to the West are given if known, along with information on the people who made the plant known to Western botany and the evolution of the plant's botanical name. The meaning of both botanical and common names often reveals something about the plant itself; wherever possible, we have included information on word origins. Most Chinese traditional herbal remedies have been used since ancient times, and we explain when the herb was first noted in the Chinese herbal literature.

A brief description of "Taste and character," important diagnostic characteristics of TCM, comes next. The terms that are used, like "hot," "cold," "neutral," "bitter," "salty," are explained in "Using Plants as Drugs in Traditional Chinese Medicine."

"Functions" indicates the purposes the plant is used for in TCM practice. Again, the introductory chapter, "A simple introduction to the theory of using plants as drugs in TCM," explains the terms used and the TCM theory supporting its use. Next comes "Uses," which explains how and for what conditions the plant is used in either TCM, or western herbal traditions. It covers, where available, the current scientific understanding of the plant's pharmacology, chemistry, and traditional applications; a review of clinical reports from the modern Chinese clinical literature; and occasionally, simple, well-known prescriptions. An understanding of the plant's use in Western herbal terms is included. If the plant is used by American herb consumers, a listing of product forms found on the American market is included. The purpose of this section is to review and report on the major—or interesting and little-known minor—uses of the plant. It is *not* to provide information on self-medication. The reader is advised to seek the services of a qualified practitioner of TCM or other health-care providers before using the herbs. If the plant is widely available in the form of herb supplement products in the United States, the reader should read the label of the product for information on dosage and use.

The "Dose" entry includes details on the amount, form, and mode of application as noted in the Chinese literature. Units of measure used in the book are all expressed in English rather than metric terms, except for the dosage information, which is best expressed in the metric weight unit of grams. If applicable, information on contraindications is listed in this section. The concept of incompatible drugs is known as *shiba-fan*. In cases where such warnings are particularly significant, cautions have been included under the headings "Warnings" or "Toxicity."

Following the information on use and dose is a "description" of the plant, representing a simple botanical description of the plant or plants treated in the chapter.

The "Distribution" section describes the habitat and occurrence of the plant in China and elsewhere. Chinese occurrence is given by listing the names of the provinces or autonomous regions where the plant occurs. Major production regions of important Chinese herb products are included under this heading, along with notes on distribution of the plant in other parts of East Asia, North America, and other regions of the world.

Details on "Cultivation" report on how the plant is grown in China, as well as how it is grown in North America. Highly practical information on habit, habitat, soil types, propagation, and management, is included. Originally most Chinese medicinal plants were collected from the wild, but today most are scarce in their native haunts and must be cultivated. Some are simply grown as ornamentals and then harvested for medicinal use as needed. China feeds one quarter of the world's population on just 7 percent of the planet's arable land. Every inch of soil is utilized not only for food, but also for medicine. Many farmers plant a few medicinal plants along fence rows and roadsides or in small plots that are not used for food production. These medicinal plants are sold at local markets and provide a small supplemental income. Each region produces medicinal plants suitable for cultivation in their particular climate. Some counties are famous for having produced certain drug plants in the same area for centuries. Nearly all plants introduced to the West from China have come to us as ornamentals. Here we learn how they are grown and how to grow them.

The "Harvesting" entries report on when and how the plant is traditionally harvested in China, or, in some instances, North America.

"Processing" entries detail any special processing methods used to produce the herbal product used in TCM. The theory and techniques of herb processing are discussed above.

The heading "Additional species" lists related plants that are used for similar purposes in Western herbal traditions, or unusual Chinese species that are accepted and used as *substitutes* for the primary source plant in local areas of China. Plants known to be adulterants to the true source plant are also included. Adulterants are spurious impurities, inferior products, or additions (either intentional or unintentional) to an herb product that adversely effects its quality. Their addition is considered unacceptable. Substitutes, on the other hand, represent related plant species or acceptable alternatives that can be used instead of the specified product.

"Other uses" includes information on plant parts that may be used as minor folk medicines in China, as well as other uses of the plant for food, fiber, material, or medicinal applications in China or other parts of the world.

We hope that *Herbal Emissaries* will help you look at familiar herbs, colorful ornamentals, or rare exotics with new eyes. It will provide you with practical information on how a plant is used in China, how it came to be known in the West, when it was first known to be used in China, what it looks like, and where it grows—as well as on how it is grown, harvested, processed, and utilized. Whether you consider yourself a lay person or scientist, gardener or farmer, health-care professional or herb consumer, Sinophile or general reader, we hope that you will find something in *Herbal Emissaries* that helps you to "weed through the old to bring forth the new."

A Note on
the Transliteration of
Chinese Names

The Chinese names of the plants discussed in this book include two primary listings, pinyin and Wade-Giles names. These represent different systems of transliterating the sounds of Chinese words into romanized or English text. The pinyin system was introduced by the Chinese in the 1950s and officially adopted by the Chinese government in the 1970s. Wade-Giles, or the "Wade" system of transliterating Chinese sounds into the Roman alphabet, was developed about 100 years ago and is used in most books on Chinese medicinal plants published before the development of the pinyin system. Most major libraries in the United States with large Chinese-language collections use the Wade-Giles system. Various books on Chinese medicinal plants use one system or the other. In particular, books on Chinese herbs published after 1980 usually use the pinyin system. In pinyin, the Chinese capital is "Beijing." In Wade-Giles, the capital is "Peking."

Primary pinyin-transliterated names used in this book follow those names used in the 1985 edition of the *Pharmacopeia of the People's Republic of China*. If a plant is not listed in the 1985 Chinese *Pharmacopeia*, the names we have used are from the Jiangsu New Medical College's *Encyclopedia of Traditional Chinese Medicine* (3 vols., 1977–1979). Wade-Giles names follow Shiu Ying Hu's *An Enumeration of Chinese Materia Medica* (1980). Chinese words in the main text of the book, including proper names of persons and places, and titles of books, in the large majority of instances follow pinyin transliterations. Sometimes we have added the Wade-Giles transliteration in parenthesis following a pinyin word.

ONE

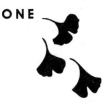

Major Chinese Medicinal Herbs

Astragalus
Huang-qi

Botanical Names: *Astragalus membranaceus* (Fisch.) Bge., and *Astragalus membranaceus* var. *mongholicus* (Bge.) Hsiao (*Astragalus mongholicus* Bge.).

Botanical Synonyms: In earlier Western works, the source plants of the Chinese herbal drug, *huang-qi*, also included *A. henryi* Oliv., *A. hoantchy* Franch. (also spelled *A. hoangtchy*, and *A. hoan tchu*), and *A. reflexistipulus* Miq. However, when the *New Chinese Materia Medica* (*Zhong Yao Zhi*) was first published in 1959, Chinese research efforts succeeded in properly identifying the source plants.

Chinese Names: Pinyin: *Huang-qi* (roots). Wade-Giles: *Huang-ch'i* (roots).

English Names: Astragalus, *Huang-qi*, milk vetch root, membranous milk vetch, yellow vetch.

Pharmaceutical Name: Radix Astragali.

Family: Leguminosae (Fabaceae)—pea family

HISTORY

If an herb can be used for numerous diseases, perhaps it has a pharmacological activity that works to help the body defend itself rather than acting on a specific disease or function. While this may be "new" information to the Western herbalist, it is common knowledge to Chinese herbal practitioners, who have recognized this fact for millennia. Astragalus is becoming one of the better-known Chinese herbs used as an immune system stimulant.

The genus *Astragalus*, primarily from northern temperate regions, is considered by botanists to be the largest genus of flowering plants, containing more than 2,000 species. In North America, for example, there are nearly 400 *Astragalus* species, mainly concentrated in the western states. Some species of *Astragalus* like *huang-qi*, are innocuous, edible, and completely non toxic. Others, like the famous "locoweeds," are poisonous to livestock if eaten over a longer period of time. Other *Astragalus* species are toxic as a result of their ability to concentrate selenium and have thus been used as indicators of uranium deposits. Still others provide important materials, like gum tragacanth, which is derived from several *Astragalus* species, including *A. gummifer*, widely used for colloidal properties in lotions, pharmaceutical suspensions, resinous tinctures, creams, jelly and even ice cream. It is native to western and central Asia, an area that harbors hundreds of Astragalus species.

The name *Astragalus* serves as both a botanical generic name and an English common name for the Chinese medicinal plant known as *huang-qi*. It was first applied to the modern botanical concept of the genus by the French botanist, Tournefort, in the early 1700s. However, the name had already been well known to botanists for centuries. It can be traced back to at least the time of the first century Greek physician Dioscorides. The word itself is even more ancient, deriving from a Greek word meaning "ankle bone." Ankle bones were once used as a form of dice. One conjecture is that *Astragalus* was applied to this plant group because the rattling seedpods of one Mediterranean species sounded like rolling dice.

The Chinese species *Astragalus membranaceus* was first described in Western terms by Dr. Alexander von Bunge, a Russian physician who explored east Asian plants in the first half of the nineteenth century. (His name is abbreviated "Bge." in the author citation of the Latin name above). Bunge produced a major monograph on *Astragalus* species, published in 1868–69.

Chinese knowledge of the plant is much older. *Huang-qi* was listed in the superior class of herbs in the 2,000-year-old classic, *Shen Nong Ben Cao Jing*. *Huang* means "yellow," from the yellow interior of the root, while *qi* means "leader," referring to the fact that this is one of the superior tonic roots in traditional Chinese medicine. In the *Medical Casebook of Shi-shan (Shi-Shan Yi An)*, published in 1531, two supplements are included that discuss *huang-qi* and its use with ginseng, still a well-known Chinese herbal prescription as a tonic for fatigue and general debility. Shi-shan is more properly known as Wang-ji (Wang Shi-shan).

TASTE AND CHARACTER

Mildly sweet, a little warm.

FUNCTIONS

Invigorates vital energy (*qi/ch'i*), strengthens the body's superficial resistance, promotes tissue regeneration, promotes diuresis, suppurates poisons, drains pus, reduces swelling.

USES

Huang-qi is used in prescriptions for shortness of breath and palpitation, lack of physical strength, collapse, spontaneous perspiration, night sweat, edema due to physical deficiency, chronic nephritis, pulmonary diseases, lingering diarrhea, prolapse of the rectum, uterine prolapse, non festering boils, and hard-to-heal sores and wounds. Honey-processed, *huang-qi* is good for the middle abdomen, fatigue from overwork, diarrhea due to spleen deficiency, urinary incontinence, vital energy (*qi/ch'i*) deficiency, bloody urine, and blood-deficient diseases.

Huang-qi has been the focus of much scientific research over the past thirty years, both in China and abroad. Laboratory studies have shown that the root has diuretic activity and confirm an experimental basis for use in nephritis. When a decoction of the root was given to mice over a three week period, their swimming duration increased, as did their body weight, suggesting the root may increase endurance. Further experiments indicated a positive result in reducing blood pressure, both by strengthening contractions of normal heart tissue and by its blood vessel dilating action, which improves blood circulation. In studies with mice, it has also been shown to augment the interferon response to viruses. No toxic side effects have been reported.

Astragalus is one of a number of herbs used in *fu-zheng* therapy. *Fu-zheng* refers to treating disease by either enhancing or promoting the host defense mechanism or normalizing the central energy. A *fu-zheng* therapy research group was initiated in China in 1975 to study the use of this ancient treatment modality in cancer patients. In the 1970s and early 1980s, Chinese scientists published a number of reports on the use of astragalus and other Chinese herbs as immune-system enhancers for patients undergoing chemotherapy for various cancers. The results showed that astragalus and other herbs acted as non specific immune system stimulants and helped to protect adrenal cortical function while patients are undergoing radiation or chemotherapy. The *fu-zheng* therapy also changed the direction of depressed bone marrow activity, while modifying gastrointestinal toxicity of patients receiving conventional cancer therapies. The end result was a significant increase in survival rates for the patients receiving *fu-zheng* therapy as an adjunct to western medical cancer treatments.

Cancer researchers have a growing body of clinical evidence indicating that cellular immune response is usually damaged in cancer patients—

advanced cancer patients in particular. Noting that immune response may be further damaged by conventional cancer treatment methods such as chemotherapy and radiation, Chinese researchers set out to find traditional drugs that might produce a positive immunological stimulation or restoration action. Their positive results attracted interest of scientists in other parts of the world, including the United States.

Researchers at several institutions in Houston, Texas, performed a number of laboratory and clinical studies on astragalus as well as on Chinese privet (*Ligustrum lucidum*). In testing the restorative effect of water extracts of *Astragalus membranaceus* on 19 cancer patients and 15 healthy persons, they found that the extracts restored T-cell function in 9 out of 10 patients. Using an assay for T-cell restoration, they confirmed that the extracts appeared to restore levels in the cancer patients to those observed in the normal healthy donors. The study showed that the herb extract had a strong immune stimulant effect, providing a rational basis for its use to modify biological response in cancer patients. Further laboratory studies revealed other mechanisms of action, as well as a polysaccharide fraction believed to be primarily responsible for the immunostimulant effects.

Unfortunately, the studies by the Houston research group were discontinued after a pharmaceutical company withdrew its financial support from the possible development of a new drug from astragalus. One of the problems experienced by the research group was difficulty in obtaining sufficient quantities of the herb to continue research or develop new products from the plant. Given the wealth of *Astragalus* species in North America, perhaps research should focus on screening native species for a possible parallel to the Chinese *huang-qi*.

Huang-qi is used in numerous Chinese prescriptions. With ginseng (*Panax ginseng*) it is used as a tonic for fatigue, general debility, lack of appetite, and spontaneous perspiration.

In combination with codonopsis (*Codonopsis pilosula*), astragalus is used to strengthen the heart. According to the tenets of TCM, a major principle used in the treatment of heart disease is *yiqi-huoxue*—replenishing vital energy while invigorating blood circulation. Pharmacological studies in China have confirmed a rational scientific basis for this method of treatment.

In Western herbalism, astragalus has been described as a diuretic, tonic, pectoral, and antipyretic. In his 1911 work, *Chinese Materia Medica*, G. A. Stuart wrote, "It is in great repute as a tonic, pectoral, and diuretic medicine. The diseases for which it is prescribed, therefore, are almost numberless." (p. 57).

The sliced root, whole root, capsulated products, teas, tinctures and other product forms of *huang-qi* are commonly available in health and natural food stores in North America.

DOSE

Normally, 9–15 g. in decoction, or sometimes larger doses of 30–60 g. Also used in pills, powder, or extract form.

DESCRIPTION

Astragalus membranaceus is an herbaceous perennial that grows to about 2 feet tall, with sprawling stems. The leaves are alternate, dividing into 12–24 oval to elliptical-shaped leaflets. Stipules are lance shaped. The small, light yellow, pea like flowers are borne on racemes extending from the leaf axils. Hard dark-brown, kidney-shaped seeds, about ⅛ inch long, are enclosed in papery, two-valved pods about an inch in length. The pods have short dark hairs on the exterior. *A. membranaceus* var. *mongholicus* is very similar but has triangular-ovate stipules, and 25 to 37 leaflets, which are shorter and wider. The flowers are dark yellow and the seed pods without hair.

DISTRIBUTION

Astragalus membranaceus grows along the margins of forests, in shrub thickets, thin open woods, and grasslands near forest margins. It has an extensive range, from the northeastern province of Heilongjiang south to the Shandong peninsula, west to mountains of Sichuan, and north to the westernmost province of Xinjiang. *A. membranaceus* var. *mongholicus* grows in sunny grasslands and on mountain sides in northeastern China.

While commonly available from sources of Chinese herbal products in North America, the source plant is very rare in Western horticulture. It is grown as a specimen plant in a handful of botanical gardens, and is in the possession of some collectors of rare plants in the United States.

CULTIVATION

The plant is generally adaptable to growing conditions, and relatively easy to cultivate—if one can germinate the seeds. It likes a deep, sandy, well-drained, somewhat alkaline soil. A well-drained soil is important, since the roots may rot in poorly drained soil. Seeds are planted after the last spring frost, or the previous fall. They should be covered with less than half an inch of soil and kept well watered. Fall-planted seed will germinate the following spring.

The seeds can be a little tricky to germinate. Like many legumes, they have a hard seed coat. Germination can be enhanced by nicking the hard coat with a small file or sand paper. Soaking the seeds overnight in warm water may also enhance germination. Using these methods, the seeds can germinate in as little as five to seven days. If planted outside with no pretreatment, they generally germinate in two to three weeks. Once young seedlings develop four to six leaves, they can be thinned to one-foot spacings.

The Chinese consider the quality of the cultivated roots to be superior to wild-harvested astragalus roots.

HARVESTING

Roots are harvested after the fourth or fifth year of growth, usually in autumn, though sometimes in spring. Lateral rootlets are removed, the crown is cut off of the root, and the main root is dried in the sun until about 60 to 70 percent dry. The roots are then sorted according to size and straightened. Next they are tied into small bundles and completely dried. Before 100 percent dry, they are usually sliced lengthwise into pieces about ³⁄₁₆ inch thick. If already dry, the roots are covered with a moist cloth until they absorb enough moisture so that they can be sliced with ease.

PROCESSING

Honey-processed *huang-qi* is used in some prescriptions. A little honey is placed in a pan and set over a low heat until the water is evaporated off, producing a brownish-yellow mass a little darker than crude honey. Using this honey, a small amount of hot water is added, mixed with the *huang-qi* slices, and then stirred frequently until the slices become a yellowish color and the honey is no longer gummy or sticky to the touch. About one part honey by weight is used for four parts dried root.

ADDITIONAL SPECIES

While *Astragalus membranaceus* and *A. membranaceus* var. *mongholicus* serve as the official source plants of *huang-qi*, according to the Chinese

Pharmacopeia a number of other species are also used as local substitutes in some parts of China. Their Chinese names often denote the region of origin. Alternative source plants include *A. chrysopterus, A. floridus, A. ernestii, A. tongolensis,* and *A. complanatus.*

A. complanatus seeds produce another traditional Chinese drug, *sha-yuan-xi.* In western Liaoning and eastern Nei Mongol, the root has been used as a *huang-qi* substitute. It is called "black-surface qi" or "iron-qi" because the root is very hard and has a blackish-brown cortex.

OTHER USES

In addition, the leaves and stems of *A. membranaceus* are used as folk medicines, to treat excessive thirst, and to reduce swelling or injuries.

Baikal Scullcap
Huang-qin

Botanical Names: *Scutellaria baicalensis* Georgi.
Botanical Synonym: *Scutellaria macrantha* Fisch.
Chinese Names: Pinyin: *Huang-qin* (roots). Wade Giles: *Huang-chin* (roots).
English Names: Baikal scullcap.
Pharmaceutical Name: Radix Scutellariae.
Family: Labiatae (Lamiaceae)—mint family.

HISTORY

Herb consumers in the United States think of mad-dog scullcap (*Scutellaria lateriflora*), a common species in eastern North America, when they hear the herb name "scullcap." The name "mad-dog scullcap" derives from historical, and presumably unsuccessful use of the leaves in the treatment of rabies. However, it has become best known as a mild nerve sedative. The plant has been poorly studied. The root of its cousin, the Baikal scullcap (*Scutellaria baicalensis*) is a traditional Chinese herb known as *huang-qin.* It is widely used in China, and has been the subject of numerous scientific investigations focusing on its traditional uses, chemistry, pharmacology, and clinical applications.

The genus *Scutellaria*, commonly known as scullcaps, includes about 300 species of herbs in the mint family. They are primarily found in the Old World, especially central Eurasia, from Syria west to the Altai Mountains and the Himalayas. The genus is also represented in central Africa, Malaysia, and Australia. In the New World there are 113 species, occurring from the Arctic Circle to the tip of South America. Mad-dog scullcap, *Scutellaria lateriflora*, is the best-known American species.

Baikal scullcap *S. baicalensis*, while known to Chinese herbalists for over 2,000 years, was first described in Western terms by a German-born botanist Johann Gottlieb Georgi (1729–1802), a professor of the Russian Academy of Sciences in Saint Petersburg. Based on collections from far eastern Russia, Georgi provided the first botanical description of the plant in a 1775 publication describing the flowering plants of the Baikal region (southeastern Soviet Union, around the Mongolian border).

Subsequently, the plant was collected by European botanists in China in the late nineteenth century. Soon thereafter, the plant became known as a rare specimen in European botanical gardens. Exactly when the plant arrived in the United States is obscure. In the United States it is sometimes grown in botanical gardens, but more often can be found in the collections of rock gardeners. Rock gardeners grow it for its showy blue flowers, and its adaptability to extreme cold and dry conditions.

The genus name *Scutellaria* derives from *scutella*, meaning a dish or platter, referring to the helmet-like form of the fruiting calyx. The species name *baicalensis* refers to the region where Georgi described the first botanical specimens of the plant.

In China, where the root harvested from the plant is known as *huang-qin*, it has been known and used for at least two thousand years. The first mention is in *Shen Nong Ben Cao Jing*, as being in the middle class of drugs. The original plant mentioned in the *ben cao* (Chinese herbals) is the same plant that is used today.

TASTE AND CHARACTER

Bitter, cold.

FUNCTIONS

Purges the fire of high fever, dispels heat, expels wet-heat, stops bleeding, detoxifies, and is soothing to a fetus.

USES

Huang-qin is used in prescriptions for all types of fevers, colds, red eyes with swelling and pain, high blood pressure, hypertension, insomnia, headaches, enteritis, vomiting of blood, nosebleed, bloody stool, for patients with vexation and thirst due to feverish conditions, cough due to lung heat, pneumonia, diarrhea, dysentery, hot urine, jaundice due to wetness and heat, hepatitis, restless fetus, uterine bleeding, threatened abortion, carbuncles, furuncles, sores with swelling, and burns. The root has also been traditionally used for the treatment of diphtheria and to prevent scarlet fever. Externally a poultice of the powdered root mixed with water was used as a folk treatment for herpes zoster (shingles).

An ancient Chinese medicinal herb, Baikal skullcap remains one of the most widely used plant medicines in traditional Chinese medicine. Over the past few decades, Chinese scientists have sought to confirm traditional uses of the plant using experimental data that show that the root is antibacterial against *Staphylococcus aureus*, has antiviral activity against influenza virus strains, and is antifungal. *Huang-qin* has also been proven to have diuretic, fever-reducing, and blood-pressure-lowering effects. In rabbit studies, the root extract has been shown to increase bile production. Clinical studies have indicated utility in chronic hepatitis, with over a 70 percent effectiveness rate. Symptoms were improved, including an increase in appetite, relief of abdominal distention, and improved liver function. Animal experiments also suggest the root may have a protective effect against toxic liver damage. The plant has also been studied for potential antiallergenic activity with promising results.

Numerous flavonoids, including baicalein, and baicalin, have been isolated from the root. Baicalein has an antibacterial effect. Baicalin is sedative, antipyretic, hypotensive, and experimentally diuretic. This substance has been used clinically in China in the treatment of infectious hepatitis. For acute and chronic hepatitis, an intramuscular injection prepared from *huang-qin* and other herbs is used once a day for a period of one month. Two milliliters of the injectable liquid is the cited dose. Other medications are contraindicated during this period. In Chinese clinics, the root has also been used as a treatment to prevent scarlet fever.

One treatment for the common cold, including upper respiratory tract infections, uses an intramuscular injection of *huang-qin*, with *Coptis chinense* (*huang-lian*), and *Phellodendron amurense* (*huang-bai*). This drug is called *san huang zhe she ye* (an injection of three yellow drugs).

A Chinese clinical report described the effect of a 50 percent decoction of *huang-qin* on children with acute upper respiratory tract infections. Fifty-one patients in the study had acute infections of the upper respiratory tract, 11 patients suffered from acute bronchitis, and one patient had acute tonsillitis. Children under one year of age were given a dose of 6 ml of the *huang-qin* decoction per day. One to five-year-olds were given 8 to 10 ml per day. For children older than five years, the dose was increased. The prescription was separated into three doses for one day's treatment. After treatment the patient's temperature was reduced to normal in all cases. In the 51 cases of upper respiratory tract infections (symptomology not specified), all had improvements of symptoms. The treatment was of no use in the cases of tonsillitis or bronchitis. The symptoms of most patients were reduced in four days.

A clinical report on the treatment of high blood pressure used a 20 percent tincture of *huang-qin*. Doses ranged from 5 to 10 ml, divided into three doses per day. Fifty-one patients were observed. Before treatment, all patients had blood pressure higher than 180/100. After receiving the treatment for one to 12 months, blood pressure levels were reduced to an average of 160/90 in 70 percent of those treated. Other clinical symptoms of high blood pressure were reduced. The report concluded that patients could take the tincture over a long period of time, for a continuous reduction of blood pressure, without reports of side effects.

In Western terms, *huang-qin* has been described as antipyretic, anodyne, astringent, stimulant to the respiratory organs, diuretic, antimicrobial, and hypotensive. The root has also been poulticed as a folk remedy for breast cancer. In the United States, the root is primarily sold through Chinatown herb shops, though is increasingly seen in products found in health and natural food stores as well.

DOSE

3–9 g, in decoction, pills, powders, poultice, or as a wash.

DESCRIPTION

Baikal scullcap is a perennial growing to about 15 inches tall. The stems are somewhat lax, mostly smooth. Leaves are opposite, lance shaped to linear, ½ to 1½ inch long, with an obtuse apex, entire, and without leaf stalks, or with very short leaf stalks. The leaf margins have small stiff hairs. Black glandular dots can be observed on the lower sides of the leaves. The flowers are blue, violet, or violet-red, in a simple raceme. The attractive two-lipped flowers are in pairs on one side of the stem. The flower calyx, once dried, has an in-curved head. It usually flowers from July to August.

DISTRIBUTION

Baikal skullcap occurs along roadsides, in fields, and in high, dry, sandy mountain soils in northeast China and the mountains of southwest China, and north of the Yangtze River in Heilongjiang, Jilin, Liaoning, Hebei, Nei Mongol, Shanxi, Shaanxi, Gansu, Henan, Shandong, and Sichuan. Major production provinces include Heilongjiang, Jilin, Liaoning, Hebei, Nei Mongol, and Shanxi. Shanxi province is the largest producer. The best quality *huang-qin* comes from Cheng-de in Hebei province. It also occurs in eastern Russia.

It is a rare plant in American and European botanical gardens. In the United States it is most commonly found in the collections of rock gardeners.

CULTIVATION

Baikal scullcap grows in full sun, is drought tolerant, and is very hardy. Good soil drainage is essential. Propagate by seeds. Two- to three-year-old plants are chosen to collect seed for propagation purposes. The seeds can be planted in spring directly in rows spaced at 1 to 1½ feet. Cover with about ¼ inch of soil. Emergence takes place in 15 to 20 days. Space individual plants at 9 inches. When the seedlings are 4 to 6 inches high they can be transplanted as necessary. Side dress with manure, once or twice during the growing season. Weed as necessary, and cultivate around the plants to aerate the soil. The flower buds are pinched back before blooming to return more energy to the roots.

HARVESTING

The roots are dug in spring or autumn. Plants three to four years of age are harvested, and the stem, leaves, and lateral roots are removed. Spring is considered the best time for harvest. The root is dried under light sunshine until half dry; then the root bark is scraped off. Alternately, when half dried, the root is cut into slices and dried completely. Strong sunlight is avoided during drying, which may turn the roots an undesirable reddish color.

PROCESSING

For alcohol-processed *huang-qin*, dried slices of the root are used. Ten pounds of yellow (rice) wine are added to 100 pounds of the root. The wine is sprinkled over the roots, covered with a moist cloth, and allowed to sit until the roots absorb the alcohol. Next they are lightly roasted (stir-fried) for a short time, then cooled.

Another method involves soaking the root in cold water for a short time, parboiling it for about one hour, and drying it.

Charcoaled *huang-qin* is made by stir-frying the root slices under high heat. The slices are turned often until they are dark brown and the inner part of the root is dark yellow. The character of the root is retained (browned but not burned). A little cool water is sprinkled on the roots and they are then taken off of the heat and cooled. Care is taken not to burn the root after water is added.

Baicalin is the main active ingredient of the plant. A recent study showed that baicalin can hydrolyze into the less active substance, baicalein, which is unstable. The highest-quality root has a higher baicalin content. Baicalin was found to be as much as 30 percent higher in boiled water extracts of the alcohol-processed *huang-qin* compared with the crude dried root. If soaked in water, baicalin content of crude root samples decreased significantly, but soaking in water had no effect on the alcohol-processed *huang-qin*. Such studies show a scientific basis for traditional processing methods.

When the root is exposed to moist air it becomes a greenish color, and the quality is greatly lessened. It should be stored in a cool, dry, dark place.

ADDITIONAL SPECIES

In Sichuan, Guizhou, and Yunnan, *Scutellaria amoena* C. H. Wright., found in mountain fields, forest margins, and very thin woods, is used as a substitute for *huang-qin*. *Scutellaria viscidula* Bge. growing in sandy fields, waste places and fields, is a substitute in Hebei, Shanxi, Nei Mongol, and Shandong. *Scutellaria rehderiana* Diels., found in stony mountain soils usually on south-facing slopes, is used in Shanxi, Shaanxi, and Gansu. *Scutellaria likiangensis* Diels., found in shrub thickets, grass fields, and pine woods, is used as *huang-qin* in Li-jiang, Yunnan province. *Scutellaria hypericifolia* Levl., which grows in grassy fields, high mountain forests, and forest margins, is a substitute used in Sichuan. *Scutellaria tenax* W. W. Smith var. *palentipilosa* (H. M.) C. Y. Wu, found in the Jin-sha-jiang river along the upper Sichuan-Yunnan border, is also used as a substitute. *Scutellaria ikonnikovii* Jus. has been used as a *huang-qin* substitute in Ningxia. The quality of these substitutes is considered to be less than that of *S. baicalensis.*

OTHER USES

The achenes (seeds) are a traditional remedy for bloody stool with pus; 4.5 to 9 g are used in decoction. This is mentioned in the 500 A.D. work, *Ming Yi Ben Lu.*

Chinese Cucumber
Tian-hua-fen and *Gua-lou*

Botanical Names: *Trichosanthes kirilowii* Maxim., *T. japonica* Regel., and *T. rosthornii* Harms.
Botanical Synonyms: *T. uniflora* Hao is a synonym for *T. rosthornii.*
Chinese Names: Pinyin: *Tian-hua-fen* (root); *Gua-lou* (fruits). Wade-Giles: *Tien-hua-feng* (root); *Kua-lou* (fruits).
English Names: Chinese cucumber, Chinese snakegourd, trichosanthes.
Pharmaceutical Name: Radix Trichosanthes (root); Fructus Trichosanthes (fruit).
Family: Cucurbitaceae—gourd family.

HISTORY

In April 1989, Steven Foster was on the phone with Yue Chongxi, who was in Beijing. As we talked, the CBS evening news was on television in the background. Dan Rather broke the news of a possible breakthrough in the search for an AIDS cure, the announcement of clinical trials on a protein called "Compound Q," derived from a plant ambiguously identified as the "Chinese cucumber." He then noted that Compound Q was a protein known as "trichosanthin." A light bulb went on in Foster's head—on the other end of the phone was a leading Chinese expert on the genus *Trichosanthes. Trichosanthes kirilowii*, better known in English as the Chinese snakegourd, which like the cucumber, a member of the gourd family, was the real identity of the plant the media deemed "Chinese cucumber."

Professor Yue Chongxi (C. H. Yueh), has specialized in the botany, histology, and morphology of Chinese *Trichosanthes* species since 1956. When he began his studies, five species were recognized by Chinese botanists. Through extensive field collections in 28 provinces of China and study of herbarium collections in China, the United States, and England, Yue Chongxi and his colleague C. Y. Cheng now recognize over 40 species of Chinese *Trichosanthes*. Extensive laboratory work has also resulted in the development of macroscopic and microscopic methods for identifying the crude drug, its substitutes, and its adulterants. In 1991 a new species of *Trichosanthes* was just discovered in China by Prof. Yue and his colleagues, and has been named *Trichosanthes mianyangensis* Yueh et R. G. Liao. In a 1987 lecture at Harvard University Professor Yue described his research:

> Thirty-six years ago, I was working on my graduate thesis on the drug *tian-hua-fen*, the root of *Trichosanthes*. The following year (1956), I began working at the Academy of Traditional Chinese Medicine. My teacher, the famous pharmacognosist Professor Lou Zhi-ching, was the consultant in our unit. After discussions with my leaders, they arranged for me to research *gua-lou*, the fruit of *Trichosanthes*. I worked on it for the last three-and-a-half months of 1956. During this period I found two problems. One problem was that two different fruits had the same name. We found that two obviously distinct fruits were used as *gua-lou*. TCM doctors in Shanghai gave the true *gua-lou* to strong adults and gave the substitute, *wang-gua*, to children or weak patients. Another problem existed with the Guangxi *gua-lou-zi* [seeds]. It is another species in the same genus with large seeds. At that point the Latin name of the source plant was unknown. A Vietnamese friend sent us some drugs including the seed, so we knew the original plants were growing in south China. I spent sixteen years trying to identify the original source plants of the drug, and finally solved the problem in 1972. The source plant of the Guangxi *gua-lou-zi* was *T. truncata* C. B. Clarke.
>
> We often use the research results of taxonomists in our work, but no one had made a systematic study of the Chinese species of the genus *Trichosanthes*, so I proceeded with that work. In 1964, the Kunming Public Health Bureau invited me

to write a handbook for their folk herbs, so I was able to study many sites in Yunnan. In North China we only have the white-flowered species of *Trichosanthes*, but there are several species with red, pink, or orange flowers in Yunnan. More important, in terms of drug research, many of the seeds and roots of the South China *Trichosanthes* species produced side effects such as nausea, vomiting, and diarrhea.

From the story you can understand the methods of our research. First, we identify the problems from the clinical situation or in production, for example, the problems of a drug plant's identity. The next step is to make a plan for the investigation. We then use methods of classification such as taxonomy, anatomy (morphology and histology), and pollen studies, as well as simple chemistry, to clarify the confused condition of the source plant or plants. We must know which species is the original plant of the drug, which one is the true species for medicinal use, and which ones may be used as substitutes or that are adulterants. Finally, we must find the details and different points of all of the above methods of identification.

My leaders asked me to research the subject for three months, but in fact, I have now researched this subject for more than 36 years. After visiting 28 provinces and autonomous regions in China, we know that most parts of China have some *Trichosanthes* species, except in the far northeastern and northwestern parts of China. A few of them are the source of the true drug, while others are substitutes or adulterants.

The genus *Trichosanthes* is the source plant of a number of official drugs in the Chinese *Pharmacopeia*. Chief among them are *tian-hua-fen*, the root of *T. kirilowii*, *T. japonica*, and to a lesser extent, *T. rosthornii*. The *Pharmacopeia of the People's Republic of China* (1985) recognizes *T. kirilowii* and *T. japonica* as the true source plants of *tian-hua-fen*. *T. rosthornii* was not recognized because its effects are considered inferior to the former two species. The fruit, known as *gua-lou*, is derived primarily from *T. kirilowii* and *T. rosthornii*. In addition, *gua-lou-zi* (the seeds) and *gua-lou-pi* (the fruit rind) are also official TCM source drugs in the Chinese *Pharmacopeia*.

In recent years, *Trichosanthes* has been catapulted into fame in the United States as the source of a potential drug for the treatment of AIDS. In January 1989, researchers at the University of California at San Francisco, Genelabs, Inc. (a Redwood City, California, biotechnology firm), and the Department of Biochemistry and Chinese Medicinal Materials Research Center at the Chinese University of Hong Kong received U.S. Patent #4,795,739 for the use of the proteins trichosanthin and momorcharin (a protein from *Momordica*, a related genus in the gourd family) in experimental HIV therapies. The patent includes a method of inhibiting HIV antigens in human blood cells with the proteins, as well as a method of screening drug agents in HIV infected humans. The chief researcher, Dr. Michael S. McGrath, M.D., Ph.D., is an associate professor of medicine at the University of California at San Francisco (UCSF), and director of the AIDS/Immunobiology Research Laboratory at San Francisco General Hospital, a UCSF affiliate. The new drug was named "GLQ223," or Compound Q, which is apparently a highly purified form of the protein trichosanthin, derived from *Trichosanthes*.

The research was funded by the Swiss pharmaceutical giant, Sandoz, Ltd., which will eventually market the product if it is approved for human use in the United States. A 13 April 1989 press release from San Francisco General Hospital and UCSF coincided with the publication of a research paper by Dr. Michael McGrath and fourteen coauthors, "GLQ223: An inhibitor of human immunodeficiency virus replication in acutely and chronically infected cells of lymphocyte and mononuclear phagocyte lineage," in *Proceedings of the National Academy of Science*, 13 April 1989. The press release stated that the drug seems to "block HIV replication in infected T-cells and kills HIV-infected macrophages—the body's scavenger cells—in cell cultures." It does so by selectively killing cells harboring the AIDS virus, apparently without affecting uninfected cells.

In a 27 April 1989 press release, San Francisco General Hospital announced that FDA approval was granted for an investigational new drug (IND) application for Phase 1 clinical trials on Compound Q. Initial Compound Q injection trials in humans have now begun. At the time of this writing, the product is in Phase 2 clinical trials. Phase 1 trials, in which the treatment was tested in patients to determine safety and tolerance, have already been completed. Results will not be announced until all phases of clinical research are completed.

While Compound Q will be sold only if positive results are obtained in the clinical trials, many in the AIDS community believe that it is the best treatment for AIDS that now exists, even though it is not a cure for AIDS. Unlike other drugs currently in use, such as AZT, Compound Q has the unique ability to destroy HIV-infected cells, without affecting surrounding healthy cells. It kills infected cells, reducing the level of HIV infection, and stops the protein synthesis of HIV in infected cells, preventing its reproduction and spreading to uninfected cells. A new book, *Compound Q: Trichosanthin and Its Clinical Applications*, by Qing-cai Zhang (1990) details what is currently known about the drug in AIDS treatment.

While trichosanthin is considered a "new drug" in the United States, it has been extensively used in clinical situations in China. Chinese clinical studies on the protein have involved more than 10,000 humans, not in the treatment of AIDS, but primarily for inducing abortions. Its use as an abortifacient has been known since 300 A.D. Proper procedures are critical in administration of the drug since it produces series side effects, including anaphylactic shock, skin rashes, nausea, and muscle spasms; if misused, it can be lethal. There have been a number of cases in which AIDS patients went to China to obtain the drug, self-administered it by injection, and then suffered seizures and high fever, requiring hospitalization. At least one such patient has died from a trichosanthin injection.

Before the breakthroughs in AIDS research with Compound Q in the United States, the Chinese snakegourd and the genus *Trichosanthes* were generally unknown except to botanists. Linnaeus established the genus name *Trichosanthes* in his *Species Plantarum* (1753). The word is derived from the Greek *thrix* or *trichos*, meaning a hair, and *anthos* (flower) referring to the finely divided petal segments of the flowers. The genus includes about 50 species of herbaceous vines native to Asia, northern Australia, and the Pacific islands. The first Westerner to collect *Trichosanthes kirilowii* was a Russian physician, Dr. P. Y. Kirilov, who traveled with Bunge to Beijing in 1830, where he stayed for 11 years. Upon his return in 1841 he collected the vine in northern China. The species name *kirilowii* honors Kirilov. It was first described in modern botanical terms and named by the Russian botanist Maximowicz in an 1856 publication.

The crude root, *tian-hua-fen*, is first mentioned in a work attributed to Lei Ziao from the later Han dynasty, *Lei Gong Pao Zhi Lun* (*Grandfather Lei's Discussions of Herb Preparation*). Later it is also treated in Su Song's *Tu Jing Ben Cao* (1061). It is still a very commonly used drug in TCM. From ancient times until now, *T. kirilowii* is the major source plant. It is now known, however, especially in south China, that many species of the same genus, some acceptable substitutes, some not, have been used as source plants for *tian-hua-fen*.

Gua-lou (*Trichosanthes* fruit) is considered by the Chinese to be a more important drug than *tian-hua-fen*. It is first mentioned in the middle class of drugs in *Shen Nong Ben Cao Jing*. In the sixteenth-century classic, *Ben Cao Gang Mu*, Li Shi-zhen placed *gua-lou* in the eighteenth volume under climbing herbs. *Gua-lou* is an ancient word. *Gua* means the fruit of a tree. In ancient times "*lou*" meant "herb with fruit." *Trichosanthes* is a vine that often climbs trees. Since the fruits of this herbaceous vine were found on plants climbing trees, the two words were combined to reflect this habit, hence the name *gua-lou*. According to the pictures and descriptions of ancient *ben-cao*, it is clear that *T. kirilowii* was traditionally the major source plant of *gua-lou*.

TASTE AND CHARACTER

Tian-hua-fen is somewhat bitter, somewhat sweet, and cold. *Gua-lou* is a little sweet, bitter, and cold.

FUNCTIONS

Tian-hua-fen promotes the production of body fluids, treats dryness syndrome by reducing fire-heat, disperses heat, disperses phlegm, nourishes the stomach, removes pus, subsides swelling, and expels toxic matter.

Gua-lou disperses toxic matter, expands the chest, clears and dissipates hot phlegm, nourishes the lungs, smooths the intestines, stimulates milk production, and disperses swelling. It has been used extensively for various lung ailments.

USES

Tian-hua-fen is used in prescriptions for thirst due to fever diseases, dry cough due to lung heat, mastitis, sores with swelling, diabetes, jaundice, and hemorrhoids. *Tian-hua-fen* protein (trichosanthin) is used as an abortifacient. Externally, the root has been used for the treatment of swellings, ulcerations of the nipple, and traumatic injuries.

Gua-lou is used in prescriptions for cough due to hot phlegm, oppressed feeling of the chest, cough with bleeding due to a withered lung, jaundice, diabetes, constipation, angina pectoris, and mastitis; externally it is used for carbuncles, swelling, and sores.

In TCM, *tian-hua-fen* has been used in compound prescriptions for thirst due to fever diseases, dry cough due to lung heat, diabetes, mastitis, and sores with swelling. Modern Chinese clinical reports include the treatment of diabetes and its use as an abortifacient in both its crude form and as an injectable drug. The protein also inhibits choriocarcinomata and invasive moles. Although the roots are reported to be one of the most frequent antidiabetic drugs in China, the decoction or extract proved hyperglycemic in experimental rabbits (Duke and Foster 1989).

In western terms, the root is considered antibiotic, antipyretic, expectorant, laxative, sialogogic, and suppurative, and is used in decoction for abscesses, boils, bronchitis, congestion, constipation, diabetes, dysuria, fever, jaundice, laryngitis, mastitis, mumps, and piles. Among 52 Chinese prescriptions for curing "excessive thirst," 23 contain Trichosanthes. A starch extracted from the roots is used for abscesses, amenorrhea, jaundice and polyuria (Duke and Ayensu 1985; Duke and Foster 1989).

The late Jonathan Hartwell (1906–1991), a National Cancer Institute researcher who documented thousands of folk cancer remedies worldwide, notes that *T. kirilowii* roots and seeds were used for breast or mammary cancers from the Ming dynasty (1368–1644) to populist mainland China in 1967 (Hartwell 1982).

In China the toxic fresh root of *T. kirilowii* has centuries of folk use as an abortifacient. The juice was expressed onto a sponge which was inserted into the vagina during the second trimester of pregnancy. An injection of the protein trichosanthin is now used to induce abortion and to kill the fetus in ectopic pregnancy. Only a tiny amount of the injection is given, separated into several doses over a period of two hours, to see if the patient adversely reacts to the drug. If the patient does not adversely react to the first administration, a large intramuscular dose is given. A report on the use of the abortant in the second trimester with over two thousand women resulted in a 95 percent success rate for inducing abortion within six days after administration. The treatment is apparently not a pleasant experience. Six to eight hours after receiving the injection, symptoms include fever, headache, throat pain, painful or sore joints, stiff neck, and sometimes hives. More serious reactions include nausea, vomiting, shortness of breath, pressure in the chest, and even shock. Altered heart, liver, or kidney function, as well as serious blood loss, were also reported.

Because of serious side effects in the use of the injection in the second trimester, its application is now primarily limited to the first trimester. While it may be a successful abortifacient when used once, patients who receive the treatment reportedly must henceforth wear a permanent bracelet warning doctors of a possible fatal reaction if the treatment is used for a second time! Sensitization to the first exposure is said to last from 10–14 years. It is used in conjunction with other Western drugs to mitigate side effects.

Gua-lou has been used in China since ancient times, and extensively researched in modern China. A tincture of the fruit has been drunk as a treatment for mastitis. The powdered fruit mixed with vinegar and applied as a poultice is a folk remedy for Herpes zoster (shingles). In modern China it is used in prescriptions to treat heart disease. One clinical study reported on the use of tablets made from 15 g of *gua-lou* and 12 g of *Allium chinense* in 25 cases of angina pectoris. The treatment was continued for 2–8 weeks. Twenty-two of the patients were said to have some improvement in symptoms. It produced stomach discomfort in some patients, however.

Experimentally, *gua-lou* is considered antibacterial against various colon bacteria, as in bacillus dysentery. Used externally, *gua-lou* soaked in water (at a ratio of 1:2) has an antifungal effect. *In vitro* experiments have shown that the peel has an inhibiting effect against certain types of cancer cells. The use of *gua-lou* may cause diarrhea.

DOSE

Tian-hua-fen: 9–12 g in decoction, pills, powders, poultice, or mixed with an oil to put on the affected area. The usual dose of *tian-hua-fen* is 9–12 g, when used in combination with other drugs that mitigate the toxicity of *tian-hua-fen*. It is, of course, contraindicated during pregnancy.

Gua-lou is used in doses of 9–12(24) g in decoction or pills; externally it is used powdered, or the juice of the fresh fruit is sometimes used.

WARNING

Trichosanthin is a dangerous sensitizing agent. Chang and But (1986) report that other severe reactions to trichosanthin have included acute pulmonary edema, brain edema, hemorrhage of brain tissue and myocardial damage. They conclude that because of severe side effects and antigenicity, there is a trend toward abandoning or minimizing the use of trichosanthin in clinical situations except for trials in the treatment of trophoblastoma (Duke and Foster 1989).

Trichosanthes products are never used in prescriptions with *Aconitum*.

DESCRIPTION

Trichosanthes kirilowii is a climbing perennial vine, with two to five divided tendrils. The alternate leaves are variable in shape but generally palmate, with 3 to 7 lobes. The base of the leaf is heart shaped. In overall outline, the leaves are broadly oval to somewhat rounded. The white flowers are unisexual; male flowers are usually in racemes, female flowers are solitary. The flowers are tubular, and 5-parted. The individual flower divisions are strongly lacerated. The orange-yellow fruits are oblong or egg-shaped.

Trichosanthes japonica (which has sometimes been treated as a variety of *T. kirilowii*) is distinguished on technical characteristics, especially its darker-colored seeds.

Tian-hua-fen (*Trichosanthes* root) is fusiform, not very cylindrical, and irregular in its form. Most producers take off the root bark; therefore the surface is white, or yellowish-white, with vertical lines. The cross section is white with a little yellow, and is quite starchy. The smell is very faint. The taste is a little bitter. *Trichosanthes japonica* root has a darker color. The root of *T. rosthornii* produced in Sichuan has many fibers. The color of *T. rosthornii* is the darkest of the three. The taste is not only bitter, but a little astringent, too.

The dark orange to orange-red dried fruits of typical *T. kirilowii* (*gua-lou*) are egg- to bowl-shaped, and from 3 to 4 inches in diameter. The peel is rather thick, more or less wrinkled, with orange pulp, and is very sticky with many seeds stuck together. The seeds are oval to elliptical, $\frac{7}{16}$–$1\frac{1}{16}$ inches long, yellowish-brown, and with a very light smell. When crushed, the seeds have a sweet, fragrant smell, with a slightly sweet and sour taste.

DISTRIBUTION

Trichosanthes kirilowii grows on mountainsides, in grass fields, and forest margins under about 50 percent shade. In mountainous areas it is usually found at lower elevations. It occurs in Hebei, Henan, Shandong, Shanxi, Jiangsu, Anhui, Zhejiang, Shaanxi, and Gansu. It is also found in Korea and Japan. *Trichosanthes kirilowii* root is mainly produced in Shandong and Henan, and it is sold throughout China as well as exported. The best quality *tian-hua-fen* is from Henan (An-yang City), and is called *An-yang hua fen*. The root is also produced in Guangxi, Gansu, Guizhou, and Anhui. The major production provinces for *gua-lou* from *T. kirilowii* are Shandong, Henan, and Hebei. The most famous *gua-lou* production areas are in Henan. There are many cultivated forms of the plant; that produced in two counties in Henan, characterized by small fruits with thick orange-red peels, high in sugar content, is considered China's finest. In Shandong *gua-lou* is the major *T. kirilowii* product. The seeds of the plant are produced in Henan, Shandong, and Anhui. Some counties in Anhui near the Henan border are the main production regions for the seeds.

Trichosanthes japonica grows in similar habitats to those above, in Anhui,

Jiangxi, Zhejiang, Hubei, Hunan, Guangxi, and Guangdong. It is primarily produced in Hubei and Jiangxi. The major production of *gua-lou* from *T. japonica* is in Hubei, Jiangxi, and Anhui, where it is used locally or sometimes sold to other regions. Seeds of *T. japonica* are mainly produced in Hubei, Jiangxi, and Anhui. The plant also grows in Japan.

Trichosanthes rosthornii is found on mountainsides, forest margins, plains, or near water in Hubei, Hunan, Gansu, Guangxi, Yunnan, Guizhou, and Sichuan. It is generally cultivated for *gua-lou* in Jiangxi, Hubei, Hunan, Guangxi, Guangdong, Yunnan, Guizhou, and Sichuan. As a source plant of *tian-hua-fen* it is mainly produced in Sichuan, where the root and seeds are consumed locally, rarely sold to other regions.

In the United States, *Trichosanthes* species are primarily rare plants grown in botanical gardens. *Trichosanthes kirilowii*, while introduced to the United States at one time, is extremely rare. When the Compound Q story broke in 1989, USDA botanist Dr. James A. Duke was only able to locate five individual plants in collections of botanical gardens in the United States.

CULTIVATION

Trichosanthes kirilowii likes warm, moist soil and is relatively hardy. The best soil is a deep, rich, well-drained, sandy loam that has been dug to a depth of 2 feet. Seeds are used for propagation. In north China the seeds are planted in April. Before planting, they are soaked in warm water for 24 hours. They are planted in rows spaced at about 2 feet, with 2 to 4 seeds planted per hole at 1½ foot centers. The seed bed is kept moist until seedlings emerge in about 20 days. After they have developed true leaves, they are thinned, so that only one strong seedling is in each hole. Root division is also used for propagation, in March or April. Male and female flowers are on separate plants. If fruit production is the desired goal, then seeds are planted. Root divisions from male plants are often used for root production. In some parts of China, roots for propagation are dug in autumn, then healed in sand for the winter months. Before they begin to produce vegetative growth the following spring, they are divided by hand into sections 3 to 5 inches long, then planted to a depth of about 6 inches, on 1½ foot centers. Two root sections are planted in each hole. They are then kept watered until leaves emerge.

Plantings are weeded and the earth cultivated 2 to 3 times during the growing season, at which time they are sidedressed with night soil. When the vines reach a length of about 3 feet, they may be trained on a trellis or other support for climbing. Plants are watered during times of drought. During the growing season, old lateral branches or thick spots are trimmed to allow for good air circulation, especially for fruit production.

HARVESTING

Roots are harvested in deep autumn when the plant is dormant. Once dug, fibrous rootlets are cut off and the bark is shaved off. The roots are cut vertically into 2 to 4 sections about 6 inches long. If a root is very large, it may be split horizontally or cut into oblique slices before drying in the sun. In some production regions the outer bark is not shaved off, but this produces a somewhat inferior product. The root is dried under the sun, or a light fire is used to bake the roots until dry. Care is taken not to char the roots. In some areas, a sulphur fumigant may be used to whiten roots that have had the bark removed.

Gua-lou is harvested in deep autumn, just before the onset of winter. The fruit should be picked when it is completely ripe, the surface begins to have a white powdery appearance, and it starts turning yellow. The fruit is harvested with its stem and several are bound together, like a girl's pony-tail, and hung under the eaves of a house to dry. They are not dried in direct sun. In some areas, the fruits are spread to dry for a couple of days before hanging them to dry for about two months. After this time the stems are removed, and each fruit is individually wrapped in soft paper. They are handled like eggs, care being taken not to bruise the surface, which will cause molding and mildewing. In the hot moist climate of Sichuan, the fruits may be cut into sections before drying.

PROCESSING

If the roots are not sliced before drying, the whole dried roots may be sorted according to size, then soaked in water until about 60 percent moist. They are covered with a wet cloth, allowed to sit until they are uniformly moist, and then sliced, and redried.

Whole fruits of *gua-lou* are preferred. In the north, in Shandong, it is not very hot, so the fruits can be dried whole. But in Sichuan, where the climate is hot and humid, the fruits are split and the peel and seeds separated before drying to prevent molding and mildewing. Depending on the production region, *gua-lou* may be the whole fruit, or the dried rinds and seeds. If a prescription calls for the whole fruits, the dried seeds and peels are combined for use. In some areas, processing consists of removing the stem, washing the fruit, and then steaming it until it becomes a little soft. It is then pressed flat and cut into small squares for market.

ADDITIONAL SPECIES

In addition to *T. kirilowii*, *T. japonica*, and *T. rosthornii*, a number of additional species are used to produce *tian-hua-fen*. *Trichosanthes damiaoshanensis* C. Y. Cheng et C. H. Yueh is distributed in Guangdong, Guangxi, Yunnan, Guizhou, and Sichuan. Some areas of Guangdong and Guangxi use this species as *tian-hua-fen*. *Trichosanthes sinopunctata* C. Y. Cheng et C. H. Yueh, found in Guangdong and Guangxi, is a local adulterant.

Melothria heterophylla (Lour.) Cogn. is used as a local substitute for *tian-hua-fen* in Fujian, Guangdong, Guangxi, Guizhou and Yunnan. In Yunnan the use of this species is very widespread. Ten to twenty years ago, this species was used as *tian-hua-fen* throughout Yunnan.

Trichosanthes cucumeroides (Ser.) Maxim grows in Gansu, Zhejiang, and Jiangxi. The pronunciation of its Chinese name is the same as *T. kirilowii*, however, the Chinese characters that designate the two species are different. To distinguish between the two for purposes of compounding a prescription, it is necessary to see the Chinese names on paper.

While the above species may be used as *tian-hua-fen* substitutes, other species of *Trichosanthes* are true adulterants that can produce unpleasant side effects such as nausea, headaches, and other problems. Many *Trichosanthes* species are included in this category, among them *Trichosanthes hupehensis* C. Y. Cheng et. C. H. Yueh. Because of its taste it is called "bitter" *tian-hua-fen*. It grows in Hubei, Sichuan, and Jiangxi. Unfortunately, this species grows very rapidly and has a very large root, so some growers prefer to produce it for its increased production.

Trichosanthes cavaleriei Levl. is found in Hubei, Hunan, Guizhou and Sichuan. It known as an adulterant to *tian-hua-fen* in Sichuan.

The seed of *Momordica cochinchinensis* (Lour.) Spreng, a type of bitter cucumber, is used as the Chinese traditional drug *mu-bie-zi*. However, the root is used as an adulterant to *tian-hua-fen* in Hubei and Sichuan. It is found in Hubei, Hunan, Guangdong, Guangxi, Sichuan, and Yunnan. In Guangxi and Guizhou, as well as Japan, it is also known as an adulterant to *Trichosanthes* fruit (*gua-lou*).

Cynanchum auriculatum Royle ex Wright is used as an adulterant to *tian-hua-fen*. It is a member of the milkweed family, with milky-juiced stems and leaves. The root cross section has "milk tubes" and can be easily identified.

OTHER USES

The seeds of *T. kirilowii, T. japonica, T. rosthornii,* and *T. truncata* are used as sources for *gua-lou-zi,* which is an official drug of the 1985 Chinese *Pharmacopeia.* The seeds of at least ten other *Trichosanthes* species have been used as substitutes in various parts of China. The traditional drug consists of the cleaned seeds removed from the ripe fresh fruit harvested from September to November, then dried in the sun. Another method involves putting whole, thin-walled fruits in a jar with water. Several days later a wooden stick is used to smash the fruits, and then the seeds are removed and dried under sun. Sometimes lime is added to the water to make the seeds separate from the fruits more readily.

The seeds are used dried or are stir-fried by heating them until the surface is a little dark in color, and they are slightly swollen. Frozen seeds are called for in some modern prescriptions. After cooling, the seeds are pulverized before use. The seed shell is cracked and the cotyledons inside are removed and then ground to a mash. They are covered with paper to absorb oils. The paper-covered pulp is put in a brick oven and heated until the oil dissipates. Then the remaining cotyledons are ground before use.

The seeds are considered slightly sweet, bitter, and cold. They nourish dryness, smooth the intestines, and disperse heat and phlegm. They are used in prescriptions for dry stool, constipation, cough due to lung heat, expectoration of phlegm, diabetes, and stimulating milk production; mixed with vinegar, the seed poultice has been used externally as a folk treatment for Herpes zoster. The dose is 6 to 12 g. The best-quality seeds are wide, rounded, very full and swollen, with a high oil content. Their use is contraindicated with *Aconitum.*

The fruit peels are yet another traditional drug officially listed in the 1985 Chinese *Pharmacopeia.* They are called *gua-lou-pi* and are primarily derived from *T. kirilowii, T. japonica,* and *T. rosthornii.* The fruit peels of other *Trichosanthes* species are used in South China. Acceptable substitutes include *T. damiaoshanensis* C. Y. Cheng et C. H. Yueh, used in Guizhou, Sichuan, and Guangxi. *Trichosanthes crenulata* C. Y. Cheng et. C. H. Yueh is used in Guizhou and Sichuan. *Trichosanthes truncata* is sometimes used in regions of Guangxi, near the Vietnam border. *Trichosanthes cucumeroides* is sometimes used as the source of the peel. Sometimes strong patients are given *T. kirilowii* while weak or old patients or children may be given the fruit peel of *T. cucumeroides.*

The fruits are collected in September or October, and the whole fruit is cut into two equal sections. The pulp and seeds are removed and the peels are dried in the sun. Care is taken to dry them quickly and evenly to avoid molding or spoilage.

Gua-lou-pi is a little sweet, bitter, and cold. It is considered beneficial to vital energy (*qi/ch'i*) and is used for coughs due to hot phlegm, sore throats, chest pains, vomiting with blood, nose bleeds, diabetes, constipation, and as an external poultice for sores or swelling. Dose is 9 to 12 g.

The stems and leaves of *T. kirilowii* are used in decoction as a folk medicine for the treatment of sunstroke.

Several *Trichosanthes* species are used as food and medicine in India.

Chinese Motherwort
Yi-mu-cao

Botanical Names: *Leonurus artemisia* (Lour.) S. Y. Hu.
Botanical Synonyms: *Leonurus heterophyllus* Sweet, *Stachys artemisia* Lour. *L. sibericus*, and *L. tarticus* are also source plants.
Chinese Names: Pinyin: *Yi-mu-cao* (whole herb); *Chong-wei-zi* (seeds). Wade-Giles: *I-mu-ts'ao* (whole herb); *Ch'ung-wei-tzu* (seeds).
English Names: Chinese motherwort.
Pharmaceutical Names: Herba Leonuri, Semen Leonuri.
Family: Labiatae (Lamiaceae)—mint family.

HISTORY

Chinese motherwort, known as *yi-mu-cao*, and the common European motherwort have been used for similar purposes, mainly menstrual and circulatory problems, for many centuries. They serve as excellent examples of plants used for parallel purposes by divergent cultures, whose uses are confirmed by modern research. This is a fascinating but still little-appreciated plant group in the West. The motherworts deserve greater attention!

The genus to which motherworts belong, *Leonurus* contains four or more species. Botanists differ on the actual number of species in this highly variable plant group, but most agree that the plant group needs close scrutiny by a discerning botanist. The Latin name *Leonurus* comes from the Greek *leon* (lion) and *oura* (tail), in reference to the perceived resemblance of the flowering stalk to a lion's tail. In 1752 *Leonurus sibericus* was the first Latin name bestowed by Linnaeus on Asian members of this plant group. In historical Western literature *L. sibericus* is the name applied to the source plant of *yi-mu-cao* as described in the Chinese medical classics. In 1960 Chinese scientists attributed *L. heterophyllus* as the source plant. The plant material referred to as *L. heterophyllus* was first described by a Portuguese missionary, Joannis de Loureiro, who resided in Macao from 1738 to 1742, and in Canton from 1779 to 1781. In 1790 he named the plant *Stachys artemisia*.

In 1825 an English botanist, Robert Sweet, saw the plant in a nursery in London. Interestingly, the plants in the nursery originated from seeds collected in Brazil, where the plant had been naturalized. In the early days of trans-oceanic trade, Portuguese traders inadvertently introduced the plant from South China to South America in the wrappings of imported Chinese goods. Two years later Sweet published the name *Leonurus heterophyllus*.

Shiu Ying Hu of Harvard University sorted through the taxonomy of source plants of *yi-mu-cao* and made detailed examinations of dozens of specimens of *Leonurus* in the mid-1970s (S. Y. Hu 1976). She recognized that Loureiro's *Stachys artemisia* and Sweet's *Leonurus heterophyllus* were in fact the same plant. According to the rules of botanical nomenclature, the two names are combined; the correct name for the source plant of the Chinese herb *yi-mu-cao* is therefore *Leonurus artemisia*. *Leonurus sibericus* is considered a distinct species.

The first mention of the plant in Chinese herbal literature comes in the first Chinese *materia medica*, *Shen Nong Ben Cao Jing*, two thousand years ago. Shen Nong noted that the seeds brightened the eyes, increased vigor, acted as a diuretic, and, over the long term, helped to maintain ideal weight and good health. The stems were noted as a wash for itching and pustules. In early times, the seeds were eaten as a substitute for sesame seeds.

Li Shi-zhen lists uses of the seeds and herb in the 1596 *Ben Cao Gang Mu*. He noted that it helped to stimulate circulation, benefit the eyes, quiet the nerves, and regulate the menses, among other uses.

Taste and Character

Whole herb: bitter, hot, a little cold. Seeds: hot, a little sweet, cold.

FUNCTIONS

The herb regulates the menses, promotes blood circulation, stimulates the development of new tissue, is diuretic, and reduces swelling. The seeds promote blood circulation, regulate the menses, and clear away liver heat to clear the eyes.

USES

The herb is used singly or in prescriptions to treat menstrual irregularities, suppressed menstrual flow, blood stasis after childbirth (stomach pain due to blood stasis), nephritis with swelling, difficulty in urinating, bloody urine, difficulty in expulsion of the placenta, uterine bleeding, and difficult childbirth. Externally, it is made into a poultice for sores with swelling. The seed is used for red eyes with pain and swelling, high blood pressure, menstrual difficulties, stomach pains due to blood stasis after childbirth, eyesight unclear with pain and a feeling of swelling in the head, and high blood pressure.

Pharmacological reports have confirmed that various preparations of the herb have a diuretic effect, antibacterial and antifungal activity, and uterine stimulatory activity; contract blood vessels to increase the volume of blood circulation, have a stimulatory effect on the central nervous system, decrease the development of ischemic cerebral edema, and reduce disorders associated with monoamine metabolism.

Numerous clinical reports in China have studied the successful use of the herb to treat acute and chronic nephritis, irregular menstruation, postpartum uterine hemorrhage, incomplete involution of the uterus, excessive menstrual bleeding, hypertension, and coronary disease.

Since 1978, intravenous drips of an extract of Chinese motherwort herb have been used in the treatment of coronary myocardial ischemia in a number of Chinese hospitals. A recent clinical study conducted at the Combined Chinese and Western Medicine Medical Ward of the Seventh Municipal People's Hospital of Shanghai provided data on the treatment of heart disease in one hundred patients. All cases had symptoms of angina pectoris, stifling sensation in the chest, palpitation, and shortness of breath. Under the tenets of TCM, patients were divided into five TCM syndrome types: block of chest yang (41 cases), stagnation of heart blood (22 cases), qi and yin deficiency (11 cases), phlegm retention (17 cases), and kidney yang deficiency (9 cases). While these divisions would not be recognized in Western medicine, those patients that were identified as having "phlegm retention" and "kidney yang deficiency" did not respond well to the treatment, therefore the divisions seem useful in identifying whether patients so diagnosed should receive the treatment in the future. Forty-five cases (45 percent) had marked improvement, 39 cases (39 percent) had moderate improvement and 16 cases (16 percent) did not respond to the treatment. The total efficacy rate is given as 84 percent.

The motherwort extract was proven to help activate blood circulation and remove blood stasis, relieving chest pain and palpitation. Other Chinese studies have confirmed the herb's efficacy in treating myocardial ischemia, helping to increase blood flow in the coronary artery, decreasing the heart rate, improving microcirculation, and preventing platelet agglutination.

While most plants in TCM are used in polyherbal combinations, Chinese motherwort has often been used alone. For example, one prescription for edema from acute nephritis calls for 180–250 g of the fresh herb, or 90–120 g of the dried herb. The herb is decocted under a light fire in 700 ml of water, simmered down to 200 ml. The decoction is divided into two doses, consumed in a day's time.

A traditional treatment for difficult childbirth included drinking the juice of the fresh herb, or in winter, decocting a "big handful" of the dried herb with seven bowls of water.

If a woman suffers from poor blood circulation after childbirth, one cup of the juice squeezed from the fresh herb has been used as a treatment.

With 9 g of *dang-gui*, 27 g of motherwort herb has been decocted, then divided into three doses to help the womb return to its original position.

Pharmacological studies have shown that various extracts of the seeds (both water and alcohol) decrease blood pressure. Syrups and injectable forms of the seed extract have been used in combination with the leaves and branches of white mulberry (*Morus alba*) in the treatment of hypertension.

Chinese motherwort is sold in Chinatown herb shops in American cities and is used by practitioners of TCM in the United States.

DOSE

Dried herb: 9–30 g, poulticed as necessary, powdered, used fresh, or as wash. Seed: 6–9 g, in decoction, pills, or powder.

Warning

Sometimes stir-fried seeds are called for in prescriptions. However, some researchers report that a 30 g (1 oz.) dose of the powdered fried seeds produced side effects in clinical trials. Four to six hours after taking the powdered seed, some patients experienced weakness, an oppressed feeling in the chest, and pain in the extremities. The leaves and seeds are contraindicated during pregnancy. Toxicological studies have also shown that the leaves have low toxicity.

Description

Chinese motherwort is an annual or biennial growing from 24–38 inches high. The erect, often branching square stems are slightly hairy. The opposite leaves have long petioles (leaf stalks). Leaves at the base of young plants are broadly heart shaped in outline, with 5–9 broad lobes. These leaves wither as the plant shoots up its flower stalk. Stem leaves are mostly three-divided, with linear to lance-shaped lobes. Leaves on the upper portion of the stem are not divided. The margins are without teeth. Leaves are somewhat hairy above and below.

The flowers are in tight whorls (verticillasters) in the leaf axils. A single flowering stalk may have 12–20 verticils (whorls of flowers). Individual two-lobed flowers are ⅜ to ⅝ inch long. The upper and lower lobes are nearly equal in length. Whitish to pinkish-purple, they are woolly on the exterior, with an incomplete ring of hairs about one third up from the base of the flower. The bell-shaped calyx has five unequal teeth. When dry, the calyx expands and the teeth become spiny, encasing four nutlike fruits. The dried ripe fruit (seeds) are elongate-triangular, ¹⁄₁₆ to ⅛ inch long, grayish-brown to black, with dark spots.

Leonurus sibericus differs primarily in having somewhat larger flowers. The leaves on the upper portion of the stem are three- to five-lobed, and the upper lip of the flower is somewhat longer than the lower lip.

Distribution

Leonurus artemisia grows in mountains and wild fields, river banks, grassy fields, moist fields, roadsides, and wet ground throughout China. It likes a sunny situation, and grows at elevations as high as 10,000 feet. Most provinces produce their own supplies of the plant. It has spread to Pacific islands, including Japan, Indonesia, and the Philippines. It is naturalized in eastern Brazil and in countries of North, South, and Central America along the Caribbean coast. It occurs along the Gulf Coast of the southern United States. While material for American collections is listed as *L. sibericus*, a Linnaean-type specimen of *L. sibericus* has been determined to be the same material now referred by S. Y. Hu as *L. artemisia*. It is likely that the material in the Caribbean basin (including the U.S. Gulf Coast) and Brazil should be referred to *L. artemisia* rather than *L. sibericus*. Motherworts are native to the northern hemisphere. Occurrence in the southern hemisphere is the result of human introduction.

L. artemisia var. *albiflora* (Migo) S. Y. Hu, a white-flowered variety, is used interchangeably with *L. artemisia*. It is distributed in Jiangsu, Jiangxi, Fujian, Guangdong, Guangxi, Sichuan, Guizhou, and Yunnan.

L. sibericus prefers gravel or sandy soils in the provinces of Hebei, Shanxi, Nei Mongol, and Shaanxi in grassy areas or under pine forests. It can be found to elevations of 4,800 feet. It is a clearly defined species, limited in natural distribution to eastern Siberia and adjacent northeastern China.

CULTIVATION

The plant likes warm, moist surroundings and will grow in an average garden soil, although it thrives best in a rich, warm, moist, sandy loam. Plant seeds about one-half inch deep in March or April. Sow directly in rows spaced at one foot. Seed germinates in 10 to 15 days. When the young seedlings have four to five leaves, thin them to spacings of about 8 inches. Weed and loosen the soil every two weeks. In China, one month before harvest, bean curds or commercial fertilizer are applied as a nitrogen source. The plant is easy to grow; Foster has had it self-sow in very poor garden soil.

HARVESTING

The whole herb is harvested in late summer or early autumn, in full bloom. The whole herb is pulled up, the roots cut off, and then the leaf stems are dried in the sun. Timing of harvest is important, since the active components are most highly concentrated when in full flower. If the plant is well into flowering and seeds have begun to form, the quality is lower. If harvested just before blooming, the herb has only a small quantity of active constituents.

For seed, the plant is harvested in midautumn, once the seeds have ripened. The whole plant is dried, and the seeds are threshed and sifted to remove foreign matter.

PROCESSING

For storage, the dried herb is simply cut into sections 6 to 8 inches long, or into one-inch lengths. If already dry before cutting, a moist cloth may be placed over the herb until it absorbs enough moisture to make cutting easy, without shattering the leaves. After cutting, it is dried in sunlight.

ADDITIONAL SPECIES

Another species in the same genus, *L. sibericus* L., is very similar to *L. artemisia*. The whole herb has the same functions. A West Asian species, *L. turkestanicus* V. Krecz. et Kuprian, is also used in some areas of China. The European motherwort *Leonurus cardiaca* is commonly naturalized in the United States. In Western tradition it is considered sedative, antispasmodic, emmenagogic, cardiotonic, hypotensive, and slightly astringent. In short, for many centuries the European motherwort has been used for parallel purposes with Chinese motherwort.

OTHER USES

The flowers, first mentioned in Li Shi-zhen's *Ben Cao Gang Mu* (1596), are used as a folk medicine. They are collected in summer when the flowers begin to open. The dried flowers are produced in Anhui and Jiangsu. It is used externally for sores with swelling, for its diuretic qualities, and to stimulate blood circulation. A dose of 6 to 9 g is used in tea for complications associated with childbirth. A decoction of the flowers increases peristalsis in the small intestines of dogs.

Codonopsis
Dang-shen

Botanical Names: *Codonopsis pilosula* (Franch.) Nannf. (*C. silvestris* Kom.); *C. pilosula* Nannf. var. *modesta* (Nannf.). L.T. Shen. (*C. modesta* Nannf.); *C. tangshen* D. Oliver; *C. tubulosa* Kom.

Chinese Names: Pinyin: *Dang-shen.* Wade-Giles: *Tang-shen.*
English Names: Bonnet Bellflower, Codonopsis, Bastard Ginseng.
Pharmaceutical Name: Radix Codonopsis.
Family: Campanulaceae—bellwort family.

HISTORY

Say the name *Codonopsis* or bonnet bellflower to rock gardening enthusiasts in America, and they will think of diminutive, cold-loving perennials with delicate bell-shaped blue flowers. The rock gardener is unaware that this plant is an "herb." Say *Codonopsis* to those who know Chinese medicinal plants in America and they may think of *dang-shen*—the root of various *Codonopsis* species. They are unaware of the fact that numerous source species of *dang-shen* grow in the collections of rock gardeners. Here is a plant group that anyone interested both in garden perennials and medicinal herbs should get to know better.

The genus *Codonopsis* includes 40 or more species of herbaceous perennials native to Central and East Asia, as far south as Malaysia. About half of these species have been used as source plants of the TCM *dang-shen*. At least 20 species of *Codonopsis* are found in American gardens, primarily in the gardens of those who collect the rare and unusual. These showy but delicate perennials first reached European gardens in the early nineteenth century and arrived in the United States during the last half of the century. *Codonopsis* means "bell-like."

Dang-shen, the dried root of *Codonopsis*, is a very important traditional drug and is often used in TCM. It is thought of as a substitute for ginseng, or a "poor man's" ginseng. Several different grades and types of *dang-shen* are available in Chinese markets, depending upon the species, whether it is cultivated or wild-harvested, and the province or county in which it is grown. Some represent typical species, while others are varieties. The major types include western *dang-shen*, eastern *dang-shen*, and Lu *dang-shen* (Lu is a county in Shanxi). These three types come from the species *Codonopsis pilosula*, including its variety *modesta* (see "Distribution" section). The fourth major type is called *tiao dang-shen*, originating from Sichuan. It is produced from *Codonopsis tangshen*. "White *dang-shen*" is derived from another species, *Codonopsis tubulosa* Kom.

Interestingly, *dang-shen* is not known to ancient Chinese herbalists. It first appears in *Ben Cao Cong Xin*, by Wu Yi-luo, published in 1751 during the Qing dynasty. It is also described in Zhao Xue-min's 1765 Qing dynasty classic, *Ben Cao Gang Mu Shi Yi* (Omissions from the Grand Materia Medica). The species mentioned in these works are the same as the cultivated forms in use today.

Taste and Character

A little sweet, neutral, or slightly warm.

Functions

Invigorates the spleen, invigorates vital energy (*qi/ch'i*), promotes the production of body fluid, and is good for the blood.

Uses

Dang-shen is used in prescriptions for the treatment of loose stool, lack of appetite, fatigue, weakness and tired feeling of limbs, shortness of breath, asthma, coughs, weak voice, vertigo due to blood deficiency, loss of body fluids causing dry mouth and thirst, excessive perspiration, hyperacidity and dyspepsia, anemia, chronic enteritis, nephritis, diabetes mellitus, and spleen deficiency.

Dang-shen is one of many Chinese herbs that crosses the perceived line drawn between foods and drugs in the United States. A decoction of the root, or even flour made from the root, given its sweet flavor, is considered a food that tonifies vital energy (*qi/ch'i*), is a blood tonic, and quells dyspepsia with hyperacidity. According to Russian researchers F. I. Ibragimov and V. S. Ibragimova (1964), *dang-shen* is one of the most important Chinese herbal medicines, with effects likened to those of ginseng. Since it is much less expensive than ginseng, it has traditionally been used by poorer Chinese patients. It is described as an aphrodisiac, general tonic, and styptic. In addition to the indications above, it has been used as an astringent in uterine bleeding, excessive menstruation, and for rheumatic and other joint pains.

Pharmacological research has confirmed that the herb promotes digestion and metabolism, helps to strengthen the immune system, stimulates the nervous system (alcohol extracts), dilates peripheral blood vessels, and inhibits adrenal cortex activity, thereby lowering blood pressure. Laboratory experiments have shown that *dang-shen* may enhance phagocytosis of the reticuloendothelial system, thereby stimulating the immune system. It has also been found to experimentally increase the respiratory rate, raise blood sugar, and increase red blood cells and hemoglobin count. It can lower the number of leucocytes in animal experiments, perhaps confirming the traditional influence of the herb on the spleen. The effects of the herb seem to reverse in a number of conditions once treatment is discontinued. Interesting yet conflicting research results to date suggest that intensive study of the herb is still required. Predictably, chemical studies have failed to reveal a single active compound responsible for the plant's broad-spectrum biological activity. Components include a volatile oil, polysaccharides, inulin, saponins, scutellarein glucoside, resin, mucilage, and trace amounts of alkaloids.

Clinical reports in the Chinese literature have reported on *dang-shen* injections for neurosis. It has been used successfully in the management of anemia and poor appetite with loose stools.

DOSE

6 to 15 g (if used in polyherbal prescriptions), in decoction, extracts or powders. If used alone, 30 to 60 g of *dang-shen* is used.

WARNING

Contraindicated with *Veratrum nigrum* (black hellebore), a poisonous plant. In China, *Codonopsis* itself is generally considered safe, and of low toxicity. Ill effects from normal dosage ranges are absent from the observed literature.

DESCRIPTION

Codonopsis species are herbaceous, often strong-smelling, mostly weak-stemmed perennials, some vinelike in habit, and most with a tuberous root. The stems have milky juice inside. The leaves are alternate or subopposite, and generally small. The flowers are bell shaped or rotate, five-divided, and blue, violet, yellowish or whitish in color.

Codonopsis pilosula is a twining, sprawling herb growing up to 6 feet long. The leaves are ovate, up to 1 1/2 inch long, with pilose hairs, and entire margins. The yellowish, purple-tinted, 1-inch-long flowers are in leaf axils (not terminal). The flower tube is as long or longer than its lobes.

Codonopsis tangshen is quite similar to *C. pilosula*, although the leaves are often smooth rather than soft-haired. The flower calyx is divided almost to the base.

Codonopsis tubulosa is a smooth perennial with twining stems. It has few lance-shaped to oval leaves, up to 2 inches in length. The 1 1/2 inch-long tubular flowers are solitary at the end of branches.

The roots are quite large and have numerous points on the crown where the stems were attached, giving the crown the appearance of a lion's mane. In Chinese herb shops, the root is called "head of lion." This distinctive feature of the root is a special identification standard. The interior of the fresh root is soft and fleshy and the fragrance strong, distinctive, and sweet. A good determiner of quality is to chew the root until it dissolves in your mouth. If only a few fibers remain, it is considered of good quality.

DISTRIBUTION

Codonopsis pilosula grows in rich soils high in organic matter on mountain sides, shrub thickets, and forest margins. Some of the root supply is from wild-harvested plants, although most is cultivated. It is found in Heilongjiang, Jilin, Liaoning, Nei Mongol, Shanxi, Henan, Gansu, Qinghai, and Sichuan.

Material harvested from Gansu, Sichuan, and Shaanxi is called western *dang-shen*. Nan-ping and Song-p'an counties in Sichuan are the major areas in which the root is collected from the wild. Wen-xian county in Gansu is another famous harvest area. Root collected from these areas is considered to be of the highest quality, and is primarily sold in the central and southeastern coastal provinces.

Codonopsis pilosula harvested from Heilongjiang, Jilin and Liaoning is known as eastern *dang-shen* (*dong dang-shen*). The supply is used in these provinces, and sold to Nei Mongol, Gansu, and Hebei, as well as being being exported.

Lu-dang-shen is cultivated *Codonopsis pilosula* root, grown primarily in Shanxi and Henan. Some of the cultivated supply comes from Nei Mongol, Henan, Hebei, and Qinghai. It is sold in Shaanxi, Hebei, Nei Mongol, Henan, Guangxi, and Guangdong, as well as being exported.

Codonopsis pilosula var. *modesta* grows in mountain fields or under the shade of shrubs and forest margins, at elevations of 4,800 to 6,400 feet. It is found in Gansu, Qinghai, and Sichuan.

Codonopsis tangshen grows at 2,700 to 6,400 feet above sea level, in mountain fields, forest margins, and shrub thickets in Hubei, Hunan, Shaanxi, Sichuan, and Guizhou. Major production is in Sichuan, Hubei, and Shaanxi. In recent years it has been extensively cultivated in China.

Cultivated material supplied from Sichuan is known as *tiao dang-shen* (*chuan-dang*). The supply is sold to Jiangsu and Zhejiang provinces.

Codonopsis tubulosa grows in mountain fields, shrub thickets, and forest margins, from 6,000 to 9,600 feet, in Sichuan, Guizhou, and Yunnan. It is known as white *dang-shen*. Most of the supply is sold to the provinces of Shandong, Jiangsu, Anhui, Zhejiang, Jiangxi, and Fujian, as well as to Hunan, Guangxi, and Guangdong.

About twenty species of *Codonopsis*, including those described above, are found in American horticulture, primarily as rare plants in the collections of rock garden enthusiasts.

CULTIVATION

Codonopsis likes a relatively cool climate. Young seedlings will not tolerate strong sunshine. Soil should be well aerated, somewhat sandy, well drained, slightly acid, rich, high in organic matter, and deeply dug, at least to one foot. The tiny seeds are used for propagation and sown in a finely prepared bed. Foster has found it best to sow the seeds in a fine soil indoors, watering from the bottom of the container or misting the soil to avoid displacing the seeds. They usually germinate within two weeks. In China the seeds are sown after the last spring frost, or in autumn, before the soil is frozen. Seeds are planted in rows about 6 inches apart, then covered with a thin layer of soil. If seeds are planted in autumn, seedlings can be transplanted the following spring. If planted in spring, seedlings can be transplanted to permanent locations the following spring. Be careful not to damage the delicate taproots at this point. Individual plants are spaced about 6 inches apart. In northern China, cultivated *dang-shen* is grown under shade in a lath shed. *Codonopsis pilosula* is trained on a trellis so that the plants will be off the ground, providing good air circulation and preventing the seed pods from touching the ground and becoming moldy. When the seedlings have become well established they are sidedressed with a liquid manure slurry to help stimulate vegetative growth. In northern climates, plants are mulched with straw over the winter, although most *Codonopsis* species are fairly hardy.

HARVESTING

Roots three or more years old are harvested in September or October. After digging they are cleaned and sorted according to size. Next, in China, the roots are pierced just beneath the crown and strung up like fish to dry. This hole can be observed on the whole dried *dang-shen* roots available on the American market. The somewhat porous spongy roots are dried under sunshine until about half dry. At this point, the roots are rubbed by hand on a board until the tissue within the root is pressed together. This evenly distributes the remaining water throughout the root, producing the best quality root. After rubbing, it is dried again until about 2/3 dry, then rubbed again. The rubbing process is repeated three or four times before completed. Once this process is finished, the root is dried under sun until 100 percent dry.

When buying the root, break it open. If there is black color in the center of the root, it means it has proably not been subjected to this rigorous processing treatment, and the quality is considered relatively low.

PROCESSING

For roasted *dang-shen*, millet is placed inside a pan and roasted until hot; clean water is sprinkled on the millet, and it is pressed (formed) at the bottom of the pan. When the millet begins smoking, the root slices are placed on top of the millet and roasted until the surface of the *dang-shen* is yellowish.

Another way is simply to roast the root slices mixed with millet. They are taken off the fire when the millet has turned dark yellow, and then cooled and the millet sifted off. For every 100 pounds of root 20 pounds of millet is used. Wheat bran may also be used instead of millet.

ADDITIONAL SPECIES

Besides the *Codonopsis* species treated above, additional species used as *dang-shen* in various localities in China include *C. nervosa* (Chiff.) Nannf., *C. clematidea* Clarke, *C. subglobosa* W. W. Smith, *C. canescens* Nannf., *C. cordiophylla* Diels, *C. subscoposa* Komar., *C. micrantha* Chipp., *C. ovata* Benth., *C. tsinlingensis* Pax et Hoff., and *C. macrocalyx* Diels.

OTHER USES

In India the roots of *Codonopsis* species have been used to prepare an edible flour. The roots and leaves have been used as a poultice for ulcers and wounds.

Dang-gui
Chinese Angelica

Botanical Names: *Angelica sinensis* (Oliv.) Diels.
Botanical Synonyms: *Angelica polymorpha* Maxim. var. *sinensis* Oliv.
Chinese Names: Pinyin: *Dang-gui*. Wade-Giles: *Tang-kuei*.
English Names: Chinese angelica, *Dang-gui*.
Pharmaceutical Name: Radix Angelicae Sinensis.
Family: Umbelliferae (Apiaceae)—parsley family.

HISTORY

As legend would have it, a young Chinese man who dearly loved his new wife left for the mountains to prove himself a man after being taunted by other men of their village. If he did not return in three years, he and his wife agreed that she should consider him lost and thus be free to marry again. Three years passed, and he did not return. Soon after, however, he came back, only to find his wife remarried. Both were heartbroken. The woman became very sick and weak. Her former husband gave her an unknown root that he had collected in the mountains, and she soon returned to perfect health. The people of the village named the herb "*dang-gui*" to honor the heart-wrenching story of the the missed husband who should have returned. In a certain context, "*dang*" means "should" and "*gui*" means "come back." The same phrase may also mean "missing the husband," and can be translated as "proper order." According to H. Y. Hsu in his *Oriental Materia Medica* (1986), *dang-gui*, in a traditional medicine context, helps to harmonize vital energy (*qi/ch'i*), and nourishes blood, returning both to their proper destination or "proper order." The name *dang-gui* therefore has several meanings, derivations, and interpretations.

If, as is often done to develop English plant names, we take the literal translation of the botanical name and call *Angelica sinensis* "Chinese angelica," few American herb consumers would know the plant. But if we call it by its Chinese traditional herb name, *dang-gui*, it is immediately familiar. *Dang-gui* is one of the best selling Chinese traditional herbal products outside of China. According to Harvard University botanist, Dr. Shiu Ying

Hu, it is also the most widely used medicinal herbs in China itself. It is used more frequently and in larger amounts than ginseng and licorice, often considered the most widely used Chinese herbs. While the herb product *dang-gui* is commonly available in North America, the source plant itself is a very rare plant in botanical gardens and is not cultivated by herb gardeners in the United States.

Dang-gui is a member of the parsley family, a plant family known for vegetables like carrot and parsnips, herbs like parsley and caraway, and its highly toxic members, including poison hemlock. The parsley family is also one of the most important plant families for producing medicinal plants. *Dang-gui* is chief among them.

The genus *Angelica* contains 50 to 100 species of herbs in the northern hemisphere. Common garden angelica, *Angelica archangelica*, a European species, is well-known in herb gardens and has long been used for health purposes, often as an antispasmodic and remedy for menstrual disorders—similar purposes to the Chinese Angelica *dang-gui*. It is also the familiar flavoring ingredient of liqueurs such as Benedictine and Chartreuse. The American species, the purple-stemmed angelica *Angelica atropurpurea*, is also widely grown in herb gardens, and is used interchangeably with its European cousin. The Cherokees used the root to relieve menstrual obstructions and as a "tonic" for nervous or "weakly" females. Several North American Indian groups used various angelicas for the treatment of headaches. In Chinese tradition, *dang-gui* is used to treat headaches due to blood deficiency. If you are familiar with uses of *dang-gui*, you soon realize that cultures throughout the northern hemisphere have used various angelicas for parallel purposes throughout recorded history.

The generic name *Angelica* derives from "angelic," referring to the cordial and medicinal properties of the root. The species name *sinensis*, of course, means "of China." *Dang-gui* was known to the Chinese thousands of years before westerners took notice of the plant. The British botanical explorer Dr. Augustine Henry collected the plant in Sichuan and Hubei, and his colleague at Kew Gardens, Daniel Oliver, named it as a new variety of *Angelica polymorpha* Maxim. var. *sinensis* in a 1891 publication. In a 1900 publication, the German botanist Ludwig Diels noted it as a distinct species, giving it the name *Angelica sinensis* (Oliv.) Diels, the botanical name used today.

The use of *dang-gui* as a medicinal plant is first recorded in *Shen Nong Ben Cao Jing*, one of the oldest Chinese herbals. It lists *dang-gui* as being in the second of three classes of traditional medicines. Shen Nong tells us that the herb was found in valleys and ravines. It cured coughs caused by "ascending adverse vital energy (*qi/ch'i*)," plus chills and fevers from springtime fever with drops of sweat on the skin. It was also noted as a treatment for women's vaginal infections, discharges, and infertility. The root was decocted in water. Externally, it was considered good for all types of skin diseases, boils, ulcers, and wounds.

Large quantities of *dang-gui* were known to be cultivated in the provinces of Shaanxi and Sichuan by 650 A.D., according to Su Jing's *Tang Ben Cao* (659 A.D.). At that time, the Shaanxi-cultivated material was considered to be the highest quality. A detailed description of the plant and its growth habit were recorded in Su Song's *Tu Jing Ben Cao* (Illustrated Classic of the *Materia Medica*) published in 1061 A.D. Li Shi-zhen's 1596 classic *Ben Cao Gang Mu* records twenty-seven formulas containing *dang-gui*.

Since ancient times, *dang-gui* has always been an important herb for women. The major production areas in China, as well as modern medicinal uses, are the same today as in the ancient *ben cao*.

TASTE AND CHARACTER

A little sweet, warm.

FUNCTIONS

Enriches the blood, promotes blood circulation, regulates menstruation, nourishes dryness, produces light diarrhea, "smooths" the intestines.

USES

Dang-gui is used in prescriptions for abnormal menstruation, suppressed menstrual flow, painful or difficult menstruation, anemia, uterine bleeding, stomachache after childbirth, constipation due to blood deficiency and dry intestines, constipation, chronic pelvic infections, headache due to blood deficiency, tenesmus, traumatic injuries, carbuncles, and sores.

Few Chinese herbs have been as extensively studied in recent decades as *dang-gui*. Laboratory experiments have shown that extracts with volatile constituents from the plant can raise blood pressure, while nonvolatile extracts reduce blood pressure. Generally, *dang-gui* is considered a blood-pressure lowering-herb. In a similar vein, volatile constituents produce a relaxing effect on the uterine muscle, while nonvolatile water-soluble constituents stimulate uterine contraction. If stimulation of uterine muscles is the desired effect, the root is decocted (simmered in water), which evaporates off the volatile constituents. Conversely, the root can be infused in hot water (herb added after water is hot) to make a tea, which captures the volatile constituents. Other experiments have shown that *dang-gui* can produce a higher rate of uterine tissue multiplication, given an increase in efficiency of glucose metabolism and an increase in DNA ribonucleic acid content. It can help to normalize or harmonize irregular uterine contractions.

Numerous animal studies have confirmed an influence on the heart and cardiovascular system, including decrease in contractions while strengthening ventricular contractility; a definite effect on arrhythmia; and an experimental ability to dilate coronary vessels, increase coronary flow, and reduce arterial blood pressure. In a number of studies, after administration of *dang-gui* extracts, an initial rise in blood pressure has been followed by a decline in blood pressure.

The volatile constituents act as an experimental brain sedative. A decoction of the whole root is considered diuretic and strongly antibacterial. Anti-inflammatory, analgesic (pain-reducing), and antispasmodic activity have been confirmed in experiments. It has been shown to increase the number of red blood cells and platelets. *Dang-gui* has hepatoprotectant, or liver-protecting, activity and helps the liver to utilize more oxygen. Preparations containing *dang-gui* are used clinically to treat hepatitis and liver cirrhosis. It is believed to help abnormal protein metabolism, raising plasma protein levels one to three weeks after treatment.

Chinese clinicians have used *dang-gui* for thrombosis, vasculitis, and other conditions resulting from poor peripheral circulation. *Dang-gui* dilates peripheral blood vessels. The powdered root has been used successfully in the treatment of shingles (herpes zoster).

An injectable *dang-gui* product is used in China for relieving muscle, joint, or nerve pain from rheumatism, sore muscles, sciatica, and pinched nerves. The injections help to reduce pain and lessen spasms. Clinical success rates (when injected at certain acupuncture points) are placed at about 89 percent. *Dang-gui* injections are sometimes used in the treatment of chronic bronchitis.

Active constituents, found at varying levels depending upon methods of preparation or processing, include butylidenephthalide, ligustilide, butylphthalide, and ferulic acid. The first three ingredients are primarily responsible for the antispasmodic action. Research confirms that traditional processing techniques for *dang-gui* actually increase their content in finished product forms. Antianemic activity of the plant has been related to the herb's vitamin B$_{12}$ and biotin content, as well as organic acids in the roots such as nicotinic acid, folic acid, and folinic acid. The herb also contains vitamin E, linking it to protection against vitamin E deficiency. Its use in TCM to produce a calming action on a fetus has been theoretically attributed to its vitamin E content.

The whole root, powdered root, sliced root, capsulated products, alcohol extracts, and other product forms are commonly available on the American market. Considered the most important Chinese herb for menstrual disorders, its blood tonic, circulation-enhancing, pain-relieving, tranquilizing, and liver-protecting qualities are less appreciated by American consumers.

DOSE

Dose 4.5–12 g in decoction, tinctured, and used in extracts, pills and powders.

CONTRAINDICATION

Patients with diarrhea are generally not prescribed *dang-gui*, as it is considered mildly laxative. It is sometimes used as a laxative and stool-softening agent for elderly and debilitated patients. It is contraindicated during pregnancy, except when administered by a qualified medical practitioner. If sold as a food ingredient on the Canadian market, a pregnancy warning is required.

DESCRIPTION

Dang-gui is an herbaceous, smooth-stemmed perennial, growing from 3 to 4 feet tall. The three divided leaves have oval, sharp-toothed segments. The long leaf stalk has a prominent sheath. Flowers are in umbels (umbrella-like structures), with 9 to 13 radial segments with numerous tiny flowers. The winged fruits, often used as an identification feature of parsley family members, are distinguished only by highly technical characteristics. The thickened, branched root is the part of the plant used.

The best quality *dang-gui* has large, long, plump roots with a yellowish-brown surface. Broken sections should be yellowish-white in color. The flavor and fragrance should be "very thick." The root is cylindrical, 4 to 10 inches long, with a yellowish-brown or deep brown surface. Near the top of the root, horizontal lenticels (for the exchange of gases) can be observed. The head of the root is swollen, and measures from ¾ to 1½ inch in diameter. The top of the root may have pieces of the stem and leaves attached (rarely seen in the American market). The main body of the root is quite short, from ¾ to 1¼ inch long, and a little larger in diameter. Two to 10 twisted, lateral rootlets are attached to the main root body. They are generally soft, not very brittle, and do not have a sharp fracture when broken. The interior is yellowish-white or a light yellowish-brown color.

DISTRIBUTION

The plant grows at sea level to mountain areas from 5,900 to 8,000 feet. It does best in very high and cold conditions in a shaded, moist location. It is cultivated in the provinces of Gansu, Ningxia, Sichuan, Yunnan, Hubei, Shaanxi, and Guizhou. The root is found wild in the deep mountains and ancient forests of Gansu. Major production counties include Min-xian county in Gansu and Wu-du county, Yunnan Province. It is also produced in Shaanxi and Hubei. In recent years, cultivation has begun in other provinces as well. The best quality *dang-gui* comes from Gansu province.

CULTIVATION

The plants likes a cool, moist environment with deep, rich, sandy soil, high in organic matter. High mountain areas are preferred. It is often grown in areas that have remained fallow for many years. Propagation is by seeds. In Gansu province, seeds are planted in June. In Yunnan, seeds are planted after ripening in August. Like seeds of many angelicas, those of *dang-gui* seem to need light for germination; therefore they are tamped into the soil surface and covered with a very light layer of straw — just enough to keep them from drying out. When growing European angelica, best results are achieved with a measure of patience. Foster has had angelica seeds take as long as six months to germinate. Fresh seed is essential. When seedlings begin to appear, a fluffed straw mulch is arranged around the seedlings, allowing for good sunshine and air circulation. The mulch is removed in late summer after the seedlings are firmly established. Seedlings are spaced at about 1 foot.

In China, first-year seedlings are carefully dug from the ground in autumn, tied into small loose bundles, and healed in light soil in a cool, dry space, usually a cellar, for the winter, then replanted early the following spring. In Yunnan the leaves of Mason's pine (*Pinus massoniana*) are placed over the seedlings instead of soil. The following spring, seedlings are placed in beds in crescent-shaped holes, with ten seedlings placed in each crescent arrangement, each plant spaced at about 6 inches. The crescent arrangements themselves are spaced around two-foot centers. Young seedlings are kept well-watered. In the first or second year, when the plants reach a height of 8 to 9 inches, any flower buds that have begun to form are pinched back. A side dressing of composted manure is then worked into the soil around the plants. Plantings are side-dressed two or three times during the growing season. Care is taken to make sure that soil is bermed up around the plants. Unless chosen to produce seeds, the buds of the flowers heads are pinched back throughout the growth of the plant. It is believed that this procedure helps return more of the plant's "energy" to the root, and is a common practice with many Chinese herb root crops. The soil around young plants is kept well watered until at least two months before harvest, when the grower is careful not to give the plants water. At this point too much water may cause the roots to decompose in the ground before they are even harvested. Growing *dang-gui* is a very painstaking process, requiring both skill and experience.

HARVESTING

Dang-gui is harvested in the autumn of the second or third year of growth, depending upon the production region. One-year-old plants are not harvested; their roots are small, their fragrance weak, and they produce an inferior product. Deep autumn of the second year is the harvest time in Gansu province.

When the roots are pulled, the dirt is shaken off, and they are placed in the shade until some of the moisture has evaporated. They are handled gently at this point to prevent bruising. The roots are not washed, since contact with water may cause them to turn an undesirable black color or even decompose. In Gansu, after the root is partially dried but still soft, it is tied into small bundles and hung from the ceiling. Next, a fire is made with *wet* wood in order to smoke the root. This process is used to give the root the color expected by the market. After smoking, a light fire is used to dry the root until 70 to 80 percent dry. During the smoking process, the roots are turned once (flipped and hung from the bottom) to get an even distribution of smoke and thus a uniform color. In Gansu, *dang-gui* is not dried in the sun because it makes the root woody and hard. The use of coal fires is also avoided during the drying process; they make the root too dark and adversely affect its medicinal qualities.

The harvest and drying process is different in various growing regions. In Yunnan, the root is harvested in the autumn of the second year and then dried in the sun, but the roots are turned frequently so that the surface does not harden. Care is taken to make sure that the roots do not freeze while drying. Roots of various sizes and forms are sorted into several lots. The "head" (rhizome), or crown of the root, and the main body of the root are separated and processed as two separate commodities.

PROCESSING

In some areas, before being dried, the roots are covered with a moist cloth and allowed to evenly absorb just enough moisture to aid in slicing the root. The root slices are then dried.

Some prescriptions call for alcohol-processed *dang-gui*. Slices of root are sprinkled with rice wine, covered with a cloth, and gently roasted under a light fire. By weight, one part wine is used to ten parts *dang-gui*.

ADDITIONAL SPECIES

The European herb lovage (*Levisticum officinale*) is known in China as European *dang-gui*, and has been cultivated as a *dang-gui* substitute. From 1960 to 1963 serious shortages of *dang-gui* were experienced in China. Since there was not enough available for clinical use, a search for substitutes was undertaken through a cooperative effort of the College of Traditional Medicine of Beijing and the Jiangsu Institute of Medical Research. A systematic search revealed that lovage had been cultivated in China since 1957. However, the quantities available were small. Cultivation then began in Hebei, Shandong, Henan, Nei Mongol, Liaoning, Shaanxi, Shanxi, and Jiangsu. Lovage had previously been used in China as a folk medicine, rather than an important medicinal plant of TCM. Chinese experiments have shown that it has a comparable antispasmodic activity to *dang-gui*. Lovage, or European *dang-gui*, has been used for amenorrhea and other menstrual conditions.

In Jilin province, Ethic Koreans of Yin-bian cultivate *Angelica acutiloba* as a substitute for *dang-gui*. It is thought to have comparable medicinal action to *dang-gui* and is known as Japanese or Korean *dang-gui*.

In Yunnan, *Ligusticum glaucesens*, called wild *dang-gui*, is used as a local substitute.

OTHER USES

None noted.

Eleuthero
Ci-wu-jia

Botanical Names: *Eleutherococcus senticosus* Maxim.
Botanical Synonyms: *Acanthopanax senticosus* (Rupr. & Maxim.)
Harms., *Hedera senticosus* Rupr. & Maxim., *Acanthopanax eleutherococcus* Makino.
Chinese Names: Pinyin: *Ci-wu-jia* (root). *Jia-pi*, the bark of *E. gracilistylus* (*Acanthopanax gracilistylus*), is the official source of *wu-jia-pi* in the Chinese Pharmacopeia; however, the bark of *E. senticosus* (*ci-wu-jia-pi*) is sometimes used as a substitute. *Ci-wu-jia*, the root of *E. senticosus*, is a separate article of *materia medica* in Chinese tradition. Wade-Giles: *Tz'u-wu-chia* (root); *chia-p'i* or *tz'u-chia-p'i* (bark).
English Names: Eleuthero, Siberian ginseng, eleuthero ginseng, ussurian thorny pepperbush.
Pharmaceutical Name: Radix Acanthopanacis senticosi.
Family: Araliaceae—ginseng family.

HISTORY

Who uses eleuthero, a shrubby member of the ginseng family? It has been used in China to help balance vital energy for over two-thousand years, but it was Russian researchers who catapulted the plant fame in the early 1960s. Now deep-sea divers, mine and mountain rescue workers, explorers, soldiers, factory workers, cosmonauts, and athletes in Russia are reported to use preparations of the plant to as a sort of "tonic" or "adaptogen," basically helping users to preform better under stress. It is also well-known among herb consumers in the West.

The plant has been referred to both botanically and as an herbal product under a perplexing number of names. The genus *Eleutherococcus* of the ginseng family includes about 20 species of shrubs from China, Russia, Japan, and Korea. Eleuthero was first described in Western botany and was named *Hedera senticosa* in a 1856 publication by the Russian botanists Franz J. Ruprecht (1814–1870) and Karl Johann Maximowicz (1827–1891). In 1859, however, Maximowicz recognized *Eleutherococcus* as a distinct genus, typified by *Eleutherococcus senticosus*. In 1894 the German botanist Hermann Harms combined the genera *Eleutherococcus* and *Acanthopanax* (originally a subgenus of *Panax*, created in 1854). Since *Acanthopanax* was published earliest, all species then placed under *Eleutherococcus* became species of *Acanthopanax*. In 1924 a Japanese botanist, Takenoshin Nakai, again recognized *Acanthopanax* and *Eleutherococcus* as distinct genera. Nakai's treatment is recognized by the Russian botanist A. I. Poyarkova in volume 16 of the *Flora of the USSR*. Unfortunately, when volume 54 of the *Flora of China* (Araliaceae) by Hoo and Tseng was published in 1978, *Acanthopanax* was recognized as the proper generic name.

Consequently, most world scientists call the plant *Eleutherococcus senticosus* and Chinese scientists refer to it as *Acanthopanax senticosus*. Publications by Soejarto and Farnsworth (1978) and S. Y. Hu (1980) both provided convincing arguments for retaining the name and position of *Eleutherococcus senticosus*, the name by which the plant should be known, and by which it is generally known in the United States and Europe. The taxonomic situation is unfortunately complex, and has caused numerous ambiguities in the scientific literature of the last century.

The common name *Siberian ginseng* has been no less controversial. In a Chinese context, "seng" is a term used by root gatherers for medicinal plants with fleshy root stocks used as tonics. In China, there is only one "ginseng." *Eleutherococcus senticosus* is not a "seng-producing" plant under the Chinese definition, and it was not known as Siberian ginseng until it was first imported to the United States back in the early 1970s. Some consider the use of the name Siberian ginseng a marketing stratagem. It has raised the wrath of traders in *Panax* (true ginseng) in the past two decades. However, it is now the name by which *Eleutherococcus senticosus* is best known in the United States. Perhaps the common name *eleuthero* would be more appropriate and less controversial. Whatever you call it, the controversies surrounding the name have probably slowed down the acceptance of the use of the plant in the United States.

Ambiguities in the Chinese names and their application to source plants for *wu-jia-pi* (bark) and *ci-wu-jia* (root) are no less prevalent, as noted under the Chinese names and additional species headings below. *Ci-wu-jia* was mentioned in the first class of herbs in *Shen Nong Ben Cao Jing*. Some scholars question whether the plant described by Shen Nong was indeed *Eleutherococcus senticosus*.

Taste and Character

Bitter, warm.

Functions

Good for vital energy (*qi/ch'i*), strengthens the spleen and kidney, useful for deficiency of yang in the spleen and kidney, stabilizes energy.

Uses

Traditionally, it has been considered good for vital energy (*qi/ch'i*), used for sleeplessness with many dreams, lower back or kidney pain, deficiency of yang in the kidney and spleen, lack of appetite, and to enhance overall resistance to disease or adverse physical influences or stress. For treating rheumatoid arthritis and making muscles and bones strong, one prescription mixes *wu-jia-pi* with sweet rice wine.

Research in Russia, China, Japan, Europe, and the United States over the past 25 years has catapulted the plant to wide use as an adaptogen and immune-system stimulant. Few if any East Asian medicinal plants have been the focus of such intensive research over the past thirty years. Studies have shown that various preparations of the plant build nonspecific immunity, improve weak nerves, increase strength and appetite, reduce incidence of heart disease, dilate blood vessels, increase cerebral blood flow, are antirheumatic, may reduce blood sugar, and may have a static effect on certain types of cancers.

Sound like a cure-all? Russian researchers call it an adaptogen, a term coined in 1947 by N. V. Lazarev to describe the action of a substance that helps to increase "nonspecific resistance of an organism to adverse influence." I. I. Brekhman, the leading researcher on the plant, defines an adaptogen as a substance that is (1) innocuous (safe), causing no or minimal side effects; (2), a substance that must have a nonspecific action, increasing resistance to a wide range of environmental or other physical factors; and (3) a substance that must have a normalizing action in the body, irrespective of a diseased state.

In the late 1940s Soviet researchers in Siberia began a search for a cheap, abundant adaptogen. Throughout the 1950s intensive research on the far eastern Soviet species *Eleutherococcus senticosus* was conducted. By 1960 human clinical trials began in earnest. In 1962, the Soviet Ministry of Health approved a 33 percent ethanol extract of eleuthero for human use. Since that time over 6,000 healthy, stressed, or diseased patients have been involved in clinical trails, measuring the effect of the eleuthero extract on exposure to increased heat, noise, motion, exercise, and work loads. Effects on mental alertness, work output, and work quality have also been measured. Results were generally positive, and side effects minimal. In Russia the 33 percent ethanol extract is used by workers in stressful jobs or jobs demanding high performance.

The dried root, extract, and tablets of *ci-wu-jia* (*E. senticosus*) are official in the 1985 edition of the Chinese *Pharmacopeia*. *E. gracilistylus* (as *wu-jia-pi*) is also official.

Information on the plant has become voluminous, although most of the studies are in Russian. For a review of the Russian studies see Farnsworth *et. al.* (1985).

Under the names of "eleuthero" and "Siberian ginseng," a wide array of products derived from the plant are available in health and natural-food markets in the United States, including capsulated herbs, tinctures, whole root (cut and sifted, whole, or powdered), teas and other product forms. Unfortunately, the high quality 33 percent ethanol extract used in Russia is unavailable in the United States.

DOSE

In China, 4.5–27 g are used in decoction, powder, poultice, or tincture. Russian studies involving healthy or stressed volunteers used doses of the 33 percent extract ranging from 2.0 to 16.0 ml, taken 1 to 3 times daily for up to 60 days, followed by a 2 to 3 week rest period. Up to five courses were administered. In patients with diagnosed disease conditions, the dose ranged from 0.5 to 6 ml, 1 to 3 times daily for up to 35 days, followed by a 2 to 3 week rest period between courses of treatment.

DESCRIPTION

Eleuthero is a shrub that grows from 3 to 15 feet in height. The crowded upright stems are densely covered with slender, sharp-pointed, usually backward-curved, bristlelike prickles. The leaves are on slender stalks 1 to 4 inches long, often covered with small prickles. The leaves are palmate, divided into five, or sometimes three elliptical-ovate to obovate leaflets. The leaflets are narrowed at the base, and from 3 to 5 inches long. The margins of the leaflets are double sharp-serrate. The veins beneath are sometimes covered with tiny bristles. The tiny five-petaled flowers are in terminal umbels, growing solitary or in groups of 3 to 4 on long stalks. The individual flowers themselves are inconspicuous. The blackish ovoid fruits are about ⅓ inch long.

DISTRIBUTION

Eleuthero occurs in mountain thickets, field edges, and sparse woods, sometimes forming impenetrable thickets in Heilongjiang, Jilin, Liaoning, Hebei, and Shanxi provinces. Major production areas in China are Heilongjiang, Jilin, and Liaoning. It is most abundant in the Xiaoxinganling Mountains of Heilongjiang. Eleuthero is often an understory shrub of bottomland mixed evergreen and hardwood forests where birches (*Betula* spp.) and alders (*Alnus* spp.) are predominant. The plant is extremely competitive in its native habitat, reportedly producing more than 10,000 plants per hectare.

In Russia, it grows from the mid-Amur River region to Sakhalin. It is said to be most abundant in the Khabrarosvk and Primorsk districts, and is abundant in the Sikhote-Alin Mountains, growing to elevations of about 2500 feet. The habitat is mixed and coniferous mountain woods, generally growing in thickets or as undergrowth. It occurs rarely in high riparian woodland and in oak groves at the foot of cliffs and ravines.

Eleuthero also grows in Japan's northern island of Hokkaido and on the Korean peninsula.

In the United States eleuthero has been a rare specimen plant in botanical gardens for more than a century. One specimen at Arnold Arboretum of Harvard University was introduced from Saint Petersburg in 1892. It is also grown in the United States National Arboretum in Washington, D.C. and other major botanical gardens. Commercial plantings in early stages of development have been established in Oregon, Washington, and Montana. Seed is now readily available in the United States, and it is likely to become more widespread in cultivation. Given its dominance in areas where it is indigenous, care should be taken to ensure that this species does not become North America's newest noxious Asian weed.

Cultivation

Eleuthero can grow in full sun or partial shade, is very hardy, and prefers a cool climate. It is not particular about soils, provided the soil is moderately rich and well drained. In China it is cultivated in fields or mountain terraces. Propagation is by seed, cuttings, or division of established clumps. Seeds are planted in spring or autumn. Cuttings are made from August through September. Branches of previous year's growth are cut into sections 6 to 12 inches long, which are then placed obliquely into the soil. Cuttings root in two to three weeks. The following spring or autumn, plants are transplanted to permanent locations, spaced at 3 to 4 feet.

In experiments with a related species, *Eleutherococcus henryi*, softwood cuttings taken in mid or late June that are treated with 3,000 ppm IBA-talc and rooted in sand and misted resulted in a 55 percent rooting rate. Another study involving *Eleutherococcus sieboldianus* used softwood cuttings taken in mid-August. Cuttings were treated with 8,000 ppm IBA-talc plus thiram, and misted.

A six-month period of warm stratification followed by three months of cold stratification has resulted in good germination of *Eleutherococcus henryi*. Root radicals emerged during cold stratification, suggesting a shorter pretreatment duration might be used for germinating *Eleutherococcus* seeds. After pretreatment, seeds should germinate in 7 to 10 days.

Harvesting

The bark is harvested in late summer or autumn. The roots are dug when the plant is dormant. Lateral rootlets are cut away and the roots are cleaned. The cortex of the root is retained, and the wood is discarded. However, on the American market most of the root material sold includes the whole cut or ground root of the shrub, rather than just the desirable cortex.

Processing

None noted.

Additional Species

Other species of *Eleutherococcus* are also used as source plants or substitutes for *wu-jia-pi*, normally supplied by *Eleutherococcus gracilistylus* (*Acanthopanax gracilistylus*). *E. gracilistylus* occurs in mountain valleys and forests in Zhejiang, Henan, Hubei, Hunan, Sichuan, Shaanxi, Gansu, Shandong, Jiangsu, Anhui, Jiangxi, Guizhou, and Yunnan.

Eleutherococcus sessiliflorus (*A. sessiliflorus*), a substitute for *wu-jia-pi*, occurs in mountains, forest edges, and shrub thickets in Heilongjiang, Jilin, Liaoning, and Hebei.

Eleutherococcus giraldii (*A. giraldii*), or *hong-mao-jia-pi*, grows in mountain shrub thickets in Hebei, Shanxi, Shaanxi, Gansu, Qinghai, Henan, Hubei, and Sichuan.

In the United States the root of a Chinese vine in the milkweed family, *Periploca sepium*, has appeared as a widespread adulterant to *E. senticosus*. This is alarming, given the fact that this milkweed family member, which has a very similar-sounding Chinese name to that of eleuthero, contains cardiac glycosides. It has recently been implicated in causing complications in fetuses, including an androgenic effect resulting in abnormal development of hair.

OTHER USES

The leaves of eleuthero are used in some herbal tea products. A number of *Eleutherococcus* species have been grown as ornamentals in Western horticulture.

Fo-ti
He-shou-wu

Botanical Names: *Polygonum multiflorum* Thunb.

Botanical Synonyms: *Helxine multiflorum* (Thunb.) Raf., *Pleuropterus cordatus* Turcz., *P. convolvulus* Thunb. ex Mat., *Pleuropterus multiflorus* Turcz. ex Nakai.

Chinese Names: Pinyin: *He-shou-wu* (root); *Shou-wu-teng* (stems). Wade-Giles: *Ho-shou-wu* (root); *Shou-wu-t'êng* (stems).

English Names: Fo-ti, nimble-Will, Chinese cornbind.

Pharmaceutical Name: Radix Polygoni Multiflori; Caulis Polygoni Multiflori.

Family: Polygonaceae—knotweed family.

HISTORY

During the Tang dynasty, there was a Chinese man named He Shou-wu. He had lived to the age of 58 without having any children because he was impotent. Feeling depressed, one day he drank himself into a stupor and fell asleep on a mountainside. When he woke up, he saw two intertwining herbs growing next to the spot where he lay. The sight of the plant sparked his curiosity. He dug up its root and took it to a an old herbalist, who told him that the roots had fabulous restorative and reviving powers. He made a decoction of the root and started drinking it every day. After several days, his virility was restored. Over the next ten years he fathered several children and his hair never turned gray. He lived to the ripe old age of 130 years. Since that time, the root of this Chinese member of the bindweed family has borne the name of *He Shou-wu*.

The source plant of *he-shou-wu* is *Polygonum multiflorum*. The root is widely known on the American herb market as fo-ti, a name given to the plant in the early 1970s by a marketer. Go to a Chinese herb shop and ask for fo-ti and you will only get a curious look. Fo-ti is not a Chinese name for the plant. Here, we will refer to the root product by the Chinese name *he-shou-wu*.

The genus *Polygonum* of the bindweed family includes about 150 species of weedy herbs primarily native to northern temperate regions. *Polygonum*, derived from *poly* meaning many, and *gonu* (knee or joint) refers to the nodes on the stems of the knotweed family. In Western botany, the plant was first described in 1784 by the Swedish botanist Carl Peter Thunberg in his *Flora Japonica*.

In the Chinese literature, *he-shou-wu* is first mentioned in the 973 Song dynasty work *Kai Bao Ben Cao*, attributed to Ma Zhi. Ma Zhi mentions two types of *he-shou-wu*, white and red. *Polygonum multiflorum* is red *he-shou-wu*. *He-shou-wu* is an official listing in the 1985 Chinese *Pharmacopeia*.

The stems, *shou-wu-teng*, are first mentioned in the 1670 Qing dynasty work *Ben Jing Feng Yuan* by Zhang Lu. The leaves, a folk medicine, are first listed in *Ben Cao Gang Mu*.

He-shou-wu is also a famous medicinal plant in Japan, where it is known as *kashuu*. It was first brought from China to Nagasaki about 1720. From there it rapidly spread throughout that country.

TASTE AND CHARACTER

Unprocessed root: a little bitter, slightly sweet, neutral. Processed root: a little sweet, astringent, slightly warm.

FUNCTIONS

Unprocessed root: relaxes the bowels, detoxifies sores. Processed root: invigorates liver and kidneys, supplements the vital essence (*qi/ch'i*), and supplements the blood.

USES

The unprocessed root is used in prescriptions for scrofula, carbuncle sores, and constipation due to deficiency of yin and blood. The processed root is used in prescriptions for deficiency of yin in liver and kidney, vertigo, insomnia, premature gray hair, lower back and knee pain and weakness, neurasthenia, anemia, weak seminal emission, white or yellowish vaginal discharges (leukorrhea), tuberculosis of lymph nodes, carbuncles, sores, and boils. *He-shou-wu* is one of the most widely used tonic herbs in traditional Chinese medicine.

Over the centuries *he-shou-wu's* reputation has bordered on the mythical for its power to produce longevity, increase vigor, and promote fertility. It has been used as an ingredient in prescriptions for premature graying, lower back pain, angina pectoris, deficiency of vital energy (*qi/ch'i*), bloody stool, malaria, night sweating, impotence, and used externally as a styptic for cuts and for treating sores and ringworm.

In laboratory experiments *he-shou-wu* has been shown to reduce blood cholesterol and slightly reduced atherosclerotic lesions in rabbits. The herb's lecithin content is believed by some researchers to help prevent the accumulation of cholesterol in the liver and the retention of fats in the blood stream. It may also help prevent the penetration of fats in the arterial lining, theoretically reducing atherosclerosis. In animal experiments, the herb has been shown to help reduce the formation of plaque and lipid deposits in the arterial wall.

He-shou-wu is considered antibacterial, and in experiments enhances animals' resistance to cold, promotes intestinal peristalsis, and promotes the growth and development of red blood cells.

Clinical studies in China have included the use of the herb in the treatment of high cholesterol, neurasthenia, and schizophrenia. It is also reportedly used in the treatment of chronic bronchitis, head injuries, epilepsy, peripheral neuritis associated with diabetes, and muscular atrophy.

For high cholesterol, a modern treatment in China uses tablets of processed *he-shou-wu*. The tablets consist of 70 percent *he-shou-wu* extract with 30 percent *he-shou-wu* powder. Each tablet weighs 500 mg. Five tablets are taken 3 times per day. The patient is given regular meals during administration of the tablets. Cholesterol levels are monitored during the treatment. The usual course of treatment is 2 to 6 weeks.

In Western terms it is considered antipyretic, hypoglycemic, experimentally antitumor, and sedative. The whole root, root slices, powdered root, root tincture, capsulated root and other products are sold as dietary supplements on the American herb market.

DOSE

6–15 g in decoction or in extracts, tinctures, pills, tablets, powders, or used as a poultice or wash.

WARNING

The unprocessed root can cause a loose stool or diarrhea, with abdominal pain, nausea, and vomiting. After processing, the root does not cause diarrhea as easily. The root is considered to have minimal toxicity, though large doses have produced numbness of the extremities. Skin rashes have also been reported.

DESCRIPTION

Polygonum multiflorum is a perennial twining herbaceous vine growing 3 to 6 feet long or more. The smooth branching stems are reddish and somewhat woody at the base. The thick tuberous rhizomes are somewhat woody, and may weigh over 6 pounds. The oval leaves, with an acuminate tip and cordate base are up to 4 inches long, and are on slender stalks up to1½ inches long. The profusely flowering branched panicles are terminal or in axils. The specific epithet *multiflorum* refers to the profusion of tiny flowers. The flowers themselves are quite small (2 to 3 mm wide). The seeds are triangular black achenes, similar in appearance to buckwheat seeds.

DISTRIBUTION

Polygonum multiflorum occur in grasslands, roadsides, forest edges, between rocks in mountains, in sunny places at the foot of mountains, and in bamboo thickets in Hebei, Henan, Shandong, Jiangsu, Anhui, Zhejiang, Jiangxi, Fujian, Taiwan, Hubei, Hunan, Guangxi, Guangdong, Sichuan, Yunnan, and Guizhou. Basically, it occurs throughout China except in the northeast.

Major commercial production of the root is in Henan, Hubei, Guangxi, Guangdong, Guizhou, Sichuan, and Jiangsu. Other regions in China where the plant occurs produce root for local consumption.

The plant also occurs in Japan and the Ryukyu Islands. Japanese material is considered naturalized from China. The material from Taiwan is *P. multiflorum* var. *hypoleucum*, differing from the typical species in that the leaves are ovate to oblong, with truncate bases.

Polygonum multiflorum was introduced to the United States as a potential ornamental in the early twentieth century, perhaps by E. H. Wilson. It persists as a rare plant of botanical gardens and collectors.

CULTIVATION

Polygonum multiflorum likes warm, moist, sandy soils, high in organic matter, with excellent drainage. Raised beds should be dug to a depth of at least one foot before planting, and liberally supplied with well-rotted manure, compost, or other organic fertilizers. It can be propagated from root divisions, stem cuttings, seeds, or layering. Seed can be sown in early spring after the last spring frost. Plant shallowly in a seed bed with rows spaced at about 8 inches. Keep soil moist and at temperatures between 60 and 68°F until seeds germinate (about 20 days after planting). Transplant young seedlings (about 6 inches high) at spacings of about 18 inches. The plant is easily propagated from cuttings taken in July and August; make cuttings about 3½ to 6 inches long, place obliquely in soil, and keep moist. It also roots easily in water, producing new roots in less than three weeks. Cuttings can be transplanted to permanent locations in the spring of the second year. The lateral tubers can be divided in late February to mid-

March to increase plantings. Plant to a depth of about 2 inches. Once plants get about one foot high, provide trellising on which the vines can be trained.

HARVESTING

The fresh root is harvested in spring or autumn, after the vine has grown for 3 to 4 years. The fall-harvested root is considered to be the best quality. The roots are cleaned and then the end rootlets are sliced off. The large roots are cut into two vertical pieces, or cut into thick pieces to be dried in sun. In some production areas, before drying the roots are first boiled in water. This helps to prevent the herb from becoming pulpy once it is dried. It also helps to evenly distribute and stabilize moisture content of the dried root and makes slicing of the roots easier once they are dried. The best quality roots are very dense and starchy. Light, porous, fibrous roots are considered of poor quality. Large roots the size and shape of a baby sell for a very high price.

PROCESSING

Before processing, the *he-shou-wu* root is cut into cube-shaped pieces about ½ inch square, or into slices about ⅜ inch thick. It is then evenly mixed with a decoction of black beans (see below). The root sections are simmered in the black bean decoction until they absorb all of the bean liquid and become brownish-red in color. A non metal cooking vessel is used for this process. About 10 pounds of the black bean liquid are used for every 100 pounds of *he-shou-wu*.

Another method uses the same process as above, adding 25 pounds of yellow wine to the mix.

The black bean liquid is made by boiling about 22 pounds of beans for four hours. The liquid is then strained off (should be about 33 pounds). Add more water to the beans and boil for an additional three hours. About 22 pounds of liquid should be produced during the second step. Once done, mix the liquid from the first and second decoctions together. This liquid is used in the processing method above.

ADDITIONAL SPECIES

Red *he-shou-wu* is *Polygonum multiflorum*. White *shou-wu* (*bai-shou-wu*) is *Cynanchum bungei*. In Jiangsu and Zhejiang, *Cynanchum auriculatum* has been used as a substitute for *bai-shou-wu*. In Liaoning, *Cynanchum wilfordi* is used. In Yunnan and Hubei, *Cynanchum otophyllum* has been used.

Polygonum cillinerve has been recorded as an adulterant to *he-shou-wu* in Gansu. In Yunnan, Gansu, and Henan, *Pteroxygonum giraldii* is recorded as an adulterant.

Note: *Polygonum multiflorum* should not be confused with *Polygonatum multiflorum*, a member of the lily family, the root of which has also been used as a medicinal plant in Chinese tradition.

OTHER USES

The stem, *shou-wu-teng*, is used for the treatment of insomnia. The stem is harvested in autumn after the leaves have fallen, or in late summer, while leaves are still on the branches. The thin branches and leaves are removed, and the stem is cut into sections about 28 inches long, tied into bundles, and dried under sun. It is considered a little sweet and neutral. Its functions include expelling wind and wetness. It is taken internally for neurasthenia, insomnia, and too many dreams; it is applied externally for aches and pains of the entire body and ringworm. Doses range from 9 to 15 g in decoction, or in a poultice or wash. The stems are official in the 1985 *Chinese Pharmacopeia*.

The leaves, *he-shou-wu-ye*, are a folk medicine used as a poultice or wash for ringworm, sores, and itching. A treatment for scrofula involves applying a poultice of the fresh leaves while the patient chews a piece of the root at the same time.

Polygonum multiflorum has been cultivated as an ornamental in gardens in India. In a 1796 publication, C. P. Thunberg noted that the starchy roots were sometimes eaten as food in China and Japan.

Garlic
Da-suan

Botanical Names: *Allium sativum* L.
Chinese Names: Pinyin: *Da-suan*. Wade-Giles: *Ta-suan*.
English Names: Garlic.
Pharmaceutical Name: Bulbus Alli Sativi.
Family: Liliaceae—lily family.

HISTORY

If your food should be your medicine, then garlic should certainly be a part of your diet. Garlic has been used as both food and medicine for as long as humans have recorded historical events. Along with ginger, no plant has been used by more cultures on more continents for such a long period of time as garlic.

Garlic is not known in the wild. It is found only in cultivation. Its wild ancestors are thought to have originated in the high plains of west-central Asia, perhaps in the Kirgiz Desert of what was the west-central Soviet Union. Its closest wild relative is believed to be a Central Asian species, *Allium longicupis*. In the Middle East, garlic was known to be under cultivation at least 5000 years ago.

The human perception of garlic, its uses, and its drawbacks seem universal, and have tended to change little over the centuries. People who like to eat garlic, are, of course, acutely aware of its effect on their breath, especially if they must deal with other people. Professor Yue has a friend from Shandong province, where garlic is a staple, who is an interpreter. He likes to eat garlic and onions. Since he interprets for foreigners, he is always embarrassed by his breath, so he was very happy when mouthwashes first became available in China several years ago. The ability of a mouthwash to suppress "garlic breath" has been championed in American advertising as a test of a mouthwash's effectiveness. However, a bumper sticker seen in the garlic-growing region near Gilroy, California, put this notion in proper perspective: it reads, "Fight mouthwash, eat garlic."

"Garlic has powerful properties, and is of great benefit against changes of water and of residence," wrote Pliny the elder, the first-century Roman naturalist (23–79 A.D.). He recommended garlic as an antidote for the poisonous bites of shrews and snakes, as well as poisoning from aconite and henbane. Like the ancient Chinese, he noted its use in the treatment of asthma, as a cough suppressant, and to expel intestinal parasites. Pliny regarded the freshly crushed seeds of coriander, mixed with garlic in neat wine, as an aphrodisiac. But there was a down side. According to Pliny, excessive use of garlic may dull the sight, cause flatulence, injure the stomach, and create excessive thirst.

Our word *garlic* is derived from the Anglo-Saxon designation "gar-leac,"or "spear-plant." Garlic is a member of the very large genus *Allium*, of the lily family. The genus has more than 700 species and includes onions, chives, leeks, and other familiar food plants. The genus name "*Allium*," is the ancient Latin name for garlic. It is believed to be derived from an ancient Celtic word "*all*," meaning hot or burning. The specific epithet "sativum" means cultivated or planted.

In China, garlic is called *da-suan*. While known as a food plant since before recorded history, the first record of its medicinal use in China comes in Tao Hong-jing's *Ming Yi Bei Lu* (*Miscellaneous Records of Famous Physicians*), published during the era of the North and South dynasties around 510 A.D. Garlic is considered a folk remedy, used by much of the population, rather than an official drug plant in modern China.

TASTE AND CHARACTER

Hot, warm.

FUNCTIONS

Promotes vital energy and circulation, relieves mass in the abdomen, kills worms, kills bacteria, detoxifies, and clears away toxic matter.

USES

The bulbs are traditionally given to people who have eaten too much and are unable to digest food or who suffer from cold pains in the stomach, lack of appetite, diarrhea, amoebic and bacillus dysentery, colds, whooping cough, and tuberculosis. Externally garlic is used to treat pinworm, carbuncles, deep-rooted ulcers and swellings, snake bites, and fungal diseases of the skin. Garlic has also been used in prescriptions for the treatment of acute appendicitis.

One of the primary uses of garlic in modern China is as a preventative for colds. To prevent bad colds the root is crushed, and one part of the juice is placed in ten parts of water, then used as a nose drop. In the Chinese *Pharmacopeia* it is recommended internally for the treatment of the common cold and bacillus dysentery, and externally for carbuncles and sores.

As a folk treatment for bacillus dysentery, as much as 9–15g of the crushed bulb is mixed with sugar water to make a cold infusion. A dose of 5–20 ml of the liquid is drunk at one time. Another method calls for 1 part of the juice of garlic bulb to be added to 20 parts water. This is used as an enema. A garlic enema is also used for the treatment of pinworm. Another method involves crushing 90 g of garlic (about three bulbs) and soaking it for 24 hours in an unspecified amount of cold water that has been boiled and sterilized. Before going to bed, an enema of 20 to 30 ml of the solution is given. The treatment is repeated for seven days.

A folk treatment for tuberculosis calls for about two bulbs of "purple-skinned" garlic. The garlic is crushed until it has a mudlike consistency. A glass bottle about 4 to 6 inches tall, with a 1¼ to 2 inch opening is chosen. The crushed garlic is spread around the walls at the bottom of the bottle. The patient then places his or her mouth above the bottle and breathes through the mouth for about 30 seconds, after which the patient takes normal deep breaths of fresh air for 30 seconds. This treatment is continued for two hours in the morning and two hours in the afternoon.

A complete review of the chemical, pharmacological, and clinical scientific literature on garlic would fill a large book, considering that over a thousand papers on various aspects of garlic have been published in the past twenty years alone. Garlic is almost a medicine chest onto itself. It is used in various world cultures to treat colds, fever, symptoms of flu, coughs, earache, bronchitis, shortness of breath, headache, sinus congestion, high blood pressure, stomachache, hypertension, diarrhea, dysentery, gout, rheumatism, whooping cough, pinworm, arteriosclerosis, snakebites, and numerous other ailments and conditions.

Garlic is well known for its antibacterial activity. Back in 1858, Louis Pasteur, best remembered for his pasteurization process universally used in dairy products, was the first to recognize garlic's antibacterial activity. Garlic is now known to have broad-spectrum antibacterial activity against gram-positive and gram-negative bacteria. The primary antibacterial component is known as allicin. A 1984 study by Indian researchers showed that garlic was a promising antibacterial agent in eight out of nine strains of clinical bacteria that were highly resistant to antibiotics.

Allicin is not actually a component of the bulb, but is produced as a chemical by-product when garlic is bruised or crushed. Alliin, a sulfur-containing amino acid, reacts with an enzyme, allinase, to produce allicin. Allicin is the substance primarily responsible for garlic's familiar flavor and fragrance. Other active components include diallyl disulfide, diallyl trisulfide, and ajoene. Ajoene, which is formed by combining allicin and diallyl disulfide, has antibiotic and antithrombotic (preventing blood platelet aggregation or clotting of blood) activity.

Research on garlic is largely determined by the needs of a culture. In Western cultures, garlic has been studied for antibacterial, antifungal, antithrombotic, cholesterol-lowering, and blood sugar-regulating activity; for the treatment of high blood pressure, hypoglycemia, and atherosclerosis; as well as its potential for colds and flu, digestive ailments, and bronchitis.

The health needs and, therefore, research interests of developing countries are different. In India and China, garlic research has focused on its potential to treat amoebic and bacillus dysentery, epilepsy, tuberculosis, and intestinal disorders; on its contraceptive properties; on its detoxifying properties, as in the treatment of industrial lead poisoning; and even as a supplemental treatment of leprosy. Indian clinical studies have shown that when administered to leprosy patients in controlled dosages, the bacteria index and the general clinical picture of the patient are improved.

One area that interests all cultures is the relationship of garlic to cardiovascular disease. This includes the blood pressure-lowering effect of garlic in hypertension, effect on blood thinning (anti-platelet aggregation), and lowering of serum triglyceride and cholesterol levels. Some researchers believe that the blood-thinning properties of garlic may hold a key to its role in reducing risk factors in heart disease. To date, however, human studies have produced results that are difficult to evaluate because of wide differences in experimental conditions. This includes the great difficulty in masking the odor of garlic, which makes performing double-blind studies very difficult—where neither the researcher or patient are supposed know whether they are getting the test substance or a placebo. The use of different garlic products also makes it difficult to analyze research results. Products can include fresh garlic, dried garlic, powdered garlic, freeze-dried garlic, and various proprietary "odorless" garlic products, all of which are commonly available on the American market.

Recent pharmacological studies in China indicate that garlic may have some immunostimulant qualities. A 1989 study by researchers in Florida and Louisiana reported on the use of garlic to enhance natural killer-cell activity in AIDS patients. Only 10 AIDS patients were included in the pilot study, and tests were available on only 7 of the participants, so the results are statistically inconclusive. The researchers measured the activity of natural killer cells and helper suppressor ratios. After taking a garlic product as a food supplement for 6 weeks, 6 out of 7 patients were found to have normal killer cell activity, which had been abnormal at the beginning of the study. Four out of 7 patients had an improved helper-suppressor ratio. The authors, T. H. Abdullah, D. V. Kirkpatrick, and J. Carter, also reported an improvement of AIDS-related conditions including diarrhea, genital herpes, candidiasis, and pansinusitis with recurrent fever. While the study is not conclusive, it certainly points the way for more intensive research in this area.

Here we have only begun to scratch the surface of the available studies and research on garlic. Despite the hundreds of studies that have already been done, not to mention at least five thousand years of human exposure to garlic, we have only begun to explore garlic's potential. The reader interested in further information is referred to Stephen Fulder and John Blackwood's excellent book, *Garlic—Nature's Original Remedy* (1991).

DOSE

9 to 15g of the fresh bulb. Poulticed as needed.

DESCRIPTION

Garlic is a perennial, although most often grown as an annual or sometimes an overwintered annual. It grows to about three feet in height when in flower. The leaves are grayish-green, flat, about 1 foot long and 1½ inch wide, growing more or less in a fan-shaped arrangement with 4 or more leaves. Atop the flower stalk, which originates from the bulb, is a globular cluster of white flowers that unfold from a beak-like papery envelope. Bulbels (miniature seed bulbs) sometimes develop in place of flowers. Nonflowering forms are also grown in some regions. The bulbous underground stem is known as the bulb. This is, of course, the part of the plant that is used. The bulb consists of five or more oblong, pointed, somewhat curved cloves. Both the bulb and the cloves are covered with papery-white to purplish skins. In some traditional Chinese prescriptions, bulbs or cloves of a specific color may be required. Large "hot" garlic bulbs are considered to be of the best quality.

DISTRIBUTION

Garlic is a cultigen, not known from the wild, but is cultivated throughout the world. It has been cultivated on a large scale since ancient times. In China it is grown in every province. Each province uses material that has been grown in that region. Garlic is known to have been cultivated in China as early as the Tang dynasty (618–907).

In the United States, garlic is commonly grown in home gardens. On a commercial scale, the bulk of garlic production is located on 18,000 acres of farmland in a five-county region in central California, where about 250 million pounds of garlic are harvested. The vast majority of the crop is used to produce dehydrated garlic products, such as garlic flakes and garlic salt. About 50 million pounds of the California crop is sold as fresh garlic. Americans consumed about 80 million pounds of fresh garlic in 1989.

CULTIVATION

Garlic is easy to cultivate. It likes a warm climate, with a moist, sandy, moderately rich, slightly alkaline soil. It requires full sun. Garlic is propagated from seed, nursery sets (bulbels), or by planting individual cloves. For the home gardener, individual cloves are the best means of propagation. Full, healthy outer cloves are chosen. The pointed end is planted up at a depth of about 1 inch. Plant on a 6 inch center. In parts of the country where the ground does not freeze in winter, garlic can be planted in late fall and harvested the following summer. In the north, plant as soon as the ground thaws in early spring.

HARVESTING

In China, the bulbs are collected in early summer, cleaned, and placed in a shaded, well-ventilated area until dry. If the weather is wet, the bulbs are baked under low heat until the skin drys. If you are harvesting garlic for personal use, dig the bulbs once the leaves begin to wither. Loose dirt can be shaken off, and the rootlets on the bottom of the bulb cut off. Let them dry outside for a day or two, then hang them up to dry, if the leaves are still attached. If you have cut off the leaves, spread the bulbs on a screen to dry. Once the outer skin on the bulbs has dried, this dirty layer can be removed, revealing a clean white or purplish layer beneath. Use as needed.

PROCESSING

No special processing is noted for normal usage. A special process is used to produce a 5 percent garlic "juice" used in some modern Chinese prescriptions. Purple *da-suan* is chosen, and juiced. The juice is set aside. Then 20 g cornstarch is mixed with cold purified water until it has a mud like consistency. Next, 300 ml sugar water is slowly mixed into this mass. 2 ml white vinegar is added to the mixture, along with purified water (up to 800 ml); then 100 ml of the garlic juice is added. The final product should be about 1 liter in volume. This 5 percent juice preparation is used in prescriptions for enemas to treat pinworm and for bacillus dysentery.

OTHER USES

Garlic is well known as a culinary herb in a wide variety of world cuisines. It is rich in various vitamins and minerals, and contains at least 17 amino acids. Garlic is high in calcium, phosphorus, iron, thiamin, riboflavin, and vitamin C; it also contains niacin, folic acid, iodine, germanium, copper, potassium, magnesium, selenium, zinc, and other nutrients. According to Indian studies, incorporating moderate amounts of garlic into the diet has a favorable effect on the microflora of the intestines and benefits lactic organisms, which helps to enhance the absorption of minerals in the diet.

Insecticides have been developed in India from garlic extracts. They have been used to kill mosquito larve, as well as houseflies and other insect pests. The dried leaves and stalks of garlic are fed to sheep and goats.

Ginger
Gan-jiang (Dried Ginger) and
Sheng-jiang (Fresh Ginger)

> **Botanical Names:** *Zingiber officinale* Rosc.
> **Chinese Names:** Pinyin: *Sheng-jiang* (fresh rhizome); *Gan-jiang* (dried rhizome). Wade-Giles: *Sheng-chiang* (fresh rhizome); *Kan-chiang* (dried rhizome).
> **English Names:** Fresh ginger, dried ginger.

Pharmaceutical Names: Zingiberis rhizoma (fresh rhizome);
Zingiberis siccatum rhizoma (dried rhizome).
Family: Zingiberaceae—ginger family.

HISTORY

Ginger is truly an herbal emissary in the broadest sense. Perhaps no other herb, except garlic, crosses all barriers, cultural, historical, and geographic—food versus medicine, Western versus Oriental, scientific versus folk tradition. Ginger is a universal herb in all respects.

Consisting of the fresh or dried roots of *Zingiber officinale*, ginger has been cultivated for so long that its exact origin is unclear. Cultivated for millennia in both China and India, it reached the West at least two thousand years ago; it was recorded as subject to a Roman tax in the second century A.D. after being imported via the Red Sea to Alexandria. The ancient Greeks and Romans thought ginger was an Arabian product because it was imported from India via the Red Sea. Tariff duties appear in the records of Barcelona in 1221, Marseilles in 1228, and Paris by 1296. About 1280 Marco Polo observed ginger production in both India and China. John of Montecorvino, a missionary friar who traveled to India about 1292, described the plant and its cultivation in that country. Commonly found in the eleventh century Anglo-Saxon leech books, ginger was known in England before the Norman Conquest. Ginger is detailed in a thirteenth century work, *Physicians of Myddvai*, a collection of recipes and prescriptions written by a physician, Rhiwallon, and his three sons, by mandate of Rhys Gryg, prince of South Wales (who died in 1233). By the thirteenth and fourteenth centuries it was familiar to English palates and next to pepper was the most popular spice. A pound of ginger was then valued at the price of one sheep. Ginger, as a product of the Far East, was indelibly imprinted on the taste buds of Europeans before they knew potatoes, tomatoes, and corn even existed.

Ginger is a member of the ginger family. The ginger family is a tropical group especially abundant in Indo-Malaysia, consisting of more than 1,200 plant species in 53 genera. The genus *Zingiber* includes about 85 species of aromatic herbs from East Asia and tropical Australia. The name of the genus, *Zingiber*, derives from a Sanskrit word denoting "horn-shaped," referring to the protrusions on the root (rhizome). The English botanist William Roscoe (1753–1831) gave the plant the name *Zingiber officinale* in an 1807 publication. The Chinese name *jiang* means to defend, suggesting that ginger helps protect the body from dampness and cold. The ginger of commerce consists of the thick scaly rhizomes of the plant. They branch with thick thumb-like protrusions; individual divisions of the rhizome are known as "hands."

In China, dried ginger (*gan–jiang*) is first mentioned in the earliest herbal, *Shen Nong Ben Cao Jing*, attributed to the Divine Plowman Emperor, Shen-Nong, who lived about 2,000 B.C. Fresh ginger, (*sheng-jiang*), was first listed in *Ming Yi Bie Lu* (*Miscellaneous Records of Famous Physicians*) and *Ben Cao Jing Ji Zhu* (*Collection of Commentaries on the Classics of Materia Medica*), both attributed to Tao Hong-jing, published during the dynasties of the North and South Kingdoms around the year 500 A.D. He considered the Sichuan-produced fresh ginger to be very hot, suitable only for medicinal use, not culinary purposes. Fresh ginger and dried ginger are considered two distinct commodities. In fact, Tao Hong-jing felt that they were so different that they must come from two different plants!

Even though in modern China, ginger is an essential ingredient in any kitchen, it is also one of the most widely consumed herbal medicines. Both the fresh and the dried root are official drugs of the 1985 edition of the Chinese *Pharmacopeia* as is a liquid extract and tincture of ginger. Ginger is used in dozens of traditional Chinese prescriptions as a "guide drug" to "mediate" the effects of potentially toxic ingredients. In modern China, ginger is probably used in half of all Chinese herbal prescriptions.

TASTE AND CHARACTER

Gan-jiang (dried root) is considered hot; *sheng-jiang* (fresh root) is hot, a little warm.

FUNCTIONS

Gan-jiang (dried root) warms the middle burner, expels cold, rejuvenates depleted yang, promotes lactation, and disperses phlegm. In cases of chronic bronchitis with thin, white, and foamy phlegm, it is used to "warm" the lungs.

Sheng-jiang (fresh root) produces diaphoresis, dispels pathogens through diaphoresis, expels cold, warms the middle burner, relieves nausea, and expels toxic material.

USES

Gan-jiang (dried ginger) is used for cold and pain in the abdomen and stomach (stomach and spleen); when legs, arms, and extremities feel cold and the pulse is light; for phlegm retention diseases with cough, asthma and cough due to cold, vomiting with blood, vomiting and diarrhea due to cold deficiency, and nose bleed.

Sheng-jiang (fresh ginger) is used to dispel pathogens via its ability to induce sweating; for colds due to wind and cold, coughs, vomiting due to stomach cold; as a detoxifier for overdoses of *Arisaema* (Jack-in-the-pulpit) or *Pinellia* (a related plant), which cause numbing, swelling, and pain of the throat, tongue, and mouth; and for poisoning induced by seafood. Pulverized fresh ginger applied as a poultice to the head two to three times a day was once used as a folk treatment for baldness. Fresh ginger rubbed on the affected area is a folk remedy for vitiligo. The juice squeezed from the fresh root has also been used in the treatment of burns.

Experimental data developed by Chinese scientists verifies the ability of dried ginger to "strengthen" the stomach while acting as a mild stomach and intestinal stimulant. It has also been shown to inhibit vomiting. Studies with fresh root showed that for the first few hours ginger tea reduced gastric secretions, followed by a longer period of stimulation. A recent study suggests that extracts of ginger may help inhibit gastric ulcers. Laboratory experiments have also shown analgesic and anti-inflammatory activity. Other scientific studies show that gingerol, one of the primary pungent principles of ginger, helps counter liver toxicity by increasing bile secretion. Ginger has potent anti-microbial and anti-oxidant (food preservative) qualities as well. A recent study, furthering ginger's reputation as a stomachic, shows that acetone and methanol extracts of ginger strongly inhibits gastric ulceration. Cotton balls soaked with the fresh juice of the root have been used in China in recent years as a clinical treatment for first- and second-degree burns. A 1984 report in a Chinese journal reported that over 400 cases had been successfully treated, allaying pain, blisters, and inflammation.

As in China, in India the fresh and dried roots were considered distinct medicinal products. Ginger has been used in India for millennia. Fresh ginger has been used for cold-induced disease, nausea, asthma, cough, colic, heart palpitation, swellings, dyspepsia, loss of appetite, and rheumatism. In short, it is used in India for the same purposes as in ancient and modern China. In nineteenth-century India, one English writer observed that a popular remedy for cough and asthma consisted of the juice of fresh ginger with a little juice of fresh garlic, mixed with honey. A paste of powdered dried ginger was applied to the temples to relieve headache. To allay nausea, fresh ginger was mixed with a little honey, topped off with a pinch of burnt peacock feathers. One modern government health guide in India suggests 1 to 2 teaspoons of ginger juice with honey as a cough suppressant. Ginger is as popular a home remedy in India today as it was 2,000 years ago.

Indigenous peoples of the Caribbean islands were quick to adopt ginger as a remedy after its introduction to the West Indies by Francisco de Mendoca. By 1547 it was being exported to Spain in considerable quantities from the Caribbean islands. In Jamaica the warm, steamy fumes of hot ginger tea are used as an inhalant to relieve head colds.

European tradition values ginger tea for digestive disturbances. The *Family Herbal* (1814) by the English physician, Robert Thorton, praises the virtues of ginger, but his statements may say more about the unsavory habits of some Britons of two centuries ago than they do of ginger. He writes: "Dyspeptic patients from hard drinking, and those subject to flatulency and gout, have been known to receive considerable benefit by the use of ginger tea; taking two or three cupfuls for breakfast, suiting it to their palate . . . as ginger promotes the circulation through the extreme vessels, it is to be advised in torbid and phlegmatic habits, where the stomach is subject to be loaded with slime, and the bowels distended with flatulency."

Thorton, though, hints at another potential benefit of ginger—help for the heart. Studies by Japanese researchers indicates that ginger has a tonic effect on the heart but may raise blood pressure by restricting blood flow in peripheral areas of the body. Further studies show that ginger can lower cholesterol levels by reducing cholesterol absorption in the blood and liver.

Ginger extracts have been extensively studied for a broad range of biological activities including antibacterial, anticonvulsant, analgesic, antiulcer, gastric antisecretory, antitumor, antifungal, antispasmodic, antiallergenic, cytotoxic, larvacidal, and molluscicidal activity. Gingerols, believed to be the active chemical component in ginger, have been shown to be inhibitors of prostaglandin biosynthesis. Danish researchers at the University of Odense have studied the anticoagulant properties of ginger and found that it was a more potent blood-clotting agent than garlic or onion. The same research group studied the potential use of ginger in the treatment of migraine, based on the long history of ginger used for neurological disorders by practitioners of the Indian traditional medicine system, Ayurveda. The researchers proposed that ginger may relieve and prevent migraine headaches without side effects.

Several human studies published in recent years have both confirmed and questioned the traditional claims for the use of dried ginger as an antivomiting agent. These studies have been widely reported in the popular press, exciting interest in the use of ginger against motion sickness. A study by D. B. Mourey and D. E. Clayson was published in the British medical journal *The Lancet* (20: 655–67, 1982). Thirty-six volunteers were given either 940 mg ginger capsules or dimenhydrinate, an antihistamine used in an over–the–counter motion sickness product. When blindfolded and subjected to a specified time period in a rotating chair, those who took ginger held out an average of five and a half minutes, while those who took the over-the-counter drug lasted about three and a half minutes.

A number of other trials have confirmed these positive results, including a study involving 80 naval cadets not accustomed to being on ships in high seas. Volunteers given a placebo (capsules with inert ingredients) developed seasickness, while those who took gingerroot capsules had reduced symptoms of cold sweats and nausea.

While these tests are promising, researchers believe that more studies should be done before coming to conclusions on the value of ginger for motion sickness. In 1988, researchers at Louisiana State University published their findings on a NASA-sponsored study. The fact that over 50 percent of space shuttle crew members experience motion sickness prompted the study. Here again, a rotating chair was used to test the effects of ginger products as a motion sickness medication in 42 men and women. This study found that dried ginger powder taken two hours before testing, or minced fresh ginger administered one hour before testing, was ineffective in relieving symptoms of motion sickness. The study did not involve a testing protocol to determine if the ginger contained appreciable quantities of what is believed to be the primary active chemical component, gingerol, found in the essential oil and responsible for the "hot" taste produced by ginger.

Based on one or two studies, ginger cannot be unequivocally touted as effective for motion sickness. Likewise it cannot be labeled ineffective until more research is done. In designing future experiments scientists should dig a little deeper into the history of the cultures who have long used ginger as an antinauseant. They may discover that *fresh* ginger root or ginger juice is more effective than the *dried* root, or that a different dose would be more effective. In the NASA study, for example, ½ to 1 g of dried root was used and only 1 g of fresh root. In traditional Chinese medicine, a single dose of fresh ginger in a medicinal herbal tea prescription ranges from 3 to 9 g. Such studies should also include analysis of the quality of the ginger used in the experiments, including levels of the active constituents. The jury is still out on whether or not ginger is a useful preventative or treatment for the symptoms of motion sickness. Scientific research often raises more questions than it answers.

Ginger is valued the world over, as a culinary herb, condiment, spice, home remedy, and medicinal agent. It is likely that ginger will be enjoyed and valued for the next millennium, and new research will undoubtedly reveal new value for this ancient herb. Given its wide availability, long history of safe use as a food and as medicine, and the recent scientific data confirming a number of historical medicinal uses, ginger could one day sit in every American medicine chest as well as the spice rack to treat the common cold and coughs and to prevent nausea.

DOSE

Gan-jiang (dried ginger) is decocted in doses of 1.5 to 9 g. *Sheng-jiang* (fresh ginger) is used in doses of 3 to 9 g in decoction, poulticed, or sometimes heated and then used as a poultice. In the United States, ginger is sold in a variety of forms. Fresh whole ginger and dried powdered ginger are widely available. Three grams of fresh ginger, the low end of the dose recommended in Chinese herbal prescriptions, is about equivalent in size (volume) to one good-sized clove of garlic—about the size of the end joint of a man's little finger. Nine grams, the high end of the dosage, is equal to about a third of an ounce by weight. In terms of relative strength or potency, one clove of garlic is again a good point of comparison. Like a little garlic, a little ginger goes along way.

For a cup of fresh ginger tea, steep about five or six thin slices of ginger root. A teaspoonful of the dried root may be used in a cup of hot water. Cover and let steep for 30 minutes. Herbalists have recommended hot dried ginger root tea in wine-glassful doses every couple of hours to help relieve menstrual cramps, allay symptoms at the onset of a cold, and relieve mild nausea or mild diarrhea. Ginger tinctures in which the root is soaked in a menstruum of alcohol and water, sometimes labeled as drops or extracts, are available in health and natural food stores. Herbalists recommend ten to twenty drops of ginger tincture in a little water with meals to counteract indigestion or help fight early symptoms of cold or flu. Some people, however, may not be able to tolerate the burning sensation it can cause in the stomach. Capsulated dried ginger root products and capsulated products with standardized amounts of the active components known as gingerols are also widely available in natural food markets. Read the product label for dosage and use information.

WARNING

In Chinese tradition, dried ginger is contraindicated during pregnancy.

DESCRIPTION

The ginger plant is an erect perennial growing from 1 to 3 feet in height. The stem is surrounded by the sheathing bases of the two-ranked leaves. The leaves are linear and lance-shaped, somewhat resembling those of irises. A clublike spike of yellowish, purple-lipped flowers have showy greenish-yellow bracts beneath. Unfortunately, ginger rarely flowers in cultivation.

DISTRIBUTION

Ginger is commercially cultivated in nearly every tropical and subtropical country in the world that has arable land for export crops. It has been cultivated for so long, its exact wild origin is not clear. In China, ginger is produced in most provinces, except cold northern regions. Supplies are often used in the region in which the plant is grown. Major commercial production is in Sichuan, and Guizhou, as well as Zhejiang, Shandong, Hubei, Guangdong, and Shanxi. Sichuan and Guizhou produce the largest quantities and highest quality ginger.

Ginger, both fresh and dried, has become increasingly popular in the United States in recent years. During the 1980s, on average, the United States imported more than 4,000 metric tons of ginger per year. Major world producers include Fiji, India, Jamaica, Nigeria, and Sierra Leone; China remains the largest producer. American imports come from China, several Caribbean islands, Africa, Central America, Brazil, and Australia. It is also grown as a cash crop in Hawaii.

CULTIVATION

In warmer regions, ginger is a plant that will grow with relatively little care provided it has a hot climate and even, abundant supplies of moisture. It likes full sun to partial shade. Ginger thrives in fertile soil with plenty of moisture, though not a saturated soil. It should have a well-drained, rich, sandy, porous soil. Drainage can be improved with moisture-retentive perlite, peat moss, or sand. In South China, beds are prepared in mid-February, double-dug to a depth of 15 to 18 inches. Compost or other soil-enriching organic matter can be added at this time. The beds are again forked in early April to prepare for planting.

The plants are propagated by root divisions, planted just beneath the soil surface. If grown outdoors, ginger needs a long growing season (about ten months), making it suitable only for southern Florida, Texas, and California. Elsewhere, when grown in containers, it can be kept indoors over the winter in relatively dry conditions at a temperature of around 50°F. After dividing the rhizomes, which is best done in spring, provide moderate watering, increasing moisture as roots become well established. In South China, the root is planted in the first 10 days of April. Fresh roots are dug from the ground and prepared for replanting at this point. The freshly dug roots are placed in a greenhouse on bamboo mats and allowed to dry out (but not completely) for two or three days. The greenhouse is kept at a constant temperature of 68 to 80°F. Over a two- to three-week period, the warm temperature forces buds at the ends of the rhizome. When the rhizomes have buds that are about ½ to ¾ inch long, they are divided into smaller sections, each with a sprouting vegetative bud. These divisions are then planted in rows spaced about 20 inches apart, with individual plants spaced at about a 16 inch distance. Each budded rhizome section is planted about 3 inches deep, with care being taken to make sure that the bud itself is planted upright. Plants may be side–dressed with compost or manure at this point. Ginger can be planted on one piece of land every other year, rotating it with a different crop on off years. It is not planted on the same piece of land two years in a row. In summer months, the plants are periodically hoed and weeded, with a side-dressing of composted manure added at least once. The soil is kept relatively moist during the growing season. When the foliage has died back in autumn, watering is reduced.

According to Madalene Hill and Gwen Barclay in *Southern Herb Growing* (1987), ginger will survive the winter in many parts of the southern United States, standing temperatures as cold as the low 20s. If you live in a cooler climate and grow ginger as an indoor container plant, water sparingly during the winter months, only enough to keep the root from completely drying out. The soil can basically remain dry during dormant periods. Cool temperatures during the plant's resting period do not seem to adversely effect it.

HARVESTING

To produce dried root, in warmer regions of China the root is harvested around the last week of December or first week of January. It is then cleaned, and either dried in the sun or baked over a light fire until dry. The fresh root is generally collected from the end of August to early December. The stems, leaves, and lateral roots are cut off, and the main root is thoroughly cleaned, and either stored in shade or heeled in sand before being shipped to market. In tropical and subtropical areas, younger roots (four to six months old) are generally harvested, since older roots tend to be fibrous and tough.

PROCESSING

Most of the dried ginger on the American market has had the cortex (outer, bark like layer) scraped or rubbed off before it is sold. That is why it has a whitish appearance.

The cortex (bark of the rhizome) itself is used as a folk remedy (see *other uses* below). To aid in the removal of the cortex, the freshly dug root is soaked in water overnight, then scraped with a knife or other sharp implement to remove the outer cortex. It is then dried in the sun.

A processed type of the dried root, *pao-jiang* is sometimes used in TCM (see *other uses* below). It is prepared by cutting the dried root into small pieces and then stir-frying them until the surface and the broken sections of the root are somewhat brownish and slightly swollen.

The fresh root is cleaned, properly stored, and cut into thin slices as needed. Sometimes Chinese prescriptions call for special preparations of the fresh root. One method involves pressing out the juice of fresh ginger, placing the liquid in a porcelain container. One or two hours later a starchy substance precipitates to the bottom. This precipitate is separated out, and dried in the sun or under low heat for future use.

Roasted fresh ginger is sometimes used. Traditionally, the fresh roots are wrapped in five to six layers of rice paper, buried in warm coals (that have mostly turned to ash), and roasted for a few minutes until the paper has blackened. The paper wrapping is removed before use.

Other Uses

The juice of the leaves, considered hot and warm, is a folk remedy first recorded in *Ben Cao Gang Mu*. It is taken as a digestive aid for dyspepsia caused by undigested food in the stomach. The leaves are called *jiang-ye*.

The bark (cortex) of the rhizome (*jiang-pi*) is considered hot and slightly warm. It is used in decoction in doses of 1.5 to 6 g to promote vital energy (*qi/ch'i*) circulation of the extremities, reduce edema (excessive water retention in the body), and for difficult urination. It is considered a diuretic.

"*Pao-jiang*," the processed or roasted dried root, is considered hot. It warms the middle burner and stops bleeding, and diarrhea. Doses of 1.5 to 9 g are traditionally used in decoction for the treatment of vomiting with blood due to cold deficiency, bloody stool, diarrhea, uterine bleeding due to cold deficiency, painful menstruation, and chronic dyspepsia.

An oil distilled from the fresh rhizome (*jiang-yu*) is sometimes used by clinicians in China in an injectable preparation for the treatment of rheumatic pains or other joint pain.

In addition to culinary and medicinal uses, ginger's essential oil and oleoresin are used as a fragrance component in perfumes formulated for men and in soaps, lotions, and other cosmetic products. If nothing else, enjoy ginger as a culinary herb. Start using a little fresh-grated ginger on a more regular basis. If you're not moved by the health claims, you will be moved by the zesty, unique flavor. Add to rice, vegetables, salads, and as a stimulant for digesting meats.

Ginseng

Ren-shen (Asian Ginseng) and
Xi-yang-shen (American Ginseng)

Botanical Names: *Panax ginseng* C. A. Meyer (Asian ginseng), *Panax quinquefolius* L. (American ginseng).

Botanical Synonyms: The use of the binomial *P. pseudoginseng* for *Panax ginseng* in *Hortus Third* (1976) has resulted in confusion, arising from the fact that in 1833 T. F. L. Nees had expressly included the earlier and legitimate *P. pseudoginseng* under his illegitimate name *P. schin-seng*. The earliest legitimate botanical name is *P. ginseng*, first used by C. A. Meyer (1843).

Chinese Names: Pinyin: *Ren-shen* (Asian ginseng), *Xi-yang-shen* (American ginseng). Wade-Giles: *Jen-shen* (Asian ginseng), *Hsi-yang-shen* (American ginseng).

English Names: Asian ginseng (*Panax ginseng*), American ginseng (*P. quinquefolius*).

Pharmaceutical Name: Radix Ginseng.

Family: Araliaceae—ginseng family.

HISTORY

If you could dig a hole to China from the Appalachians or the Ozarks you just might end up in a forest that looks very similar to the one where you started. For more than 200 years, plant geographers have recognized a phenomena known as the "disjunct eastern Asiatic—eastern North American range." There are about one hundred genera of plants that only occur in eastern Asia and eastern North America, including well-known plant groups such as sassafras, witch hazel, hickory, blue cohosh (*Caulophyllum*), and the most famous example, ginseng (*Panax* spp.). These patterns of plant disjunctions, where plant populations are separated by dozens, or even thousands of miles, are believed to be remnants of an ancient forest that covered much of the northern hemisphere about 70 million years ago. Surviving plants in these groups have survived in much of eastern Asia as well as eastern North America, especially in the Appalachians and the Ozarks.

In 1709, Petrus Jartoux (1668–1720), a Jesuit missionary, was on a mapping expedition for the Emperor Kangxi in North China, near the Korean border. Four roots of the Asian ginseng (*Panax ginseng*) were brought to him in a basket. He recorded its uses and tried the root himself, observing its effects on his pulse and general energy. Jartoux's observations became the first authentic account of ginseng by a westerner. In 1713 his comments were published in English in the *Philosophical Transactions of the Royal Society of London*.

> As to the place where this root grows; it is in general between the 39th and 47th deg. of north latitude and between the 10th and 20th deg. of east longitude from the meridian of Pekin [Beijing]. There is a long tract of mountains, which the thick

forests, that cover and encompass them, render almost impass-
able. On the declevities of these mountains, in thick forests, on
the banks of torrents, or about the roots of trees, and amidst
a thousand different sorts of plants, the ginseng is found. It is
not to be met with in plains, valleys, marshes, the bottoms of
rivulets, or in places too much exposed and open. If the forest
take fire and be consumed, this plant does not appear till 2 or
3 years after; it also lies hid from the sun as much as possible;
which shows us that heat is an enemy to it. All which makes me
believe, that it is to be found in any other country in the world,
it may be particular in Canada, where the forest and mountains, according to the relation of those that have lived there,
very much resemble these here.

In 1715 Joseph Francois Lafitau (1681–1746), a Jesuit missionary who
worked above Montreal in Canada from 1711–1717, read Jartoux's words
and began a search for ginseng in Canada. In 1716 Lafitau, strolling in the
woods near his cabin, found the red-berried plant. American ginseng
(*Panax quinquefolius*) was discovered. That year he apparently sent specimens to the French botanist, Michel S. Sarrazin (1659–1734), who described American ginseng and its discovery. Lafitau sent samples of the
root to Jartoux, who showed them to Chinese merchants and arranged to
have the roots imported to China. Thus, exports of American ginseng to
China began around 1720.

Both American and Asian ginseng are members of the genus *Panax* in
the ginseng family. There are about six species in the genus. In 1753
Linnaeus named American ginseng *Panax quinquefolius*. The name *Panax
ginseng* was established in an 1843 publication by C. A. Meyer. The word
Panax comes from Greek, *pan* meaning "all," and *akos*, "cure," which refers
to the traditional "cure-all" or "panacea" effect attributed to the plant. The
species name quinquefolius means "five-leaves," referring to the five leaflets on each leaf division of American ginseng.

Ginseng, jen-seng, schin-seng, and *ren-shen* are all different transliterations
of the same Chinese ideograms. It means "essence of the earth in the form
of a man." According to Harvard botanist Dr. Shiu Ying Hu, *sêng* is a term
used by Chinese medicinal root gatherers to described fleshy roots used as
tonics. The word *sêng* is preceded by modifiers that help describe the
source plant, the region in which it was harvested, or its medicinal uses.
She notes that all species of *Panax* do not produce *sêng*, and all *sêng*-
producing plants are not members of the genus *Panax*. Dr. Hu uses this

metaphor: "A horse is a mammal, but not all mammals are horses. Likewise, ginseng is a *seng* but not all *sengs* in Chinese medicine are ginseng." Dr. Hu has documented over 60 species of "seng-producing" plants in at least 20 plant families. However, there is only one "gin-seng."

Prior to its discovery in the early seventeenth century, American ginseng had been used by native Americans for purposes quite similar to the use of Asian ginseng by the Chinese. It was among the five most important medicinal plants of the Seneca tribe, and was primarily given to the elderly. According to Crow legend, the wife of Gray Bull learned in a dream that the leaf or root tea would aid in pain-free childbirth. The Penobscots, who referred to it as "man root," prescribed the root tea to increase female fertility. Ginseng was regarded as a universal remedy for children and adults by the Meskwaki (Fox) tribe of Wisconsin. It was combined with other medicinal plants to render them more powerful. The Menominee considered the root to be a tonic and strengthener of mental prowess.

American ginseng never became an important medicinal plant in American medicine, although the root was an official listing in the *United States Pharmacopeia* from 1842–1882. It was regarded as a mild stimulant and soothing to an upset stomach. Its first mention in a Chinese work was in *Ben Cao Gang Mu Shi Yi* (*Omissions from Ben Cao Gang Mu*) by Zhao Xuemin, published in 1765 during the Qing dynasty.

The earliest reference to Asian ginseng is in *Shen Nong Ben Cao Jing*, compiled in the late Han dynasty (approx. the first century A.D.).

In her translation of the account, Dr. Shiu Ying Hu writes: "It is used for repairing the five viscera, quietening the spirit, curbing the emotion, stopping agitation, removing noxious influence, brightening the eyes, enlightening the mind and increasing the wisdom. Continuous use leads one to longevity with light weight," (1977a, p. 289).

In the 1596 classic of the Chinese *materia medica*, Li Shi-zhen's *Ben Cao Gang Mu*, ginseng is listed in the superior class of herbs. Small amounts were said to lead to light weight while improving vitality (S. Y. Hu, 1976).

The first Western description of the plant was that of Père Jartoux, whose 1709 observations were first published in 1711. Attesting to the past and present potential of the herb, the Jesuit Jartoux wrote:

> Nobody can imagine that the Chinese and Tartars would set so high a value on this root, if it did not constantly produce a good effect. Those that are in health often make use of it, to render themselves more vigorous and strong; and I am persuaded that it would prove an excellent medicine in the hands

of any European who understands pharmacy, if he had but a sufficient quantity of it to make such trials as are necessary, to examine the nature of it chemically, and to apply it in a proper quantity, according to the nature of the disease for which it may be beneficial (1713, p. 56–57).

TASTE AND CHARACTER

Asian ginseng: sweet, bitter, warm. American ginseng: sweet, slightly bitter, cool.

FUNCTIONS

Asian ginseng is considered a tonic and adaptogen to replenish vital energy (*qi/ch'i*), increase strength, increase blood volume, promote appetite, quiet the spirit, and give wisdom. American ginseng benefits vital energy, nourishes yin, nurtures the lungs, promotes fluid production, and disperses heat.

USES

Asian ginseng is used alone or in prescriptions for general weakness, deficient vital energy patterns, anemia, lack of appetite, shortness of breath with spontaneous perspiration, nervous agitation, forgetfulness, thirst, and impotence (S. Y. Hu, 1976). American ginseng is considered less potent than Asian ginseng, and is often preferred for older or weak patients. It is primarily used to for lung conditions such as a dry cough with heat, and for nourishing lung yin with heat, fevers, weakness, irritability, and thirst.

American and Asian ginseng are considered to be distinct medicinal plants. In Chinese traditions, American ginseng is considered to be more *yin*, helping to reduce the heat of the respiratory and digestive systems. Asian ginseng is stronger, and more *yang*—a heat-raising tonic for the blood and circulatory systems, as understood in TCM. Since American ginseng is a cold or mild tonic that will reduce "heat" in the system, while acting as a general tonic, it is often preferred by ginseng users in subtropical and tropical regions of Asia.

Over the past 50 years there have been nearly 3,000 scientific studies published on all aspects of ginseng. The vast majority have focused on Asian ginseng rather than American ginseng. Chinese researchers, as is the case with medicinal plants in general, have focused on *how* ginseng works, whereas western researchers focus on *if* it works. This reflects a fundamental difference in research approaches between the East and the West. In Asia, the efficacy of an herb is already established in a cultural context. In the West we presuppose that traditional or folk uses have no rational scientific basis.

The focus of pharmacological research on ginseng has included diverse applications, including for radioprotective, antitumor, antiviral, and metabolic effects; antioxidant activities; nervous system and reproductive performance; effects on cholesterol and lipid metabolism; and endocrinological activity. Studies have also looked at the adaptogenic and performance-enhancing effects of ginseng, including adaptation to dark, high and low temperatures, and work efficiency. Ginseng's antifatigue activity has been demonstrated by the swimming capacity of mice. Stimulation of the adrenal cortex has been suggested as a possible mechanisms of action for ginseng's purported ability to help animals (including humans) cope with stress. Used in some cosmetic products, ginseng has been reported to help in the skin regeneration process and reduction of wrinkling. In initial experiments *Panax ginseng* extracts have been shown to have hypoglycemic activity, providing a basis for the traditional use of ginseng in the treatment of diabetes.

Saponins are regarded as the primary active components of *Panax* species. The major saponin group in *Panax* are termed *ginsenosides* or *panaxosides*. Of the 13 or more ginsenosides in ginseng, those that have been best studied as isolated compounds include ginsenosides Rg_1 and ginsenoside R_{b-1}. Sometimes results were opposite with different chemical fractions. Rg_1 has been shown to slightly stimulate central-nervous-system (CNS) activity, to counter fatigue, aggravate stress ulcers, and slightly increase motor activity. In behavioral tests it has produced an acceleration of discrimination in pole-climbing tests and Y-maze tests in laboratory animals. Ginsenoside Rb_1 works as a CNS depressant; is anticonvulsant, analgesic, tranquilizing, hypotensive, fever-reducing, antipsychotic, ulcer-protective, and weak anti-inflammatory properties, and increases gastro-intestinal motility. Review of the pharmacological literature of pure ginseng saponins can be found in S. Shibata *et al.* (1985).

Several European clinical studies, involving extracts standardized to 4 to 7% of ginsenosides, have shown interesting results, among them a shortening of reaction time to visual and auditory stimuli, increased respiratory output, increased alertness and power of concentration, a better grasp of abstract concepts, and increases in visual and motor coordination.

Clinical trials have focused on the effect of red ginseng powder on diabetes, excessive fat in the blood, performance and stress, postoperative gynecological patients, and other conditions.

Despite over two thousand years of use of Asian ginseng, and over two hundred years of documented use of American ginseng, both in the West and the East, the interpretation of the modern scientific literature yields mixed results. There are many variables to consider including the identification of the type of ginseng, the product form, different procedures in preparations, lack of active components in products, differences in plant and animal species studied, and differences in route and dose administered. A bewildering number and forms of ginseng products from China, Korea, Japan, and other Asian countries are available on the American market. Their evaluation is beyond the scope of this book. Consumers are advised that whole roots or products standardized to 7 percent ginsenosides will have the most predictable results. For the future, clinical studies may need to involve products with defined levels of active components.

To cover all of the data on ginseng would require at least one book. Several authors have provided such works. Stephen Fulder's The *Tao of Medicine* (1990) has extensive information on the traditions, pharmacology, and clinical aspects of ginseng. Botanist James A. Duke's *Ginseng: A Concise Handbook* (1989) provides detailed information on all aspects of ginseng biology, culture, history and use.

DOSE

Asian ginseng: 1 to 9 g. American ginseng: 2 to 9 g.

DESCRIPTION

Asian ginseng is a glabrous (smooth) perennial herb growing up to 24 inches tall. A single stalk arises from the roots. The above-ground portions of the plant are actually a single compound leaf dividing into 3 to 5 fronds, each producing 3 to 5 leaflets. The middle leaflet is the largest, with two slightly smaller leaflets on either side. Two much smaller leaflets are beneath. The margins are finely serrated, and tiny bristly hairs are scattered on the veins. The single flowering stalk, 3 to 8 inches long, is topped by an umbel of relatively small inconspicuous pale yellowish-green flowers. The berrylike bright red fruits enclose two hard seeds.

In overall appearance, American ginseng differs little from its Asian counterpart. The flower stalk of Asian ginseng is usually much longer than that of American ginseng, although this characteristic is not always stable. In *Ginseng: A Concise Handbook* (1989), Duke says that he is not sure how to distinguish between the two, and that perhaps the most reliable differences are in the seedlings. He notes that the leaflets of American ginseng seedlings tend to have many sawlike teeth, and that the teeth on Asian ginseng seedlings tend to be less conspicuous and more irregular.

DISTRIBUTION

Panax ginseng occurs in rich mountain slopes in the northeastern provinces of Heilongjiang, Jilin, and Liaoning, as well as in adjacent Korea and Russia. Most of the Chinese cultivated supply is produced in Jilin and Liaoning. It is also a major commercial export from Korea. In the United States, *Panax ginseng* is a rare plant in botanical gardens or private collections—exceedingly rare. As little as three pounds of wild Asian ginseng are harvested each year. A single root may sell for tens of thousands of dollars.

Panax quinquefolius occurs on rich, rocky, shaded, cool slopes, preferring sweet soils. It is found in eastern North America from Quebec to west Manitoba, and south to northern Florida, Alabama, and Oklahoma. Its peak abundance is in the Cumberland Gap region of the southern Appalachians. Elsewhere it is rare (Eastman 1976). While never a common plant in its range, American ginseng is found less frequently than it once was and is considered to be rare, threatened, or even endangered in some areas, due to over harvesting. The trade of American ginseng is regulated under an international treaty, CITES (Convention on International Trade in Endangered Species), as well as by state agencies, the U.S. Fish and Wildlife Service, and the USDA. Permit requirements have been developed for imports, exports, and reexports of American ginseng. Over 500 acres of American ginseng are now under cultivation in China.

CULTIVATION

Ginseng cultivation is a specialized art and a risky business. The cost of ground preparation and providing shade for an acre of American ginseng in the United States is estimated at more than $10,000. First, it takes a very specific habitat, requiring very rich, deeply dug, well-drained, moist soil, and deep shade. The soil should be a friable, well-textured loam, high in humus. Heavy clay or sandy soils are not suitable. The pH should be between 5 and 6. Shade is provided with lath shade or screen cloth. In China, ginseng is often grown under lath shade made of bamboo. Ginseng is also grown under natural tree canopies in the United States. The shade structure has to be designed so that it allows rain to reach the crop.

Propagation is by seeds. The seeds have a long period of dormancy after they ripen. They may take from six to 24 months to germinate. Stratified seeds are used for planting. The seeds are placed in sand or other stratification medium and kept in a refrigerator for four months before planting, or allowed to stratify outdoors over the winter months. First or second year seedlings are called "strawberry leaf" ginseng, because the small seedlings only have three leaflets, much like a strawberry leaf. Ginseng is not propagated vegetatively. Plants are spaced at 6 to 12 inches, depending upon the growing conditions. In China the flowers are pinched back, except in plants saved for seed production, to send more energy to the roots.

Ginseng culture can also be a risky business, because the sensitive plants are subject to attack by leaf and root blights, insect infestations, root rot (fungal disease), and are a favorite treat of rodents.

Abraham Whisman of Boones Path, Virginia, established the first commercial cultivation of American ginseng in the 1870s. In 1895 there were about 20 growers. Now there are several hundred growers, most of whom are in Marathon County, Wisconsin, where 90 percent of the cultivated American ginseng crop is reportedly produced. In 1989, 2,359,510 pounds of cultivated ginseng root was exported from the United States—about a $54 million export. In the same year 203,440 pounds of wild-harvested root worth about $18 million was exported.

No figures on Chinese production of Asian ginseng are available.

HARVESTING

Both Asian and American ginsengs are harvested in the fall, usually after the fifth year of growth. Roots are carefully removed from the ground and handled so that they remain completely intact. Loose soil is removed by spraying with a hose or carefully cleaning by hand. They are then spread on a rack to dry and closely monitored to ensure proper and complete drying. Wild ginseng is harvested only after the red berries have ripened, so that seed can be collected or dispersed to regenerate the species. This is the only ethical time to harvest ginseng, and it is a time-honored practice. When the Ojibwa people dug the root of American ginseng, they always planted the ripe fruiting tops in the same hole from which the roots were dug.

Traditionally, cultivated or wild ginseng is harvested only after the plant is at least five years old. The timing of the harvest has been shown to be related to amounts of the active ginsenoside content. According to

James A. Duke (1989), citing research of Soldati and Tanaka (1984), the highest yields of ginsenosides in Asian ginseng were found in the roots at the end of the fifth summer of growth. The root reportedly doubled in weight at this time. Growth as well as ginsenoside content were less marked after the fifth year.

PROCESSING

At least fifteen different crude root products of Asian ginseng whole root, primary root (with rhizome and rootlets removed), the rhizome ("neck," with annual scars from which the age of the root can be approximated), and rootlets, are commonly available in Chinese markets. Whole "white" (unprocessed) ginseng is simply the carefully dried root. Red ginseng is hard, brittle, and has a translucent reddish coloration. It is made by steaming the roots for three hours, and then drying them over a low fire or in the sun. Branch roots and rootlets are removed and sold as separate products. Sugared ginseng is made by taking the clean fresh roots, and parboiling them for 3 to 7 minutes, after which the roots are pricked with needles. The roots are dried in the sun and then soaked in a thick sugar syrup for 10 to 12 hours. The entire procedure is repeated three times before the product goes to market. For more detailed information on these and other procedures, as well as the use and processing of ginseng by-products, see the excellent publications on ginseng by Dr. Shiu Ying Hu, listed in the bibliography.

Certain glycoside fractions of processed (red) *Panax ginseng* have antioxidant activity. In TCM, decocting ginseng in iron vessels is contraindicated. Ng and Yeung (1986) present a rational scientific explanation for this tradition in their review of antioxidant experiments with ginseng.

ADDITIONAL SPECIES

Besides *P. quinquefolius*, there is one other American species, *P. trifolius*, known as "groundnut." The globe-shaped root is considered edible. The plant is little researched and seldom used. A tea of the whole plant was used by American Indians for colic, indigestion, gout, hepatitis, hives, rheumatism, and tuberculosis. The root was nibbled for treating headaches, fainting, and nervous conditions (Foster and Duke 1990).

There are a number of species of Asian ginseng, between 5 and 10, depending upon the botanical authority. Among the best known is *Panax notoginseng* (Burk.) F. H. Chen. Called *sanqi* (*tienchi*), the dried root is used to stop bleeding and allay pain by dispersing blood stasis. It is used for reducing swelling of wounds, soft tissue injuries, and bleeding; to treat angina pectoris; and is listed as an official drug in the 1985 Chinese *Pharmacopeia*. It is grown in Yunnan province, where the leaves and flower tops are enjoyed as a beverage tea.

Zhu-jie-shen is the rhizome of *Panax japonicus* C. A. Meyer. *Zhu-zi-shen* is the rhizome of *Panax japonicus* var. *major* (Burk.) C. Y. Wu et. K. M. Feng (*P. major*) or the rhizome of *P. japonicus* var. *bipinnatifidus* (Seem.) C. Y. Wu et K. M. Feng. Both *zhu-jie-shen* and *zhu-zi-shen* are official drugs in the Chinese *Pharmacopeia*. *Zhu-jie-shen* is used as a ginseng substitute for strengthening the stomach and as a tonic. *Zhu-zi-shen* is used in prescriptions for cough, asthma, and to benefit vital energy (*qi/ch'i*).

OTHER USES

In Missouri folk tradition, as in China, the leaves of ginseng, as well as the roots, have been used as a tonic tea. The leaf tea has also been used in Ozark folk traditions for fevers. The Oriental ginseng's leaves have been used for fevers in Chinese folk tradition (Foster and Yueh 1991).

Licorice
Gan-cao

> **Botanical Names:** *Glycyrrhiza glabra* L. (*G. glandulifera* Walst. & Kit), *Glycyrrhiza uralensis* Fisch., and *Glycyrrhiza inflata* Bat.
> **Chinese Names:** Pinyin: *Gan-cao*. Wade-Giles: *Kan-ts'ao*.
> **English Names:** Licorice.
> **Pharmaceutical Name:** Radix Glycyrrhizae.
> **Family:** Leguminosae (Fabaceae)—pea family.

HISTORY

Most of us associate licorice with a flavor, but that flavor is not actually "licorice," but rather, the flavor of anise. Licorice itself, known to the civilized world for thousands of years, has a very sweet, somewhat musty flavor.

Licorice root, derived from the Mediterranean native species (*Glycyrrhiza glabra*) was known to the ancient Greek and Roman writers. The first century Roman naturalist Pliny mentions that licorice is native to Sicily. Theophrastus notes the sweet flavor of the roots and says it is used for asthma, dry cough, and all diseases of the lungs. Until about a thousand years ago, most of the European licorice supply was harvested from the wild. Licorice was a well-known herb in Germany by the eleventh century. Cultivation was first recorded in Bologna in the thirteenth century. Licorice was extensively cultivated in Bavaria by the sixteenth century and in the north of England, cultivation was known by the end of the sixteenth century. In the year 1305, a duty was levied on licorice by Edward I to help finance the repair of the London Bridge.

The English name licorice is derived from *liquiritia*, itself a corruption of the ancient name *Glycyrrhiza*, which now serves as the scientific generic name for the plant group.

Licorice is a member of the genus *Glycyrrhiza* of the Leguminosae (pea family). The genus includes about 20 species native to Eurasia, North and South America, and Australia. Five species are native to Europe. One species, *Glycyrrhiza lepidota*, is native to the United States, though the common European licorice, *G. glabra*, has escaped from cultivation and become naturalized in North America. China has at least six species, three of which are source plants of the Chinese licorice, known as *gan-cao* (sweet herb). The European licorice *G. glabra* grows in China where it is known as *guang-guo-gan-cao* (glabrous or smooth-fruited *gan-cao)*. Another name for it is *ou-gan-cao*, meaning European *gan-cao*. Another species used in China is *G. inflata*, or *zhang-guo-gan-cao*. The species name *inflata* refers to the swollen seed pods, as does the Chinese name for the plant (*zhang* means "swollen"; *guo* means "fruit").

The major source plant of Chinese licorice is *G. uralensis*, the most widely distributed licorice species in northern and western China. All three species, but especially *G. uralensis*, are listed as official source plants of licorice or *gan-cao* in the 1985 edition of the Chinese *Pharmacopeia*. Licorice solid extract and liquid extract are also official drugs in the Chinese *Pharmacopeia*.

Licorice is first mentioned in the superior class of herbs in *Shen Nong Ben Cao Jing*. Chinese herbals from every dynasty in Chinese history give the plant prominent recognition. From the ancient *ben cao* it is clear that the form, production regions, collection methods, and quality, of the *gan-cao* of ancient texts is the same as is used today.

As in the past, licorice is still one of the most commonly used traditional herbs of China. The root and the rhizome are the part that are used. In recent years the European licorice (G. *glabra*) has begun to be widely produced in Gansu and Xinjiang and is used throughout China. *Glycyrrhiza inflata* is also produced in these two provinces in large quantities. The quality is acceptable, but it is not considered as good as G. *glabra* and G. *uralensis*. The 1977 edition of the Chinese *Pharmacopoeia* notes that in addition to use as a source plant for the traditional drug *gan-cao*, the plant is also a source of food sweetener and a coloring agent used for manufactured food products in China. It is very widely used in China.

Taste and Character

Sweet, neutral.

Functions

Gan-cao invigorates the spleen, benefits vital energy (*qi/ch'i*), stops cough, expels phlegm, clears away heat, detoxifies, relaxes spasms and convulsions, stops pain, and mediates the medicinal character of other herbs. Processed *gan-cao* is also used to invigorate the spleen and benefit vital energy (*qi/chi*). It is considered a demulcent for the lungs and throat, and is an expectorant.

Uses

Gan-cao is used in prescriptions for cases of weak spleen and stomach energy, for coughs, sore throats, asthma, carbuncles, swelling with pain, sores with toxic matter, stiffness inside of the abdomen with pain, stomach ulcers, duodenal ulcers, hepatitis, hysteria, and as a detoxicant for food or medicine poisoning, as well as to "mediate" or "harmonize" the poisonous character of toxic medicinal plants.

Numerous Chinese studies on the effect of the plant provide evidence that licorice extract as well as the powdered root are effective in the treatment of stomach and duodenal ulcers. Acute or newly formed ulcers respond better than chronic cases. This is confirmed in both animal and human studies. The flavonoids liquiritin, isoliquiritin, liquiritigenin, and isoliquiritigenin contained in the root, are thought to be responsible for the anti ulcer activity. Clinical reports indicate that a 90 percent success rate can be achieved using licorice preparations for the treatment of stomach and duodenal ulcers.

Another important constituent of licorice is the very sweet, foaming, triterpene glycoside glycyrrhizin (glycyrrhizic acid), which is 50 times sweeter than sugar. It occurs in quantities of 5 to 20 percent of the weight of the root. It stimulates the excretion of hormones by the adrenal cortex and has been suggested as a possible drug to prolong the action of cortisone. Glycyrrhizin is considered to be similar in chemical structure to corticosteroids released by the adrenals. It has been used in injectable forms in China for the treatment of mild cases of Addison's disease. The hormone like activity of licorice may in the future prove useful in reducing clinical dependence on cortical hormones, and improve the withdrawal symptoms of patients taken off hormones as well as improving the function of the hormone drugs themselves. Licorice has also shown estrogenic activity in laboratory animals.

Glycyrrhizin and another important triterpene, glycyrrhentinic acid, both have anti-inflammatory activity, which has been suggested as the reason for the efficacy of the herb in the treatment of asthma. Research has also confirmed antirheumatic activity.

In controlled dosages, the root is used in the treatment of high sodium levels and water retention in Chinese clinics. Above a certain dosage, however, licorice can induce sodium and water retention.

The cough-suppressing activity of licorice is likened to codeine in its level of efficacy. Preparations adjusted to 1 mg of the root per kg of body weight inhibit coughing in up to 80 percent of cases studied. The antitussive (cough-suppressing) effect is reported to last longer than with codeine. Evidence suggests that the antitussive activity is the result of an antispasmodic effect on the central nervous system.

Licorice root extract is also used as a stomach antacid. Laboratory experiments and clinical use confirm the antacid activity of licorice. It also serves as an antispasmodic for the smooth muscles of the stomach and the intestines. Anticoagulant activity is also reported in the Chinese literature. Extracts are antibacterial and antimicrobial against *Staphylococcus aureus*, tuberculosis, colon bacilli, amoebas, and trichomonads. In China, licorice is used as a detoxicant for food, medicine, and poisonous substances.

Licorice has been used in modern China for the treatment of chronic viral hepatitis with over a 70 percent success rate. Preparations are given over a period of two to three months, resulting in improvement of symptoms such as malaise, anorexia, abdominal distention, nausea, and vomiting. Improvement of liver function tests and a reduction in the size of an enlarged liver or spleen has been observed. An antioxidative action may be involved in the liver detoxifying activity of licorice root. Side effects have included such symptoms as edema, hypertension, and headache.

In India, licorice is not indigenous, but it is also revered as a venerable medicinal plant. Ancient Hindu works describe it as a demulcent, cooling herb useful for coughs and hoarseness. As in other parts of the world, it was also used as a flavoring agent because of its sweet taste.

In the ancient Arab world, the root was considered hot and dry, and a demulcent for coughs and relieving thirst. It was also considered a diuretic, emmenagogue (bringing on menstruation), and a useful treatment for asthma and irritation of the bronchial passages.

In a Western context, it is considered to be a demulcent, anti-inflammatory, expectorant, antitussive, detoxicant, and spasmolytic. Licorice has stood the test of time as a safe and effective medicinal substance if used in appropriate dosages for a reasonable period of time. It has been used for millennia by peoples throughout Europe and Asia for parallel purposes, most notably for the treatment of cough, stomach ulcers, asthma, sore throat, liver disease, swelling and inflammation, and thirst. Dozens of modern clinical, pharmacological, toxicological, and chemical studies have substantiated many of the traditional uses of the herb, while revealing new applications for the plant.

In the United States, licorice is available for flavoring and health purposes in a wide variety of product forms, including whole dried root, sliced root, cut and sifted root, powdered root, capsulated products, liquid and solid extracts, and products standardized to certain levels of the active components. The extract is used as an ingredient in cough syrups and drops and as a flavoring agent for laxatives.

DOSE

1.5–9 g of the root is used in pills and powders, poulticed or applied as a wash. In Chinese tradition, if the herb is to be used to "disperse heat" it is used fresh. For strengthening the vital energy of the middle burner, honey-processed licorice is used (see "Processing").

CONTRAINDICATIONS, TOXICITY, AND CAUTIONS

Large doses of licorice taken over a long period of time have produced side effects such as edema (swelling of the limbs and face), hypertension, and headache. It can also produce cardiac disfunction and sometimes severe hypertension. Glycyrrhizin can increase extracellular fluid and plasma volume, causing the retention of sodium and potassium loss. Therefore, it is appropriate to use moderate amounts of the herb on a short-term basis. Licorice should be avoided by persons with a history of cardiac and kidney problems, hypertension, and obesity; it is best avoided during pregnancy.

While licorice is used to counteract the toxic effects of some medicinal plants, it is also contraindicated for use with certain plants, including with the root of *Euphorbia pekinensis*, the flower buds of *Daphne genkwa*, the root of *Euphorbia kansuii*, and *Sargassum pallidum*.

DESCRIPTION

Glycyrrhiza species are perennial herbs or subshrubs with alternate, odd-pinnate leaves. Some or all parts of the plant have glandular, often sticky hairs. The flowers grow either in racemes from the leaf axils or in spikes that are usually shorter than the leaves themselves. The small pealike flowers are whitish-violet, and rarely, yellow, depending upon the species. Flowering is usually in June through August. The flowers possess ten stamens, nine of which are united, while one stands alone. The fruits are flat, plump, oblong, either straight or curved legumes with 1 to 8 seeds. The seed pods often serve as the most efficient means of distinguishing between species. The roots are cylindrical and branched, with numerous burrowing horizontal underground stems that travel six feet or more away from the mother plant in the second year and send up new shoots. The underground stems provide the licorice root that is used for commercial purposes.

Fen-gan-cao (*fen* means powder) is licorice root with the root bark removed. This is used for making powdered licorice. The highest quality *fen-gan-cao* is characterized by being smooth, light yellow in color, and fibrous, with vertical lines or wrinkles. If the bark is retained, the highest quality licorice has a very thin, firm bark with wrinkles and a reddish-brown color on the exterior, and will be dense, hard, and starchy. Broken sections should be yellowish-white in the interior. If the bark is very rough, a greenish-brown color, or dense, not starchy, with broken sections exhibiting a deep yellow color, it is considered to be of inferior quality. If the bark is brownish-black, very hard, and the broken sections are brownish-yellow, with a bitter taste, this is a sign of very poor quality licorice and it should not be used as medicine. Licorice root without root bark (*fen-gan-cao*) is considered to be of higher medicinal quality than that with the bark.

DISTRIBUTION

Glycyrrhiza uralensis, the primary source plant for *gan-cao*, is found in dry grassy plains, and sunny mountainsides from Heilongjiang, Jilin, and Liaoning in the northeast, and to the west and south in the provinces of Hebei, Shanxi, Nei Mongol, Shandong, Shaanxi, Ningxia, Gansu, Qinghai, and Xinjiang. It also occurs in Mongolia and Soviet Siberia. It is produced mainly in Nei Mongol, Gansu, and Xinjiang. Depending upon where the supply is produced, it is known in Chinese markets as eastern *gan-cao* or western *gan-cao*. Western *gan-cao* is produced in Nei Mongol, Shaanxi, Gansu, Qinghai, and Xinjiang. Eastern *gan-cao* is produced in Heilongjiang, Jilin, Liaoning, Hebei, and Shanxi. The best quality comes from Nei Mongol and the borders of Gansu and Ningxia near Nei Mongol. In recent years the greatest quantity has been produced in Xinjiang, followed by Nei Mongol and Ningxia. It is sold throughout China, and large quantities are exported as well.

Glycyrrhiza glabra occurs in wild desert regions, dry plains, grassy plains with salty alkaline soil, and fallow wastelands that were once used for producing rice, wheat, and millet. The distribution center of the plant is in the Mediterranean region. It is the major source plant of licorice in Western herbal traditions and Russia, occurring in many parts of Eurasia to northern Africa. In Europe it occurs in dry open habitats in the southern and eastern regions of the continent. It has been cultivated throughout Europe and is naturalized in almost all of Europe except Scandinavia. In the wastelands of northwestern China, it acts more like a weed than a wild native plant. It is found in the provinces of Xinjiang, Qinghai, and Gansu.

Glycyrrhiza inflata is found in salty alkaline soils of grassy plains and moist depressions in the southern parts of Xinjiang and some parts of Gansu.

Glycyrrhiza glabra and *G. inflata* are mainly produced in Xinjiang and Gansu. They are both considered acceptable source plants of *gan-cao*.

CULTIVATION

Glycyrrhiza uralensis is a calciphyte; that is, it likes soils high in calcium. It thrives in sunny, cool, dry regions, such as grassy plains and on the sandy banks of rivers, and tolerates somewhat salty, alkaline soils. However, heavy saline (salty) alkaline soils will not produce a good crop. The soil should be relatively rich, sandy, deep, and with good drainage. It will not tolerate soggy soils.

Licorice can be propagated by seed, root division, or rhizome cuttings. Seeds are harvested in August or September from healthy three-year-old plants with plump, firm seeds. Seeds can be planted in October or the following spring, usually in March. Like many legume family members, licorice seeds have a hard seed coat that must be softened before planting. If seeds are used for propagation, they should be soaked in water at 85° F for two to three hours before planting. Another method is to scarify the seeds, scratching the hard seed coat with sandpaper or a sharp implement so that water can penetrate into the embryo and initiate germination. Once pretreated, seeds are planted directly in the field in rows and covered to a depth about two times the seed's diameter. Plants are spaced at 1 to 1½ feet.

The rhizome can also be used for propagation. In early spring or late autumn, when the plant is dormant, strong healthy rhizomes are chosen and cut into individual sections about 4 to 6 inches long, each with one or two buds, or "eyes." These rhizomes are planted in rows spaced at 20 inches apart, with individual rhizomes planted at a spacing of about 18 inches. Once planted, cover the rhizomes and tamp the soil.

Young seedlings are thinned to proper spacings. The crop should be kept well weeded, with frequent shallow cultivation beneath the plants. Composted manure can be used as a side-dressing one or two times during the growing season each year.

HARVESTING

The roots of cultivated plants can be dug when the plant is dormant in spring or autumn. Spring-harvested roots are considered to be the best. The quality of fall-dug roots is somewhat lower, and roots harvested in summer are of very poor quality. Cultivated plants are harvested after three to four years of growth. Wild-harvested licorice root is best collected in autumn. The root and lateral rhizomes of the plant are harvested. The main beds are left undisturbed, and the long-traveling rhizomes are carefully harvested from between the rows and plants so that the root is not damaged.

While roots are still fresh, young buds and lateral branches are cut off. The roots are washed and are then graded into several lots according to diameter. They are then tied into small bundles and placed in an area with good air circulation to dry. After drying, they are wrapped in paper for shipment to market. The roots may also be placed in the sun to dry. The cortex or root bark can also be scraped off when the root is still fresh. This type of root is called *fen-gan-cao* and is used for making powdered herb products.

During drying and storage it is important to make sure that the roots do not become wet, since they are susceptible to mildew and insect infestations. The root is very sweet and is liable to attract both insects and rodents.

PROCESSING

Processed *gan-cao* is made by placing slices of the dried root in preheated honey. The honey is mixed with a little hot water, then poured over the root in a roasting pan. It is then stir-fried for a short period until the root's color becomes dark yellow and it is no longer sticky to the touch. For every 100 pounds of the root, 25 to 30 pounds of the heated honey is used.

To slice the dried root, it is soaked in a little water until the roots are about 80 percent moist. It is then cut into slices and dried again.

Licorice extract (inspissated, or thickened juice) has been used in Western traditions to make pomfret cakes, which are used for flavoring purposes or confections. The extract is a tarlike, solid, dark brown, plastic mass. To make it the roots are bruised, cut up into small pieces, and then boiled in water until the sweet mucilaginous juice is extracted. This decoction is allowed to rest and, after straining, it is evaporated down to the proper consistency. A special process is used to boil and mix the juice, after which the material is rolled out by a machine into thin sheets, placed on trays, and then left in a warm room (about 100°F) overnight. The next morning, the sheets are stamped, pressed, or rolled into their finished form. The resulting cakes are again subjected to high temperature to "skin over" the exterior, and sent to market.

ADDITIONAL SPECIES

Several additional *Glycyrrhiza* species are used locally in China. *Glycyrrhiza korshinskyi* Grigoriev (*G. kansuensis* Chang et Peng mss), known as *huang-gan-cao* or yellow licorice, is very similar to *G. uralensis* but has a curved, somewhat swollen, flattish fruit. The flowers are in a loose raceme rather than a head. It is used locally in the southern part of Xinjiang and Gansu. It occurs eastward as far as southeastern Russia.

Glycyrrhiza aspera Pall. (*cu-mao-gan-cao*, or rough-hair *gan-cao*) is sometimes used in Xinjiang as a substitute for *G. uralensis*. The plant is quite similar and the root and rhizome are very thin, with a slightly sweet taste.

It also occurs in southeastern Russia and the Asian steppes.

Yunnan-gan-cao (*Glycyrrhiza yunnanensis* Cheng f. et L. K. Tai) grows in Yunnan province, where it is used as a folk medicine.

Glycyrrhiza echinata L., which is found in Hungary and southeastern Europe east to Korea, is sometimes used in northern China.

Glycyrrhiza lepidota (Nutt.) Pursh, the wild American licorice, occurs in prairies and fields from western Ontario to Texas, and from Missouri west to Washington. It was used by various native American groups to reduce fevers in children and as a treatment for toothaches; the leaves were applied as a wash for earache.

OTHER USES

Pumpkin seeds can be roasted with licorice root to give the seeds a sweet flavor. In China, licorice is also used to produce natural dyes for cloth and as a coloring agent in food.

In ancient Persia, the wood of the European licorice was used by glassmakers for melting their materials, because it was said to create more heat than any other fuel.

In nineteenth-century Western pharmacy, licorice root was used to disguise the flavor of vile-tasting medicines. The powdered root was added to pill mixes to impart stiffness, and once dried, pills were dusted with licorice powder to prevent them from adhering to one another.

In India, the leaves were used as a treatment for a scalded head and to quell the odor of foul feet or armpits.

In Nei Mongol, the leaves have been used as a tea substitute.

Licorice is also used as a flavoring in confectionery, plug tobacco, and for flavoring stout beer. If 1 pound of glycyrrhizin is added to 100 pounds of sugar, it will double the sweetness of the sugar.

Licorice sticks were for many centuries a popular chewing stick in Europe, as well as the West Indies, after its introduction by European explorers. Licorice chewing sticks were responsible for turning Napoleon's teeth black.

According to the *Wealth of India*, spent pulp remaining from the manufacture of licorice extract has been used as an ingredient in foam stabilizers for fire extinguishers. It has also been used as a wetting and foaming agent in ore refining and as a wetting, spreading, and sticking agent in insecticide formulations.

Red Sage
Dan-shen

Botanical Names: *Salvia miltiorrhiza* Bunge.
Chinese Names: Pinyin: *Dan-shen* (root). Wade-Giles: *Tan-shen* (root).
English Names: Red sage root.
Pharmaceutical Name: Radix Salviae Miltiorrhizae.
Family: Labiatae (Lamiaceae)—mint family.

HISTORY

When Americans hear the word *sage* they generally think of the common garden sage (*Salvia officinalis*). This group in the mint family, however, is very large, containing dozens of plants used for culinary, fragrant, and medicinal purposes worldwide. The genus *Salvia* of the mint family contains more than 750 species of herbs and shrubs, mostly from tropical and subtropical areas.

Red sage, or *dan-shen* (*Salvia miltiorrhiza*), is one of many Chinese species in the genus. It received its Latin name from the Russian botanist Alexander von Bunge (1803–1890) in an 1833 publication. The generic name *Salvia* is derived from a Latin word root, *salvare*, which means "to heal," referring to the medicinal qualities of the common garden sage. The specific epithet *miltiorrhiza* is derived from the Greek *miltos*, meaning "red lead," and *rhiza*, "root," and refers to the reddish-purple color of the root.

Seed of the plant was introduced from Beijing to Paris by the French Jesuit, Pierre d'Incarville (1706–1756) in the eighteenth century, where it was cultivated as a rare botanical specimen. The plant, not very showy, persists as a rare specimen in a few Western botanical gardens and in the hands of several collectors in the United States. Live plant material is not available in the American horticultural trade.

This is a very commonly used Chinese herbal medicine, first mentioned in the primary class of medicinal plants in *Shen Nong Ben Cao Jing*. The source plant mentioned in the ancient *ben cao* is the same plant that is used today. Accepted substitutes, such as *Gansu dan-shen*, have a short history of use (see "Additional species").

Taste and Character

Bitter, a little cold.

Functions

Promotes blood circulation, removes blood stasis, subsides swelling, stops pain, tranquilizes the mind by nourishing the heart, promotes growth of new tissue, and regulates menstruation.

Uses

Dan-shen is used in prescriptions for abnormal menstruation; painful or difficult menstruation; suppressed menstrual flow; a mass in the abdomen, or blood stasis after childbirth; blood stasis and pain in the chest, abdomen, or arms and legs; palpitation; swelling of the liver and spleen; and chronic hepatitis, angina, joint pains, carbuncles, swelling, sores, and insomnia.

The dried root of *dan-shen* is used in traditional Chinese medicine. It is used in numerous prescriptions to relieve pain after childbirth and regulate menstruation. Combined with *dang-gui*, it is used to regulate suppressed menstrual flow. A tincture of *dan-shen* and schisandra fruits are used to treat sleep loss due to weak nerves. A decoction of the two herbs is also used to treat weak nerves. If menstruation is irregular (late or early every month), with unpredictable flow, accompanied by lower back and joint pain, the root (with the crown removed) is powdered and prescribed with alcohol before meals. If the patient experiences sudden chills or fever, it might be prescribed to her as needed.

In traditional terms *dan-shen* helps to promote blood circulation and eliminate blood stasis. Because of the perceived positive effect on circulation, it is also traditionally used to treat of angina pectoris. A clinical study of angina pectoris reported on the use of *dan-shen* tablets. The daily dose of two tablets, three times per day, equaled an extract of 60 g of the crude drug. The course of treatment was 2 to 4 weeks. Patients involved took the drug for 1 to 9 months. In the treatment of 323 cases, the effective rate was placed at 82.3 percent. Over 20 percent of patients showed marked improvement. The treatment was most effective in patients with mild or moderate cases of angina, and when it was carried out for two months rather than one month. Most patients did not experience side effects.

Additional clinical studies on *dan-shen* for angina have experimented with various modes of administration, drug forms, or traditional combinations, generally reporting positive results. It is used clinically in China for myocardial infraction or other myocardium damage. It has also been successfully used in chronic hepatitis, cerebrovascular disease, and skin disease; externally, it has been used to treat surgical infections.

In recent years, the plant has been the subject of much research by Chinese scientists. Experimentally, *dan-shen* (or its components) dilates coronary blood vessels and peripheral blood vessels, increasing blood flow and lowering blood pressure. It is considered antibacterial and anti-inflammatory. Cryptotanshinone, the main antibacterial agent, is used as an isolate in tablet or ointment form for the treatment of tonsillitis, infected sores, or other ailments involving *Staphylococcus aureus*. Active components of the plant are primarily water soluble, and its water extracts are antifungal. Various components have been shown to be mildly sedative. Animal experiments suggest that the extracts of *dan-shen* prevent intramicrovascular coagulation, relieve local anemia or lack of blood flow to affected tissue, and accelerate repair of liver lesions while aiding in enriching liver-cell nutrition.

In Western terms, red sage is considered alterative, antispasmodic, antiarthritic, astringent, tonic, sedative, and vulnerary. In the American herb market it is used as an ingredient in some Chinese herb combination products. Capsulated powdered root and whole roots are sold, though they are primarily prescribed by TCM practitioners.

DOSE

Dose 5–15 g (up to 30 g if used alone).

WARNING

In Chinese medicine, the use of *Salvia miltiorrhiza* is contraindicated with the highly toxic black false hellebore (*Veratrum nigra*).

DESCRIPTION

Red sage is a branched or unbranched perennial growing from 1 to 2 feet in height. The stem is densely covered with spreading hairs, except on the flowering stalks. The opposite leaves, prominent at the base of the plant, are divided into 5 (or occasionally 3–7) ovate, round-toothed leaflets, from

1 to 3 inches long and about half as wide. They are pubescent above and pilose-hairy beneath. The leaf stalks are up to 1¹/₂ inch long. The reddish-purple flowers grow in terminal or axillary racemes up to 8 inches long, with 3 to 10 flowers in whorls.

The best-quality root is strong purple-black within, with many medulary rays and white points or dots in cross section. Cultivated roots tend to be larger, with longitudinal wrinkles. The outer layers of the root bark tend not to peel. Wild roots tend to be thinner, more divided, with a cortex peeling, and often have rootlets attached. The cultivated root is more desirable.

DISTRIBUTION

Red sage occurs on sunny mountains, in roadside ditches, fields, forest margins, and near streams throughout most of China, except in Heilongjiang, Jilin, Nei Mongol, Xinjiang, Qinghai, Yunnan, and Xizang. Most of the supply is from wild-harvested plants, though it is cultivated commercially on a relatively large scale in Sichuan. Major production is in Sichuan, Shanxi, Hebei, Jiangsu and Anhui. It is also produced in Liaoning, Shaanxi, Henan, Hubei, Zhejiang, Fujian, and Shandong. The best quality is considered to be the cultivated material grown in Sichuan.

CULTIVATION

The plant likes moist sandy soils and is tolerant of cold. Seeds or root division are used for propagation. Seeds can be sown indoors in early spring and transplanted after the last frost. Seeds emerge in 15 to 20 days. When the seedlings are 3 to 5 inches high, they can be transplanted to permanent locations. Plants are spaced at about 1 foot apart. If direct-sown, they can be planted in April or August. Clump division is best done in autumn or early spring before the leaves appear. The plant is dug, cut into 2 to 3 sections, and then replanted. The planting is side-dressed with well-rotted manure or night soil 2 to 3 times during the growing season. While red sage does best in a relatively moist, rich sandy soil, good drainage is important. Plants are watered during periods of drought.

HARVESTING

The root is collected from November to the following March, while the plant is dormant. The first ten days of November is considered the best time for harvest. Sometimes the root is harvested during the growing season as well, though the quality is not as good. After harvest, the stems and lateral rootlets are cut off. The short rootstock, or rhizome, at the crown of the root, which is attached to aerial stems, is sometimes removed. The roots are washed, and then dried in the sun.

PROCESSING

After cleaning the root crown is removed; the roots are then covered with a moist cloth and left to sit until the roots become uniformly moist. They are then cut into sections and dried in the sun.

Roasted dan-shen is made by stir-frying the roots over a light fire until the surface of the root is covered with about 5 percent "charcoaled points." It is then taken from the heat source and cooled.

ADDITIONAL SPECIES

Two other species are relatively widely used as source plants of dan-shen in China. These include Salvia bowleyana Dunn, known as nan-dan-shen (southern dan-shen), and Salvia przewalskii Maxim. (Gansu dan-shen).

Nan-dan-shen grows on mountains, along forest margins, and near rivers in Zhejiang, Jiangxi, Fujian, Hunan, Guangdong, and Guangxi. Nan-dan-shen is produced in Hunan, Jiangxi, Zhejiang, and Fujian. It is often confused with and mixed with lots of Salvia miltiorrhiza.

Gansu dan-shen grows in high mountains, forest margins, roadsides, ditches, and shrub thickets in Gansu, Qinghai, Sichuan, Yunnan, and Xizang. Salvia przewalskii var. mandarinorum (Diels) Sieb., is known as brown-hair Gansu dan-shen. It occurs in Gansu, Qinghai, Sichuan, Yunnan, and Xizang. Major production areas are in Gansu and Yunnan. It is sold to markets in Beijing, Shanghai, Ningxia, Gansu, Qinghai, and Yunnan.

In various parts of China there are a number of Salvia species used as "folk" dan-shen or substitutes, including Salvia yunnanensis, which is distributed in Xi-nan and Yu-gui-chuan counties in Yunnan. It is used as a folk medicine in several areas of Yunnan. Salvia trijuga is used as a folk substitute in Sichuan, Yunnan, and Xizang. Salvia plectranthoides, from Hubei, Shaanxi, Sichuan, Yunnan, and Guizhou, is used as a dan-shen folk substitute. Salvia digitaloides is used in Yunnan. Salvia miltiorrhiza var. alba, produced in Shandong, and Salvia kiaometiensis f. pubescens from Sichuan, are also used in some areas.

Other indigenous Chinese *Salvia* species containing the primary active components of *dan-shen*, known as tanshinones, include *S. evansiana*, *S. brachyloma*, *S. prattii*, *S. aerea*, *S. castanea*, *S. bulleyana*, *S. flava*, and *S. mekogensis*.

OTHER USES

None noted.

Rehmannia
Di-huang

Botanical names: *Rehmannia glutinosa* (Gaertn.) Libosch. ex Fisch. et Mey.

Botanical Synonyms: *Digitalis glutinosa* Gaertn., *Rehmannia chinensis* Libosch. ex Fisch. et Mey.

Chinese Names: Pinyin: *Di-huang* (dried root), *Sheng-di-huang* (unprocessed, fresh root), *Shu-di-huang* (prepared or processed root). Wade-Giles: *Ti-huang* (dried root); *Shêng-ti-huang* (fresh unprocessed root), *Shu-ti-huang* (prepared or processed root).

English Names: Chinese foxglove, rehmannia.

Pharmaceutical Name: Radix Rehmanniae.

Family: Scrophulariaceae—figwort family; some botanists place it in the Gesneriaceae—gesneria family.

HISTORY

Rehmannia, or *di-huang* ("earth yellow"), is a very commonly used herb in traditional Chinese medicine. Before Westerners first became aware of this herb, it had been extensively cultivated in China for many centuries, resulting in the evolution of numerous forms. The plant has many cultivated varieties and is produced in many parts of China. Yue compares the variations in flavor among *di-huang* roots to apples: some are sweet, some sour, others have a bananalike taste. The size of the root, habit, and size of the plant are extremely variable, based on local environmental conditions. The many varieties and forms of rehmannia, however, are believed to belong to a single species, *Rehmannia glutinosa*. *Rehmannia glutinosa* form *hueichingensis* (Chao et Schih) Hsiao is often used in China as well. *Hueichingensis* denotes the origin of the form, from Hueiching in Henan province.

Three separately prepared products from the root are used as *di-huang*. *Gan-di-huang* (*sheng-di-huang*), or dried rehmannia root, consists of freshly harvested roots that are baked slowly until nearly dry, and then kneaded into round balls. *Xian-di-huang*, or fresh *di-huang*, consists of the crude newly harvested,and cleaned roots. *Shu-di-huang*, or prepared rehmannia root, refers to the dried roots that have been steamed to a black color and then redried.

The genus *Rehmannia* is now placed by some botanists in the gesneria family, though it has often been placed in the figwort family as well. There are about 10 species of *Rehmannia*. Another species, *R. elata* is the most commonly grown ornamental from the genus, although *R. glutinosa* is cultivated for ornamental purposes as well.

While the plant has been known to the Chinese for several thousand years, it did not come to the attention of Westerners until the eighteenth century. A dried pressed specimen of *Rehmannia glutinosa* was collected by the French Jesuit, Pierre d'Incarville (1706–1756), in the mid-1700s. In 1770 J. Gaertner, a botanist in Saint Petersburg, published the first botanical description from a living specimen, which he named *Digitalis glutinosa*. A Frenchman, Pierre Martial Cibot, is believed to have sent the seeds to Gaertner a few years earlier from Beijing.

Joseph Liboschitz, a physician who lived in Saint Petersburg in the early 1800s, is responsible for naming the plant *Rehmannia*. Liboschitz possessed a private herbarium; after his death in Vienna in 1824, a specimen was found in his collections labeled *Rehmannia*. He had segregated the plant as a new genus, but had never published the name. The genus name refers to a Dr. Josef Rehmann (1779–1831), who served in the Russian embassy in China during the early 1800s. The generic name *Rehmannia*, as proposed by Liboschitz, was published in an 1835 work by F. E. L. Fischer and C. A. Meyer describing *R. chinensis*. While known to be cultivated in European botanical gardens as early as the 1760s, it is unclear when the plant arrived in the United States.

Di-huang is first mentioned in *Shen Nong Ben Cao Jing*. In ancient times, smaller forms of the plant were utilized. In recent centuries, the plant has become somewhat larger in habit through the selection of improved varieties, but it is the same species that was used by the ancient Chinese. The use of the fresh root is first mentioned in a Qing dynasty work. The use of the leaves was first noted in *Shi Liao Ben Cao*, a seventh-century Tang dynasty work by Meng Shen. Prepared *di-huang* is mentioned in the 1061 Song dynasty work, *Tu Jing Ben Cao* (Illustrated Herbal) by Su Song. Su Song was a government official who served as the major author in preparing this 21 volume work by order of the emperor. His herbal was the first to contain detailed illustrations of all the plants treated in the work. *Di-huang* is an official drug in the 1985 edition of the Chinese Pharmacopeia.

TASTE AND CHARACTER

Dried rehmannia: A little sweet, bitter, cold. Fresh rehmannia: a little sweet, bitter, very cold. Prepared rehmannia: a little sweet, warm.

FUNCTIONS

Dried rehmannia: nourishes yin, dispels heat, cools the blood, stops bleeding, and nourishes the blood. Fresh rehmannia: dispels heat, cools the blood, increases saliva. Prepared rehmannia: nourishes yin, enriches the blood, and regulates menses.

USES

The action and use of the drug depend on the type of processing the roots have received. Dried rehmannia is used for vexation due to febrile diseases, measles, low fever due to yin deficiency, diabetes, nosebleed, bloody urine, uterine bleeding, dry mouth, thirst, vomiting of blood due to blood with heat, restless fetus, and constipation due to damaged yin. It is believed to nourish and replenish depleted vital energy (*qi/ch'i*).

Fresh rehmannia is used for febrile diseases with damaged yin; to treat very high temperatures that cause vexation, thirst, red tongue, blurred thought, or loss of consciousness; and coughing with blood, diabetes, uterine bleeding, measles, vomiting with bleeding, nosebleeds, bloody urine, sore throat, constipation, and bloody stool.

Prepared rehmannia is used for loss of blood, yin deficiency, lower back pain with kidney deficiency from overwork (it replenishes the vital essence of the kidneys), lumbago, cough, hectic fever, diabetes, urinary incontinence, deafness, uterine bleeding, vertigo, tinnitus, and for regulating menstrual flow.

Di-huang is among the 50 most important herbs of Chinese medicine. It is very often used in polyherbal prescriptions for the treatment of diabetes, as well as for gynecological disorders. The crude root is used in the treatment of anemia and as a blood tonic. Externally, the juice of the fresh root is applied to cuts and wounds to help stop bleeding. The powdered dried root, combined with powdered mint leaves, has been decocted and then drunk as a traditional treatment for nosebleeds.

The fresh or the dried root have been shown to have an experimental protective effect on the liver, helping to prevent the depletion of glycogen stored in the liver. Laboratory experiments show that the fresh root has an antifungal effect. Over the last 60 years, various research groups have studied the ability of the herb to lower glucose levels. While initial experiments showed that the root can lower serum glucose levels, subsequent experiments have produced conflicting results. In experiments on heart-related disorders, injections of an extract of the herb in relative small dosages have produced a cardiotonic effect. Larger doses produce a cardiac-inhibiting effect slowing down the heartbeat. Injectable forms of the herb combined with Chinese licorice have been used clinically in China for the treatment of infectious hepatitis and have produced improvement in symptoms and liver function parameters in most cases. Injectable preparations have been used in China for the treatment of rheumatoid arthritis in children and adults.

According to Chinese clinical studies, the prepared or steamed root has proven useful in the treatment of hypertension. It helped to reduce blood pressure and serum cholesterol levels while improving blood flow to the brain. Its cardiotonic action also produces a diuretic effect by dilating blood vessels to the kidneys. Oral extracts given to laboratory animals has induced a reduction in blood-sugar levels.

In Western terms, *di-huang* and its various prepared root forms are considered to be cardiotonic, diuretic, hemostatic, and hypoglycemic. Active constituents are believed to include mannitol, beta-sitosterol, catalpol, and rehmannin, as well as vitamin A. Experimentally, various preparations of the root have been studied—with conflicting results—for their hyperglycemic, antiradiation, hemostatic, diuretic, anti-inflammatory, and antifungal activity, as well as their ability to protect the liver. Clinical studies have included the effect of various root preparations on rheumatoid arthritis, infectious hepatitis, hypertension, and dermatitis.

In the United States, *di-huang* has not become widely known as an herb product. While various preparations containing *di-huang* are sometimes sold in health and natural food markets, TCM practitioners are the major users of the plant.

DOSE

Dry *di-huang*: 9–15 g, (up to 30–60 g), used in decoction, extracts, pills, powders, or poultice. Fresh *di-huang*: 12–30 g, decocted, juiced, extract, or poulticed. Prepared *di-huang*: 12–30 g, in decoction, pills, powders, extracts, or tincture.

CONTRAINDICATIONS AND WARNINGS

Various animals studies have shown the relative safety of the herb. However, any member of the figwort family attributed with cardiotonic properties should be used cautiously. If used in large doses over a long period of time, the herb is known to cause loose stools and abdominal distention.

DESCRIPTION

Rehmannia, or Chinese foxglove, as it is sometimes known in the horticultural trade, is a hardy, pubescent-hirsute, herbaceous perennial growing 6 to 12 inches in height. The leaves are in a basal rosette (alternate leaves on flowering stalks), obovate to elliptical, up to 4 inches long and 1½ inches wide, tapering to a short stalk, with irregularly, wavy, or sharp toothed margins. The leaves are often purplish underneath. The tubular, five-lobed flowers, about 1½ inches long, are densely covered with resinous glandular hairs. Flowers are yellowish to purplish-brown, with purple veins. The calyx, often purplish, is inflated, with five up-curving segments.

DISTRIBUTION

Found in waste places in mountains, fields, and roadsides; often cultivated in China. It occurs in Liaoning, Hebei, Nei Mongol, Shanxi, Shaanxi, Shandong, Jiangsu, Anhui, Zhejiang, Henan, Hubei, Hunan, and Sichuan. In Liaoning, Hebei, Shandong, and Zhejiang, wild plants are harvested for the fresh root. While the plant is grown throughout China, the highest quality comes from Henan province, which is also the largest producer.

The outskirts of the city of Hangzhou in Zhejiang province was once a famous *di-huang* production region, but there is no longer significant commercial production from this area.

It is occasionally grown as an ornamental in the United States, primarily as a specimen plant in botanical gardens and in the gardens of specialty plant collectors.

Another variety, *R. glutinosa* var. *purpurea* Makino, known in Japan as *akayajio*, is cultivated in Japan, Korea, and some parts of China. In Japan it is primarily grown in Nata prefecture. The Japanese call the typical species (*R. glutinosa*) *kaikeijio*.

CULTIVATION

Most of the root supply is cultivated. Rehmannia, a heavy feeder, prefers full sun and a rich, friable, well-drained sandy soil. The soil should be cultivated to a depth of at least one foot. Well-rotted horse or cow manure is liberally added as fertilizer. The plant does not do well in high alkaline or poorly drained soils. In China, it is not commercially produced on soils planted the previous year in cotton, corn, or soybeans. Likewise, a rehmannia crop is not planted on the same ground twice until it has been fallowed or rotated with other crops.

The rhizome is used for propagation from April through the first of May. Sections of the rhizome with two or three buds or eyes, each about 1¼ to 2¼ inches long are cut for planting. They are planted in rows spaced 1 to 2 feet apart, with 6 inches between plants. The rhizome cuttings are covered with 1 to 2 inches of soil. The leaves appear in about 20 days. Rehmannia can also be propagated from seeds or stem cuttings made from basal shoots. The shoots develop after the flower stalks die back in older plants.

Plants are kept well weeded and cultivated. They are watered every 3 to 4 days during dry seasons. The soil is always kept moderately moist. The flower buds are pinched off as they develop to return more energy to the roots. If planted in spring, the roots can be harvested in late autumn of the same year.

After rain, the plant is more susceptible to fungal infections. Rain may splash microorganisms on the lower side of leaves, causing infestations. In China the lower side of the leaves are sometimes rinsed off after a rain. This potential problem can also be prevented with an appropriate mulch.

HARVESTING

The roots of cultivated plantings are harvested from the end of September to November. Wild-harvesting is done in spring. Harvested roots are sorted according to size. The rhizome, or root crown is cut off and the tiny lateral rootlets are removed. Then the main root is washed.

In order to maintain a high-quality product, when digging the root, care is taken not to puncture the cortex. The fresh roots are heeled in sand, then covered with dry soil. Roots can be stored in this manner for up to three months. As needed, they are washed, and sliced for use.

PROCESSING

To prepare dried rehmannia root, the larger roots, covered with a gunny sack, are slowly heated under a light fire on a bed of bricks. They are baked until the middle part of the root is dry and black (about 80 percent dry). The roots are turned often so that the color remains uniform without burn marks. Once 80 percent dry, the roots are rubbed into rounded masses, then cut into slices, and dried in the sun.

Prepared *di-huang* is made by mixing the dried root with rice wine (30 percent by weight). The roots are placed in a steamer and steamed until the inside and outside of the root are dark black and moist. The blackening of the root is the result of the decomposition of one of the active components, catalpol. They are then cooled and dried in the sun. Another method involves steaming the dried roots for eight hours. They are then removed from the heat and covered with a wet cloth for one night. The next day they are steamed for another 4 to 8 hours, and again covered with a wet cloth for another night. The next morning they are dried to 80 percent, sliced, and dried completely.

An old method to make prepared or steamed *di-huang* is to boil the root in the top of a double boiler in 50 percent rice wine until the roots have absorbed the alcohol and the surface becomes very sticky. The root is then taken from the heat, cooled, cut into slices, and sun-dried.

A new method is simply to wash the roots, steam them until the interior is moist, and cut into slices and dry them completely.

For charcoaled *di-huang* the roots are sorted according to size. Larger roots are placed in the bottom of a pan, with the smaller roots toward the top. A piece of paper is placed over the roots, which are heated until the paper turns dark yellow. At this point the roots are removed from the fire, sorted according to size, and stir-fried until "charcoaled," while still retaining the character of the root, i.e., without burning.

ADDITIONAL SPECIES

Rehmannia glutinosa var. *lutea* has traditionally been grown outside of the city of Hangzhou in Zhejiang province. However, in recent years production of this variety has ceased.

OTHER USES

The leaves, flowers, and seeds are used as well as the fresh, dried, and steamed rhizomes. The leaves, called *di-huang-ye*, have traditionally been used as a folk remedy poultice for bad sores or ringworm of the hands and feet. The fresh juice of the leaves was used, or the bruised leaves were rubbed very lightly on the affected area. For sores caused by leprosy, the sores were first washed with salt water, and then the bruised leaves were applied as a poultice.

The flowers of rehmannia (*di-huang-hua*) have been used as a folk remedy for diabetes and for lower back pain due to kidney deficiency. For diabetes, the flowers are dried in the shade, and powdered. Using a measure the size of a fifty-cent piece, three measures of the powder are added to two cups of millet porridge and boiled. After the porridge cools, it is eaten.

The seeds of rehmannia (*di-huang-shi*), dried in the shade and powdered, are used as a folk substitute for the root.

Rhubarb
Da-huang

Botanical names: *Rheum palmatum* L.; *R. tanguticum* Maxim. ex Balf., and *R. officinale* Baill. are also official source plants of *da-huang* in the 1985 edition of the Chinese *Pharmacopeia*.
Chinese Names: Pinyin: *Da-huang* (roots and rhizome). Wade-Giles: *Ta-Huang* (roots and rhizome).

English Names: Chinese rhubarb, medicinal rhubarb, turkey
rhubarb.
Pharmaceutical Name: Radix et Rhizoma Rhei.
Family: Polygonaceae—buckwheat family.

HISTORY

Most Americans are familiar with the common garden rhubarb (*Rheum* x
cultorum Hort.), which is grown for the use of the leaf stalks (petioles) for
jam, pies, wine, sauce, puddings, etc. This species is now considered to be
a cultivar that became established in European gardens in the eighteenth
century. It probably arose in cultivation as a cross between *R. undulatum*
and *R. rhaponticum*, perhaps involving *R. palmatum* as well. It is sometimes
known as *Rheum rhabarbarum* L., or erroneously called *R. rhaponticum*.
The leaf stalks of various rhubarbs are also used in Chinese cuisines. The
leaves themselves are considered highly toxic. See "Warnings."

The genus *Rheum* (rhubarb) of the buckwheat family includes about 70
species of stout, large-leaved perennial herbs native to temperate and
subtropical Asia and Europe. The generic name *Rheum* is derived from
Rha, an ancient Greek name for rhubarbs. The section *palmatum* of the
genus *Rheum* contains the medicinal species. In addition to *Rheum palmatum*,
R. officinale and *R. tanguticum* are used as source plants for the Chinese herb
root *da-huang*. *Da-huang* means "big yellow." Another traditional name
for the root means "army general." The herb is given the name because
it is fast acting—like an army general, its action is swift.

The roots of various rhubarb species have been used as strong laxatives
for at least 5000 years. There is still much worldwide interest in rhubarbs.
Under the direction of the symposium secretariat, Dr. Hu Shi-lin, the first
International Symposium on Rhubarb was held in the city of Cheng-de in
China, in May 1990. A total of 278 scientific papers were presented at the
symposium by participants from China, the United States, Japan, and
Italy. All aspects of rhubarbs were covered, including ethnobotany, pharmacology, clinical medicine, horticulture, biochemistry, and food use. In
the future, a second international rhubarb symposium will be held in Italy.

As further indication of international interest in the plant group, a
USDA researcher, Dale Marshall, has recently produced *A Bibliography on
Rhubarb and Rheum Species* (1988), containing 3,385 references.

The name *Rheum palmatum* is a Latin binomial created by Linnaeus in
1759. Through Chinese merchants, seeds of the plant were brought to
European botanical gardens around 1750. A specimen and seeds were

received by Linnaeus from de Gorter in 1758. Apparently the young plants perished. A live flowering specimen was eventually grown, which enabled the younger Linnaeus to describe the plant in a 1767 publication. Seed of the plant was introduced to British botanical gardens as early as 1762.

The scientific name *Rheum officinale* was established by the French natural historian Henri-Ernest Baillon (1827–1895) in an 1872 publication. Dabry de Thiersant introduced the plant to France. He obtained living plants in 1867, and sent them to France, where they were successfully cultivated.

Seeds of a medicinal rhubarb were collected by the Russian botanist N. M. Przewalski in 1872–73 when he visited the alpine regions of Gansu. This area produces high-quality *da-huang*. He sent seeds to Saint Petersburg where in 1875 Przewalski's contemporary Maximowicz published a paper on the plant. He named it *Rheum palmatum* var. *tanguticum* (*R. tanguticum*). Przewalski himself took great interest in medicinal rhubarb and wrote on the Chinese methods of production, gathering, and preparation.

While actual botanical or live specimens of the source plants of Chinese rhubarb were apparently unknown in the West until the eighteenth century, the use of the drug in Europe is ancient. It is known that Chinese rhubarb root produced in Shaanxi was imported via caravans from northern China as early as 114 B.C. The root drug is described by Dioscorides, as well as Pliny in the first century A.D. In 359 A.D., importation of rhubarb is mentioned by Ammianus Marcellinus, a Mesopotamian historian, and emissary to the Satrap of Corduene. Marco Polo, the thirteenth-century Venetian traveler-merchant, imported the drug to Europe. Chinese rhubarb is mentioned in a number of eleventh- and twelfth-century Arabian works, which note its superiority to rhubarb obtained via Turkey.

The designations Russia, Turkey, and India rhubarb as used in European commerce of previous centuries, arose from the trade route for rhubarb produced in China, rather than specific types of rhubarb. Chinese-produced rhubarb was variously imported through the Asian steppes via Turkey, over the Caspian Sea to Russia, and from India via the Persian Gulf and Red Sea to Egypt, Syria, and Asia Minor. Before 1842 it was also shipped from Canton, the only Chinese port trading with Europe before that date. In eighteenth-century Britain, material designated India rhubarb was Chinese rhubarb imported through Canton.

Prior to the mid-seventeenth century, most rhubarb arrived from the East via Turkistan. As early as the 1630s, however, Chinese rhubarb reached Russia through Mongolian merchants. In 1653, China opened her borders with Russia to trade. By 1657 Russia began to monopolize the trade of rhubarb root, and did so intermittently until 1731 when monopoly was asserted through the creation of the Kiakhta Rhubarb Commission, or "Rhubarb Office," on the Siberian-Mongolian border. Established by decree of the Russian minister of war, the Kiakhta Rhubarb Commission not only monopolized trade in the root, but took pains to assure high quality, so that material which came directly from Chinese ports was generally considered inferior to the Russian-supplied product.

From 1731 until 1782 the Russian state exercised its monopoly on the rhubarb trade through the Rhubarb Office. Up until the last caravan of 1755, which carried very little rhubarb, imperial Russian caravans brought the drug from the high Gobi, via Lake Baikal and Irkutsk, to Moscow, where supplies were shipped to Saint Petersburg for distribution to European points west. The Rhubarb Commission contracted for large, regularly scheduled shipments of rhubarb root. Occasionally they attempted to obtain seed as well. In 1782 the state monopoly was abolished, allowing private competitive trade, which resulted in the introduction of seed material to western Europe. However, the Kiakhta Rhubarb Commission continued to regulate selection and quality control over shipments, rejecting or burning adulterated or spoiled root. Russian overland trade in rhubarb continued until 1863, when the monopoly-controlling Rhubarb Office was closed. By this time, Chinese ports had "opened" to the West, and the drug was exported from a number of Chinese ports. The root was also cultivated, at least on a small commercial scale, in Germany, Austria, France, and England.

By the late 1780s the Russian monopoly on trade had already become a moot point, at least in the mind of the prominent English physician William Cullen, writing in his *Treatise on the Materia Medica*. Cultivation in Britain had begun.

> Much pains have been taken to ascertain the species of this genus that gives the root which the physicians of Britain have considered as the species of greatest value, and such as has been imported under the name of Turkey Rhubarb. Whether this may be exactly determined or not, I cannot clearly judge; and in the mean time, I do not think it necessary to prosecute the matter farther with any anxiety, as we have now got the seeds of a plant whose roots, cultivated in this county, show all

the properties of what is considered as the most genuine and valuable rhubarb; and which, properly cultivated and dried, will, I believe, in time supersede importation of any other.

(Cullen 1801, pp. 296–7)

Given the high price of the Chinese root imported via Russia and the low-quality adulterated material that came from Chinese ports of the day, cultivation of *Rheum palmatum* in Britain was vigorously pursued in the late eighteenth century. Seeds of *Rheum palmatum* was first introduced into Great Britain by Dr. Mounsey in the year 1762. They were also cultivated by Dr. John Hope and Sir Alexander Dick of Edinburgh in the following year. Plants were raised in the botanic garden at Cambridge from Mounsey's seeds. The seeds, obtained from Saint Petersburg, proved to be those of *R. palmatum*. The questions were then raised whether a drug equaling the quality of the Chinese-produced material could be achieved in Britain and, once successfully cultivated, whether skill in processing the drug for medicinal purposes could be developed.

By 1784, it was asserted that most of the apothecaries in Edinburgh held stock of Scottish-produced *Rheum palmatum*. In the last quarter of the eighteenth century the Society for the Encouragement of Arts, Manufacture, and Commerce devoted great effort to successfully promoting the cultivation of *Rheum palmatum* in England.

This success is detailed by Robert Thorton in his *Family Herbal*:

> Sir William Fordyce, so early as the year 1780, took up three roots, six years old. . . . He stripped off the bark from the smaller roots, and cut off most of it from the larger parts; and hung them up in festoons on a packthread, three or four inches from each other, at a moderate distance from the fire. From these roots he made one pound four ounce of rhubarb, as fit for the market as any imported from Russia, Turkey or China; he obtained likewise one pound more, fit for private use, or to be powdered. The roots should be cleared entirely of the rind, for the parts which are covered with it will be apt to turn mouldy. Large pieces should have a perforation made through the middle, that they may dry more perfectly, with less fuel and in less time. (Thorton 1812, p. 405)

The 1789 *Edinburgh Dispensatory* claimed that the drug cultivated in Britain was equal to any that was then imported. It is also noted that the

Chinese material was considered inferior not only to domestic material but to the Turkey and Russia rhubarbs as well. Unless kept very dry, the root was subject to becoming moldy and infested with worms. Some industrious merchants, if holding worm-eaten material would fill-up the worm holes with inert materials, and color the outside of the root with a powder made from high-quality rhubarb in order to hide the defects. Rhubarb buyers had to examine the root with great care before purchasing it.

In China, the root has been used since at least 2700 B.C., the time of the Five Rulers. *Da-huang* was first mentioned in the third class of drugs in *Shen Nong Ben Cao Jing*. Shen-Nong placed the herb among those having poisonous characteristics. It is also treated in Su Jing's *Xin Xiu Ben Cao*, also known as *Tang Ben Cao*, the world's first official pharmacopeia, published during the Tang dynasty in 659. The *Xin Xiu Ben Cao* notes that *da-huang* produced in Hebei province is smaller and of poor quality compared with the root which was at the time produced in Sichuan.

Da-huang is a very commonly used traditional Chinese drug. In Chinese tradition, species and varieties of *Rheum* with lobed leaves are considered to have the active anthroquinones in the roots that can cure diarrhea, without causing cramping. If the leaves of a rhubarb species are rounded, nearly entire, or only slightly wavy, the anthraquinone content is said to be low; this species would not be useful as *da-huang*. According to the tenets of traditional Chinese medicine, the direction of high-quality *da-huang* is vertical. Poor-quality *da-huang* has a horizontal function, and thus causes abdominal cramping.

TASTE AND CHARACTER

Bitter, cold.

FUNCTIONS

Purges fire, relaxes the bowels, relieves retention of or stagnation of undigested food, and expels blood stasis. Externally, poultices can disperse heat, expel toxic matter, and reduce swelling.

USES

Da-huang is used in prescriptions for constipation due to heat (not due to deficiency), delirium, accumulations of food in the stomach, abdominal pain, first stages of dysentery, headache, acute appendicitis, acute infectious hepatitis, conjunctivitis, swelling and pain of gums, sores of the mouth or tongue, toothache, vomiting of blood, nosebleed, suppressed menstruation, blood stasis after childbirth, mass in abdomen, jaundice, edema, and for urine that feels hot. Externally it is used in a poultice for burns, skin diseases with pus, carbuncles, swellings, sores, and traumatic injuries.

The strong laxative or purgative action of the roots is the result of the action of stimulant anthraquinones, including sennosides a–f, rhein, emodin, and aloe emodin. The anthrone glycosides stimulate peristalsis, and at the same time stimulate the bowel-reflex nerve of the colon. The quality of chemical components and ratios of various anthraquinones are very important to the pharmacological activity of the root. The root is considered both astringent and cathartic. The astringent action is due to tannins in the root.

Experimentally, the root has been shown to stimulate bile and pancreatic secretions, and is antibacterial, especially against staphylococcus and streptococcus bacteria. It is astringent, and in small doses stomachic. A number of *Rheum* species have been investigated for anticancer potential.

In addition to its widely accepted use as an astringent cathartic, the root has been used for numerous applications in Chinese folk medicine. For example, in folk tradition, after fried *da-huang* has been macerated in alcohol, a cotton ball is soaked in the tincture and applied for five minutes to an aching tooth. The ground, processed root, mixed with water, was once used as an externally applied treatment for herpes zoster (shingles). A gargle of the infused root has been used in Chinese folk medicine for treating inflammations of the oral cavity. The treatment was limited to two days' use.

Another traditional use was for the treatment of minor burns. A modern clinical report for the treatment of burns (*not* recommended) uses *da-huang* fried until it is black in color. The root was then powdered, mixed with sesame oil, and applied to first-degree burns. In the treatment of 415 cases, all patients were reported to have some improvement. The course of treatment was very short. No side effects were reported, and there was no scarring of tissue.

Another clinical report discussed the use of powdered *da-huang* in the treatment of six patients with intestinal gas. The powdered root, mixed with vinegar, was applied to a certain acupuncture point on the bottom of the foot. The poultice remained in place for two hours. After one hour, the patients reported abdominal movement. Gas was expelled by the end of the treatment.

While still a very important pharmaceutical laxative in Asia, in the West rhubarb has largely been replaced by other plant-derived and synthetic laxatives.

DOSE

Dose 3–12 g, in decoction, poultice or powder. The fresh root is very powerful. Processed, the function is rather neutral, not as strong, and slower-acting. The charcoaled root is used to stopping bleeding. *Da-huang* is not suitable for a long decoction. If used in a decoction, the root is decocted for a short period of time.

WARNING

Da-huang is a powerful plant drug that should only be administered under the care of a qualified medical practitioner. It is not a plant for general self-medication. The herb has a complex action and, in different dosage forms, produces different actions. Only a person knowledgable in the drug's action in various quantities, dosage forms, and combinations can be expected to reasonably predict the plant's action. Weak, pregnant, or postpartum patients should avoid this drug. Overdose can result especially from ingestion of the fresh root, causing nausea and vomiting, jaundice, vertigo, cramps, and other problems. Like most laxatives, long-term use should be avoided.

The large leaves of rhubarbs are well known to be highly toxic to humans because of the calcium oxalates and anthrone glycosides they contain. Over the centuries their ingestion has resulted in many deaths worldwide.

DESCRIPTION

Rheum palmatum is a stout perennial herb with large leaves, rounded in outline with a heart-shaped base and deeply palmate lobes. The lobes themselves may have further divisions. The small flowers bloom in a panicle, on a stout hollow stem up to 6 feet tall.

Rheum tanguticum (*R. palmatum* var. *tanguticum* Maxim. ex Regel.) has deeper sinuses between the leaf lobes.

Rheum officinale has rounded- to elliptical-shaped leaves measuring up to 3 feet across. They have 3 to 7 notched lobes. The whitish flowers are in a spreading panicle up to 10 feet tall.

The best quality *da-huang* is hard and firm, not porous; the fragrance is clean and the flavor bitter, with an astringent aftertaste.

DISTRIBUTION

Rheum palmatum is found in very high cold mountains, forest margins, and wet soils in grassy hills in Shaanxi, Gansu, Qinghai, Sichuan, Yunnan, Ningxia, and Xizang. Major wild-harvested supplies are from Qinghai, Gansu, Xizang, and Sichuan. It is cultivated in Hebei, Shanxi, and Nei Mongol. In recent years there have been supply shortages. Traditionally the root is wild-harvested, but such supplies have been nearly exhausted. In the past 20 years the plant has been cultivated more extensively. *Rheum tanguticum* (*R. palmatum* var. *tanguticum*) is found in shaded moist soils, on forest margins in mountains, and on grassy hills in Gansu, Qinghai, Sichuan, and Xizang. It is morphologically and chemically similar to *R. palmatum*. While sometimes considered a separate species, it is given varietal status in many modern works. It is mainly produced in Qinghai, Gansu, Xizang, and Sichuan.

Rheum officinale is found in moist and heavy but well-drained mountain soils in Hubei, Henan, Shaanxi, Guizhou, Sichuan, and Yunnan. It thrives in full sun. It is produced in Sichuan, Guizhou, Yunnan, Hubei, and Shaanxi. Production of this species is minimal. It is not often seen in Chinese markets, and is probably not exported.

CULTIVATION

Rheum palmatum likes cool climates, and full sun, and can bear very cold weather. The average yearly temperature should be about 50°F. Foster has had very little success "summering" the plants in Arkansas. They burn up, even if protected from hot sun and kept well watered. In China it is often cultivated in high mountain areas. The soil should be silty with some sand, deep, and calcareous. Seeds are used for propagation. In the South, it is better to plant the seeds in autumn. If they are planted in spring, the earlier, the better. A Chinese technique to sprout the seeds before planting consists of soaking the seeds in water at 65–68°F for six to eight hours. Strain off the water, and cover seeds with a wet cloth, turning the seeds once a day. Rinse once or twice daily. When 1 to 2 percent of the seeds begin to sprout, they are planted in rows spaced 3 feet apart, with individual hills spaced about 2 feet apart. Five to eight seeds are planted in each hole, at a depth of about ½ inch.

In preparation for planting, the soil is worked to a depth of 1 to 2 feet, with half-burned herbaceous material (scorched grass) added as a fertilizer. Night soil or well-rotted barnyard manure is thoroughly worked into the soil. After planting, seeds are covered with rice straw or other suitable mulch.

Another method for propagation is to divide an old plant with many root buds. Ashes are spread on the cut roots of the mother plant to prevent disease infestation and to prevent loss of moisture. This method is used to establish a planting more rapidly. Flowering stalks are pinched or cut back in summer and autumn, before buds form. This method is said to make the roots much stronger.

HARVESTING

Plants three or more years old are dug in September or October, after the leaves and stems have withered and yellowed. It is also harvested early in spring before new leaves appear. The roots are cleaned, lateral rootlets and the crown are removed, and the roots are graded according to different standards and sizes.

The rough outer cortex is removed. The roots are then cut into horizontal slices or cut into cubes. During processing, they are formed into cylindrical or egglike shapes. If the root is too large to dry easily, it is cut into several sections, strung on a wool line, and then hung to dry inside a well-ventilated building or under the eaves of a roof. The hole thus created in the root is a sign that the drug has come from an important production area.

The root is dried very slowly, in "cool" sun or over the heat of a "dark" fire (a fire with little red flame). If it is to be exported, it is put inside a bamboo basket or burlap sack filled with sharp rocks or broken glass or porcelain. Two people take hold of either end of the container and shake it back and forth until the lateral rootlets are worn away and the surface of the root becomes smooth.

Processing

Recently picked *da-huang* is prepared by sprinkling water on the root or soaking the roots in water for a short period to soften it. When the root becomes soft it is cut into slices or small cubes and dried in the sun.

Processed or "ripe" *da-huang* is made by sprinkling yellow wine on roots slices or cubes and mixing them together. The roots are placed in a loosely covered container and heated in a double-boiler until the root absorbs all the wine. The root is then dried. For every 100 pounds of root, 30 to 50 pounds of yellow wine is used. Traditionally this process was sometimes repeated two or three times before the root was dried. Another method that was used involves cutting the *da-huang* into small squares and placing it in a loosely covered jar. The jar is put in hot water, and steamed until the interior of the root loses its white color.

Alcohol *da-huang* is made by sprinkling yellow wine on the root slices, covering them with a wet cloth for a short time, frying them in a pan for a few minutes over a light fire, and drying them. For every 100 pounds of root slices, 14 pounds of yellow wine is called for.

Charcoaled *da-huang* is produced by stir-frying *da-huang* slices under a strong fire until the surface is blackish-brown, but still retains its character. A little water is sprinkled on the roots to cool them, and they are dried then in the sun.

Additional Species

In addition to the above species used as official drugs, various *Rheum* species are used locally in China as folk medicines, adulterants, or substitutes.

Rheum emodi Wall. is used as a substitute in the provinces of Sichuan, Yunnan, and Xizang (Tibet). In Xizang it is used as *da-huang*. This species is widely grown in India, producing what is called Himalayan or Indian rhubarb.

Rheum hotaoense C. Y. Cheng et. C. T. Kao is sometimes produced in Shaanxi, Gansu, and Qinghai for commercial markets. The leaf margin of this species is wavy or entire, rather than lobed, so it is not traditionally considered suitable for medicine. It may cause severe abdominal cramping, and is thought useful for animals, but not humans.

Rheum franzenbachii Munt. is found in Hebei province in Weichang and Anguo, the latter of which has for centuries been famous for a large herb market held there twice a year in spring and fall. While its exact source plant has not been determined, some speculate that *R. franzenbachii* is probably the source plant of Chinese edible rhubarb (Weichang rhubarb), the leaf stems of which are cooked in a special sauce and served as a famous local culinary specialty. Over 2 million pounds of the stem are produced each year. Local people refer to it as "native rhubarb." The leaf stalks have been found to be very high in carotene, thiamin, and riboflavin.

This species is also found in Shanxi and Nei Mongol. It is cultivated in Hebei and Shaanxi and harvested from the wild in Nei Mongol. Large amounts of it are reportedly produced primarily for export. The extract is thought to make the stomach strong. It is also known as mountain *da-huang*, or bitter *da-huang*. The root is not fragrant and the taste is bitter and astringent. As a drug-producing plant, traditionally the quality of the root is considered poor, and it may cause abdominal cramping. It is also used as a dye plant.

In the northwestern most province of Xinjiang, *Rheum wittrochii* Lundstr. is found on two famous mountains, Tian-Shan and A Er Tai Shan, where it is used as a folk substitute for *da-huang*. It is not considered very effective against diarrhea.

Many rhubarb species are used in various parts of China as folk medicines for dispersing toxic heat, as anti-inflammatory agents, or to stop bleeding and invigorate blood circulation.

OTHER USES

The stems and young seedlings of *Rheum*, first mentioned in the *Tang Ben Cao*, are considered sour (some authors say bitter), and without poison. They are traditionally used to sober up a drunk. The fresh stem clears away heat. Too much should not be used. The fresh stems will also relieve constipation. *Rheum x cultorum*, garden rhubarb, is commonly grown for its edible stalks in American and European gardens. Extracts of the plant are sometimes used commercially for flavoring beverages. Zucca rhubarb liquor has been produced in Italy for over 150 years. Old and new rhubarb liquors have been, and are produced in China in Chengde. Tanguticum wine is a rhubarb beverage available throughout China.

Schisandra
Wu-wei-zi

Botanical Names: *Schisandra chinensis* (Turcz.) Baill. and *Schisandra sphenanthera* Rehd. et Wils.

Botanical Synonyms: *Maximowiczia sinensis* Rupr., *Kadsura chinensis* Turcz.

Chinese Names: Pinyin: *Wu-wei-zi* (fruit), *Bei-wei-zi* (fruit of *S. chinensis*), *Nan-wu-wei-zi* (fruit of *S. sphenanthera*). Wade-Giles: *Wu-wei-tsu* (fruit), *Pei-wei-tzu* (fruit of *S. chinensis*), *Nan-wu-wei-tzu* (fruit of *S. sphenanthera*).

English Names: Schisandra, magnolia vine, Chinese magnolia vine, northern schisandra (*Schisandra chinensis*), southern schisandra (*Schisandra sphenanthera*).

Pharmaceutical Name: Fructus Schisandrae.

Family: Schisandraceae—magnolia vine family (sometimes placed in the Magnoliaceae—magnolia family).

HISTORY

It is a memorable pleasure to stroll through a garden in the United States or Europe and see a lush, fruiting trellis of Chinese schisandra, draped with clusters of the miniature red berries, as if they were bunches of grapes. Schisandra is a rare ornamental vine in Western gardens. The herb user is more likely to find the dried fruits, known as *wu-wei-zi*, in a Chinese herb shop or, increasingly, in Western-style herb products in natural or health food stores. The fruits have an unusual tart flavor. The Chinese name *wu-wei-zi*, meaning "five taste-fruits," derives from the fact that the fruits are sweet, sour, bitter, pungent (hot), and salty. The herb is considered "balanced" by virtue of this distribution of flavors.

The genus *Schisandra* of the magnolia vine family includes about 25 species, all of which are native to eastern Asia except for one species, *Schisandra coccinea*, which is a rare vine of the southeastern United States.

The genus *Schisandra* was first established by the French botanist André Michaux (1746–1802), who spent ten years of his life in North America. In 1803, his name *Schisandra coccinea* was published in reference to the single American species, which he first encountered in 1786. Also known as southern magnolia vine, smooth magnolia vine, bay star vine, or star vine, this rare plant occurs in undisturbed stream and creek bottoms, rich woods, and ravines in North Carolina, Tennessee, Georgia, Florida, Louisiana, and Arkansas. It is considered a threatened species, but sufficiently established in its range to keep it off the federal endangered species list. The name *Stellandria glabra* was published for the same plant in 1803 by John Brickell (1749–1801), an Irish botanist and physician who settled in Georgia in the 1770s. The two names were later combined by Alfred Rehder, becoming *Schisandra glabra* (Brickell) Rehder. The name *Schisandra coccinea* is the preferred name used in most modern botanical works, though *Schisandra glabra* is still seen. The names are synonymous.

In Western botany the Chinese source plant of *wu-wei-zi* (*Schisandra chinensis*) was first named *Kadsura chinensis* in an 1832 publication of the Russian botanist Nikolai S. Turczaninov, who died in 1864. In an 1856 publication, another Russian botanist Franz J. Ruprecht (1814–1870) created a new genus called *Maximowiczia*, to honor his colleague, Karl Johann Maximowicz (1827–1891), one of the most famous of all Russian botanists. Ruprecht called the plant *Maximowiczia chinensis*. In 1866 the French botanist, Henri Ernest Baillon (1827–1895) transferred the plant to the genus *Schisandra*. Since that time the plant has been known as *Schisandra chinensis* (Turcz.) Baill.

The generic name *Schisandra* (sometimes spelled *Schizandra*) is derived from the Greek *schizein*, meaning to "cleave," and *andros*, "man," referring to the cleft or separate anther cells on the stamens of *S. coccinea*.

This hardy deciduous, perennial vine was introduced to western botanical gardens in the late 1850s. It is occasionally grown for the ornamental effect of the bright green leaves and brilliant scarlet fruits the vine produces in autumn.

The fruit is a very commonly used herbal product in China. *Wu-wei-zi* is first mentioned in the primary class of herbs in *Shen Nong Ben Cao Jing*. In his 1596 classic, *Ben Cao Gang Mu*, Li Shi-zhen was the first to distinguish between species of *Schisandra* used in the north and south of China.

TASTE AND CHARACTER

Sour, warm.

FUNCTIONS

The fruits are considered to be astringent and nourishing; they promote the production of body fluid, stop diarrhea, stop coughs, allay sweating, and nourish the kidneys.

USES

The fruits are used in prescriptions for coughs due to lung deficiency, asthma, kidney ailments, chronic diarrhea, neurasthenia, nonjaundiced types of infectious hepatitis, for depleted body fluids that cause thirst, spontaneous perspiration, and night sweating.

Primary traditional uses of *wu-wei-zi* include the treatment of nervous conditions, coughs, and liver conditions. One traditional prescription for neurasthenia, for example, calls for 9 to 15 g of schisandra in decoction. A tincture made by macerating 30 g of schisandra in 300 g of 66 percent alcohol for seven days has also been used for neurasthenia in doses equivalent to one shot glass per day. For the treatment of coughs, pills are made combining 2 parts of poppy seeds with 1 part of *wu-wei-zi*. The pills are taken with water before the patient goes to bed. The fruits have been used in folk medicine as well as in TCM. A folk treatment for ulcerated skin sores uses *wu-wei-zi* that has been stir-fried until it is black; the powdered fruits are then applied as a poultice.

Recent laboratory and clinical studies by Chinese researchers have explored the experimental basis of the fruit's activity. Laboratory experiments and clinical experience suggests that *wu-wei-zi* may help to improve brain efficiency, increase work capacity, and build strength. It may have a calmative effect, work to sedate the central nervous system (in ether extract) or conversely have a stimulating effect on the central nervous system, and counteract the stimulatory effect of caffeine.

Schisandra is believed to have an adaptogenic function, increases non-resistant immune response, reduces tiredness and sleeplessness, and may help enhance vision. It has an obvious expectorant and antitussive effect.

Water or low-percentage alcohol extracts are used to help stabilize blood pressure. In China an injectable form of the roots of dwarf lily turf (*Ophiopogon japonicus*), ginseng (*Panax ginseng*), and *wu-wei-zi* is a famous treatment for shock. In laboratory experiments, schisandra extracts also have an ulcer-preventative effect, inhibit stomach acidity, are antibacterial, promote bile secretion, and stimulate rhythmic contraction of uterine smooth muscles.

Alcohol extracts have helped to regenerate liver tissue, and thus have been used clinically in China for infectious hepatitis. Chinese researchers have isolated a number of lignans from the fruits of *Schisandra*. At least 13 lignan compounds from five species of schisandra have shown the ability to lower elevated levels of serum glutamic pyruvic transaminase (SGPT), an indicator of hepatitis. The drug has been tested in over 5,000 cases of hepatitis patients with success rates from 84 to 97.9 percent in lowering SGPT levels. The lignans also act as a central nervous system depressant.

In treating nonjaundiced infectious hepatitis, the dried baked powder of the fruits is made into pills that are taken in specified doses for a period of one month. Clinically, in modern China, SGPT levels are monitored during the treatment. When levels return to normal, the treatment is continued for an additional 2 to 4 weeks. A clinical study of the treatment of nonjaundiced infectious hepatitis reported using baked, dried, powdered schisandra fruit in 3 g doses 3 times per day for 30 days. In 102 cases, the treatment was helpful in 85.3 percent of patients. More than 76 percent of patients were reported to have significant improvement. After some patients improved, the treatment was discontinued. If symptoms returned, the treatment was resumed at a larger dose.

In one clinical trial, a decoction of schisandra to which sugar was added was used for acute intestinal infections. In the treatment of 33 cases of acute bacillus dysentery, 29 patients improved; one patient died.

Given its long history of safe use, along with confirmation of traditional uses by modern research, *wu-wei-zi* should certainly be further studied for its potential applications in world health care. Schisandra fruits are becoming increasingly available in Western herb markets. Capsules, the powdered fruits, whole fruits, tinctures, and other products are seen in health and natural food stores in North America.

DOSE

Dose 1.5–15 g.

DESCRIPTION

Schisandra chinensis is a climbing perennial vine with alternate, deciduous leaves that are narrowly obovate to circular in outline and smooth above, about 2½ inches long and 1 to 1½ inches wide. The margins have 5 to 10 teeth along the edge, and the midrib beneath is impressed on the upper side of the leaf blade. The leaf stalks are up to half as long as the leaves themselves. The solitary nodding, cream-white flowers are in the lower axils of young shoots. Male and female flowers are produced on separate plants. Plants of both sexes must be present to produce fruits. The berry-like, roundish, smooth scarlet fruits are in drooping clusters. The seed within is kidney-shaped. Fruits appear from September to November. The best quality dried fruit has a bright red color, is large (¼ to ⅜ inches wide), plump, quite oily, with a shiny surface.

DISTRIBUTION

Schisandra chinensis grows in mixed forests under shade in the mountains of Heilongjiang, Jilin, Liaoning, Hebei, Shanxi, Nei Mongol, Shaanxi, Shandong, Jiangxi, Hubei, Sichuan, and Yunnan. It also occurs in the mountains of Hokkaido and Honshu in Japan, as well as in Korea, Sakhalin, and adjacent regions of Russia. It is grown as a horticultural specimen in the United States and Europe. *Schisandra chinensis* is mainly produced in Liaoning, Heilongjiang, and Jilin, as well as in Hebei and Nei Mongol. It is sold throughout China and exported as well.

Schisandra sphenanthera, which produces *nan-wei-zi* (southern *wei-zi*), occurs in fields, shrub thickets, and along roadsides, streams, and banks of rivers in Henan, Jiangsu, Zhejiang, Jiangxi, Hubei, Shaanxi, Gansu, Sichuan, Yunnan and Guizhou. It is primarily produced in Henan, Shaanxi, and Gansu, as well as Yunnan and Sichuan, and is sold throughout China but not exported.

CULTIVATION

Schisandra chinensis likes moist rich, shady conditions and can bear very cold temperatures. The soil should be rich, loose, somewhat sandy, deeply cultivated, and well drained. Schisandra is propagated by cuttings, layering, or seeds.

March, before the leaf buds unfurl, is considered the best time to take cuttings. Cuttings can also be made in July and August. Strong healthy branches are selected and cut into 4 to 5 inch lengths. Cuttings, spaced at 5 inches, are placed obliquely in beds. The cuttings are kept moist until roots develop in 2 to 3 weeks.

In spring before the buds open, the plant can also be propagated by layering. The layer is cut from the parent plant in autumn after it has rooted and is transplanted to a permanent location.

If seeds are used for propagation, they are planted either in the fall soon after ripening or in the following spring. If seeds are sown at the end of March or early April, they are soaked in water overnight before planting. Since the seeds have a hard coat, in China acid scarification is sometimes used as a pregermination treatment. Rows of seedbeds are spaced at about two feet, and seeds are covered with about ¼ inch of soil. Young seedlings are supplied with plenty of moisture and shade. In China, seed beds are covered with a rice-straw mulch until the seedlings are transplanted to permanent locations. When seedlings are 6 to 8 inches high, they are transplanted to permanent locations.

HARVESTING

After frost in late October or early November, the fruits are harvested, stems and foreign matter are removed, and the fruits are then dried in the sun. Adequate ventilation is provided to prevent mildew or spoilage.

PROCESSING

To make yellow wine schisandra the cleaned fruits are evenly mixed with yellow wine. They are placed in a covered double boiler and "steamed" until the fruits absorb all of the wine. The fruits are then dried under well-ventilated conditions or in the sun. Twenty pounds of wine are used for each 100 pounds of fruit.

Steamed schisandra is made by steaming the fruits in a double boiler until the middle part of the seeds is no longer white, and dried in the sun.

ADDITIONAL SPECIES

Besides the two species above, eleven additional species of schisandra are used as substitutes in China, including *S. rubriflora* Rehd et Wils.; *S. neglecta* A. C. Smith; *S. lancifolia* (Rehd. et Wils.) A. C. Smith; *S. henryi* Clark; *S. propinqua* (Wall.) Baill. var. *sinensis* Oliv.; *S. pubescens* Hemls. et Wils.; *S. viridis* A. C. Smith; *S. spherandra* Stapf.; *S. glaucescens* Diels; *S. bicolor* Cheng; and *S. micrantha* A. C. Smith.

The American *S. coccinea* (*S. glabra*), known as smooth magnolia vine or bay star vine, is a rare climbing understory vine that grows in deep woods in bottomlands, creek bluffs, rich draws, or river banks with rich sandy silt-loam. It was formerly under review for possible endangered species status but was determined abundant enough not to be in immediate danger of becoming extinct.

Many authors have discussed the need to protect endangered plants as a possible source of new drugs. Since the fruits of most species of schisandra are aromatic, and since at least half of the Chinese species are used in medicine either locally, regionally, or as an export, intensive research on the chemistry and pharmacology of the single American species could reveal interesting data.

OTHER USES

According to the German botanical worker Philipp Franz von Siebold (1796–1866), a Western pioneer of Japanese botany, the fruits and branches, abundant in viscid mucoid material, were used by Japanese women to dress their hair. It is also said to have been used as a sizing for making paper from *Broussonetia papyrifera* (the paper mulberry).

The fruits of various *Schisandra* species have been eaten for their pleasant sweet-and-sour aromatic flavor.

TWO

Garden Flowers

Balloonflower
Jie-geng

Botanical Names: *Platycodon grandiflorum* (Jacq.) A. DC.
Botanical Synonyms: *Campanula grandiflora* Jacq., *C. glauca* Thunb., *C. gentianoides* Lam., *P. grandiflorum* var. *glaucum* (Thunb.) Sieb. et Zucc., *P. chinense* Lindl. et Paxt., *P. glaucum* (Thunb.) Nakai
Chinese Names: Pinyin: *Jie-geng* (root); Wade-Giles: *Chieh-keng* (root).
English Names: Balloonflower, Chinese bellflower, Japanese bellflower, platycodon.
Pharmaceutical Name: Radix Platycodi.
Family: Campanulaceae—bellflower family.

HISTORY

Of the hundreds of garden flowers introduced to Western gardens from Asia, few plants are as attractive as the balloonflower—or as underappreciated for their ornamental, food, and medicinal potential. The balloonflower is unique.

The genus *Platycodon* of the bellflower family is monotypic—that is, it includes only one species. The balloonflower's scientific name, *Platycodon grandiflorum*, was published by the Swiss botanist Alphonse Louis Pierre Pyramus de Candolle (1806–1893), son of Augustin Pyramus de Candolle, both important figures in nineteenth-century botany. The younger de Candolle published the scientific name in an 1830 monograph on the Campanulaceae (bellflower family). The plant had previously been placed in the genus *Campanula* in a 1776 publication by N. J. von Jacquin (1727–1817), a Viennese botanist. Heinrich Adolph Schrader (1767–1836) had also placed it in the genus *Wahlenbergia*.

Although the plant had been observed by Europeans in East Asia as early as 1696, the first knowledge English botanists had of the plant was dried specimens collected by the Rev. G. H. Vatchell near Macao in December 1829. Robert Fortune (1812–1880), a Scottish botanist, opened a new era of Western botanical exploration of China in 1843. During the following eighteen years he made four trips to China and Japan (in 1843–45, 1848–51, 1853–56, and 1861), traveling to remote areas of Fujian,

Anhui, and Zhejiang—regions not previously seen by Europeans. Prior to Fortune's collections, most European botanical collections from China came from Beijing and coastal port cities. Fortune published several books on his Chinese ventures. In the beginning of 1844, Fortune sent roots of the plant to the Horticultural Society at Chiswick, introducing the first live balloonflower plants to England. He collected a semidouble white-flowered variety, which was described by the eminent English botanist John Lindley (1799–1865) in 1846. In an 1853 publication, Lindley called the balloonflower (under the name *P. chinensis*) the finest herbaceous specimen that Fortune had sent from China. The plant is a popular ornamental in American gardens, although it is little known as a medicinal and food plant.

The name *Platycodon* is derived from the Greek *platys* meaning broad, and *kodon*, a bell, referring to the shape of the flower. The species name "grandiflorum" of course, refers to the large, grand flowers.

The plant was well known in Chinese and Japanese gardens long before Europeans arrived on their shores, and double-flowered and white forms had already been selected for cultivation. It is an ancient drug plant, listed in the third class of *Shen Nong Ben Cao Jing*.

TASTE AND CHARACTER

Bitter, hot, neutral.

FUNCTIONS

Opens inhibited lung energy, eliminates phlegm, promotes the throat, and drains pus.

USES

Balloonflower root is used in prescriptions for cough, excessive phlegm, feeling of oppression in the chest, sore throats, hoarseness, lung abscesses, vomiting with pus, coughs due to a cold, difficulty in expectorating phlegm, pleurisy, tonsillitis, dysentery, abdominal pain, and for stopping bleeding and skin diseases.

Balloonflower root is primarily associated with use in lung- or throat-related ailments. The root is sometimes combined with licorice roots and then decocted to treat cough and throat ailments. Twice as much licorice root is used by weight than balloonflower root. In Indochina the root is chewed along with licorice as a sedative for coughs and throat ailments. For gum ulcers with foul-smelling breath, equal amounts of *jie-geng* and fennel seeds were traditionally stir-fried so that the outer part is charcoaled, but still retains its character. The herbs were then ground, and the powder poulticed on the affected area.

Recent pharmacological studies confirm the root's expectorant, antitussive, and antibacterial effects. Studies show *jie-geng* inhibits gastric secretions. Additional studies have shown that the crude root works as a mild tranquilizer, analgesic, antipyretic, anti-inflammatory agent, and vasodilator, and reduces high blood pressure and blood sugar. In animal studies, preparations have had a beneficial effect on cholesterol metabolism, while they decrease liver cholesterol levels. The root contains a saponin. When hydrolized it splits into two sapogenins, polygalacic acid and playcodigenin.

Clinical studies have involved cases of lung abscesses, pharyngitis, carbuncles, furuncles, and the promotion of gastric function in postpartum patients, with generally positive results.

In Western terms, balloonflower root is considered astringent, carminative, expectorant, slightly sedative, tonic, and antiasthmatic. It has also been used as a folk cancer remedy; extracts of the roots have proven to have antitumor activity in animal experiments. Several Japanese patent medicines employ root extracts for the treatment of bronchitis. In the United States, the plant is primarily grown as a garden ornamental; however, the roots are available from sources of Chinese herbs. The packaged dried roots are also commonly available at Asian groceries in the United States.

DOSE

3–9 g in decoction or powder.

DESCRIPTION

Balloonflower is a tap-rooted, branched perennial growing 15 to 40 inches tall. The alternate leaves are narrowly to broadly ovate, 1½ to 3 inches long and ½ to 1½ inch wide, with an acute apex; they are smoothish beneath, and without petioles (leaf stalks). Lower leaves are sometimes opposite. The rich violet-blue flowers are shaped like a balloon before expansion, from whence the common English name, balloonflower. The bell-shaped, mostly terminal, showy flowers are 1½ to 2 inches across, five-lobed, usually blue or violet-blue, and sometimes white. It flowers from June through September. Fruits are five-lobed, obovate, papery capsules. Seeds are oblong, flat, and about 2 mm long.

DISTRIBUTION

In the wild, balloonflower occurs on grassy slopes on hills and mountains, ditches, and fields in much of Japan, Korea, north and northeast China, and adjacent Russia. Originally, all of the drug material was wild-harvested, but in the past twenty years the drug has been commercially cultivated in China, improving both quantities available and the general quality of the herb. Most parts of China have commercial production of this plant, especially Heilongjiang, Jilin, Liaoning, Hebei, Shanxi, Nei Mongol, Anhui, Jiangsu, Jiangxi, Zhejiang, and Fujian. The best-quality root comes from the eastern coastal provinces. The finest-quality root is strong, large, rich in color, white, with very few cracks in cross section, and has a bitter taste.

CULTIVATION

The plant has been popular in American and European flower gardens for over a hundred years. It is easy to grow, adaptable to various growing conditions, and hardy. Numerous cultivars (cultivated varieties) are available in American horticulture. The plant likes cool, moist surroundings. Deep, well-tilled beds should be prepared the previous fall or winter before planting. A sandy, well-drained loam, high in organic matter, is suitable. Propagate by seeds. Plant seeds directly in late April (or after the last frost), at rows spaced 1 foot apart. Scatter seeds evenly, covering with about ½ inch of soil, and then water. Seedlings emerge in 15 to 20 days. When they are about three inches high, thin plants to 6 to 12 inch spacings. The root crown can also be used for propagation. In March or April, dig up the root, cut off the crown in sections about 2 inches long, and place them in holes about 3 inches deep that are 18 inches apart. Cover with earth and then water. In June or July, before the flowers bloom, the Chinese side-dress plantings with night soil. An additional side-dressing with compost or manure can be made later in the season. Keep weeded and well cultivated.

HARVESTING

In spring or autumn, after 2 to 3 years' growth, the root can be collected. Autumn-harvested roots are considered to be of somewhat better quality. Very dense, full, heavy roots with few cracks are best and store well.

PROCESSING

The traditional processing method is to use broken pieces of porcelain or a bamboo knife (not a metal knife) to remove the rough outer bark and then dry the root in the sun. Recently some Chinese production regions have been retaining the cortex (outer bark), cleaning the root, cutting it into slices, and then drying it. This change from traditional methods saves hand work and labor, but the form of the drug is not as attractive as the traditionally processed root. If harvested during a rainy season, the roots are baked dry rather than dried in the sun. Another method is to cover the half-dried roots with wet cloth overnight, slice them, and dry the slices in the sun. The peeled roots, roots derived from wild plants, and those with violet flowers are traditionally considered to be stronger in action. However, recent research suggests that the peeled and unpeeled root are similar in their expectorant effect and content of active constituents.

OTHER USES

In Japan and Korea, balloonflower is cultivated as a food plant for its edible roots. The blanched young leaves are eaten as a salad in mountainous regions of Japan. Dried, packaged balloonflower roots for making soup are widely available in Asian groceries in the United States. They are primarily used in Korean cuisine. The roots, with the bark removed, are also pickled or preserved in sugar. It is asserted that the reason that the root is eaten by Koreans as a tonic and energizing food is because of the resemblance of the dried root to that of ginseng.

Balloonflower is also grown in Asia for cut flowers.

The rhizome (upper portion of the root that meets the stem) of *jie-geng* is a folk remedy to treat the "upper abdomen with wind heat and phlegm." It is ground into powder and taken with hot water in a dose of 3 g. Forced vomiting is employed with the treatment to expel phlegm.

Blackberry Lily
She-gan

Botanical Name: *Belamcanda chinensis* (L.) DC.
Botanical Synonyms: *Ixia chinensis* L., *B. punctata* Moench.,
Gemmingia chinensis (L.) O. Kuntze, *Pardanthus chinensis* Ker-
Gawl., *Moraea chinensis* Thunb.
Chinese Names: Pinyin: *She-gan* (rhizome); Wade-Giles: *She-kan*
(rhizome).
English Names: Blackberry lily, leopard flower.
Pharmaceutical Name: Rhizoma Belamcandae.
Family: Iridaceae—iris family.

HISTORY

Blackberry lily occurs sporadically in roadside ditches in the southern
United States. It is listed in many wildflower books, and most people are
surprised to learn that it is not a native wildflower, but a garden introduction that has escaped cultivation, establishing itself in suitable habitats.
Though commonly referred to as "blackberry lily," *Belamcanda* is not a lily,
but a member of the iris family. The genus includes two species from East
Asia.

Seeds of the plant were collected by Jesuit missionaries in China and
sent to Europe by the 1730s. Linnaeus identified the plant as *Ixia chinensis*.
It was cultivated in the botanical garden in Uppsala by 1748, and in
English gardens by at least 1759. Various botanists have placed the plant
in at least five different genera. The genus name *Belamcanda* was first
published in 1763. In 1802 the Swiss botanist Augustin Pyramus de Candolle
(1778–1841) named the plant *Belamcanda chinensis*, the name used in virtually all modern works. The plant was known in American gardens as
early as 1825. It had become widely naturalized in the eastern United
States by the late nineteenth century. The name *Belamcanda* derives from
an East Indian name for the plant. The specific epithet *chinensis*, of course,
means of China.

She-gan is listed in the third class of drugs in the ancient *Shen Nong Ben
Cao Jing*, one of the oldest Chinese *materia medica*. Shen Nong mentions
she-gan in the treatment of laryngeal tumors. The root is listed as an official
drug in the 1985 Chinese *Pharmacopeia*.

Taste and Character

Bitter, cold, poisonous.

Functions

Clears away heat and toxic materials, stimulates the pharynx to expel phlegm, and reduces swelling by "promoting blood."

Uses

She-gan is used in prescriptions for swelling and pain in the throat, coughs with asthma, wheezing, chronic bronchitis, mumps, coughs with excessive phlegm, irregular menstrual cycle, and swollen breasts. Externally, it is poulticed for traumatic injuries such as a twisted or sprained ankle and for dermatitis caused by working in rice fields; historically it is also used for boils, contusions, rheumatism, and goiters.

Pharmacological studies have shown that ethanol extracts of *she-gan* lower the blood pressure of rabbits yet increase the strength and frequency of their pulse. Extracts also have an experimental antifungal, antibacterial, and antiviral effect. A wash made from the roots has traditionally been used for dermatitis resulting from overwork in rice fields. The root is decocted in water for an hour, and salt is added to it. Once it cools to room temperature, it is applied as a wash.

In Western terms, *she-gan* is considered antipyretic, detoxicant, expectorant, deobstruent, carminative, diuretic, and resolvant. It is also used for tonsillitis, laryngitis, stomachache, swollen liver and spleen, and dysuria. The root is a traditional folk cancer remedy for breast cancers, and is reportedly purgative. It was once used as an antidote for arrow poisons. The root is rarely sold in American herb markets outside of Chinatowns in major cities.

Contraindications and Warning

Use is contraindicated during pregnancy. *She-gan* contains potentially toxic iridoid components, such as belamcandin and iridin. Other components include flavonoids like tectoridin and tectorigenin. Most members of the iris family, including *Belamcanda*, are considered potentially poisonous. The root should be used only under medical supervision.

DOSE

2.5–9 g decocted, or in powder for a poultice. A paste for a poultice is made by mixing the powdered root with water.

DESCRIPTION

Blackberry lily is a short-lived perennial herb growing 1 to 2 feet tall. The sword-shaped leaves are two-ranked on the stems, producing a fan-shaped arrangement. The showy flowers grow in loose terminal branching cymes, arising from the base of the plant. The plant flowers for several weeks at a time from June to July. Each flower, 1 1/2 to 2 inches across, has six petaloid (false petal) segments, or "tepals," and is bright orange or yellow-ish in color, mottled with reddish or purplish spots. The fruits consist of capsules that open to reveal tight clusters of fleshy, shiny black seeds. These black seed clusters have the appearance of blackberries, hence the common name blackberry lily.

DISTRIBUTION

The plant occurs in most of China, Japan, Indonesia, northern India, eastern Russia in the Ussuri region, and other parts of East Asia. It is thought to be native to North China, but is now widely naturalized throughout the country. It grows in dry grasslands, open slopes, sandy meadows near the sea, and near small streams in mountain valleys, often in partially shaded areas, from sea level to 6,000 feet. Blackberry lily is sometimes cultivated as an ornamental in China. Major production provinces include Henan, Hubei, Jiangsu, and Anhui. Henan province is the largest producer of *she-gan*. The best quality comes from Hubei province.

It is naturalized in much of the eastern and southern United States along roadsides, thickets and open woods, and is commonly grown in flower gardens in America and Europe.

CULTIVATION

The plant is not particular about soils and is very easy to grow. It prefers a relatively poor dry soil, but it will become most luxuriant in a well-drained soil with a fair content of organic matter. Propagation is achieved by dividing the rhizome in March or April. Once dug up, each root can be divided into 3 to 5 sections, with 1 or 2 buds or eyes each. The ends of the cut sections are dried before planting to avoid fungal infections. The rhizome divisions are planted 3 to 4 inches deep, with plants spaced at about 8 to 12 inches. Tamp the soil after planting, and then water. Plants emerge in about 10 days. Blackberry lily is also easily grown from seed. In China the flowering stems are pinched back in July or August to prevent flowering, returning more energy to the root.

HARVESTING

The root is harvested in May through September, but usually in autumn; it is washed, and then dried. Stems and leaves are removed before drying. Roots are placed in the sun until half dry, after which they are placed between two screens and heated over a small fire, and are turned often until the root hairs and lateral rootlets have burned off.

PROCESSING

If the root is to be cut into slices, the roots are soaked in water for a short time, covered with a wet cloth, and cut into pieces. After slicing, the roots are dried in the sun.

ADDITIONAL SPECIES

Iris tectorus has similar components to *Belamcanda chinensis* and has been used as a widespread substitute to *she-gan* in China. It has been investigated as a possible bona fide substitute, due to shortages of *Belamcanda*.

Belamcanda flabellata, another Asian species, is sometimes grown in flower gardens. It has yellow flowers that are without spots or only faintly spotted.

OTHER USES

Belamcanda root has itself been used as a substitute for *Polygonum aviculare* in China. In Guangdong and Guangxi, the stem and leaves of *Belamcanda* have been used as a substitute for the root.

After the branches are cut, the shiny black seeds do not drop for a long time after the pods have opened. Therefore, the dried fruiting branches are useful for dried arrangements and bouquets.

Bletilla
Bai-ji

Botanical Name: *Bletilla striata* (Thunb.) Reichenb. f.
Botanical Synonyms: *Limodorum striatum* Thunb., *Epidendrum tuberosum* Lour., *Cymbidium hyacanthinum* J. E. Smith, *Bletia hyacinthina* (J. E. Smith) R. Br.
Chinese Names: Pinyin: *Bai-ji* (tubers). Wade-Giles: *Pai-chi* (tubers).
English Names: Bletilla, hardy orchid.
Pharmaceutical Name: Rhizoma Bletillae.
Family: Orchidaceae—orchid family.

HISTORY

Orchid enthusiasts know bletilla as one of the few hardy terrestrial orchids that can be grown by a novice with no previous experience in orchid culture. What is more, it is hardy and can be grown outside in many parts of the United States, if given a mulch to protect it during the winter or planted in a sheltered situation. Bletilla can also be grown as a house plant and can be forced to bloom in the winter months to add floral color to an otherwise drab season. It is one of the easiest and most rewarding orchids anyone can grow, novice or expert. Few orchid enthusiasts, however, are aware of the fact that this hardy orchid is also the source plant of a traditional Chinese herbal medicine, *bai-ji*.

The genus *Bletilla* of the orchid family contains about nine species native to China, Taiwan, Japan, and adjacent Pacific islands. The first Westerner to name the plant was the Swedish botanist Carl Peter Thunberg, (1743–1822) an early European explorer of the flora of Japan and author of *Flora Japonica* (1784). He published an early western description of the plant in this book. In an 1878 publication, Heinrich Gottlieb Reichenbach, the son of a famous German botanist of the same name, transferred the plant to the genus *Bletilla*, which he had created in an 1853 publication. The generic name *Bletilla* is the diminutive of *Bletia*, another genus in the orchid family named after Blet, a Spanish botanist. *Bletilla* had once been placed in the genus *Bletia* creating some confusion on the taxonomy of the plant. *Striata* refers to the white striations in the leaves.

The Chinese name *bai-ji*, meaning "spreading the white color," refers to the notion that the white striations of the leaves spread from the white-colored root. According to S. Y. Hu (1977), however, the Chinese name, transliterated as *Bo-ji* (*Po-chi*), means "white chicken," using the sound of a vernacular name for the orchid from Sichuan and Guizhou. She notes that cultivated forms of this orchid in western and central China have a fleshy tuber that resembles a small white chicken. A Chinese name *Bo-ji-er* (*Po-chi-êrh*) is used as a local vernacular name for the plant.

The plant was introduced to English gardens by Thomas Evans around 1802, where the species proved hardy, unlike most subtropical orchids. It has been grown in American gardens for at least 100 years.

Bai-ji is listed in the third class of drugs in *Shen Nong Ben Cao Jing*. The source plant has been used since ancient times without confusion of identity. *Bai-ji* is an official entry in the 1985 Chinese *Pharmacopeia*.

TASTE AND CHARACTER

Bitter, astringent, a little cool, somewhat sweet (bitter at first, then becoming a little sweet upon prolonged chewing).

FUNCTIONS

Reduces swelling, promotes new tissue (promoting granulation), and stops bleeding.

USES

Bletilla is used in prescriptions for chronic cough due to lung deficiency, including tuberculosis and inflammation of the trachea associated with bronchitis; it is also used for expectoration of blood from the lungs, vomiting of blood (caused by ulcers), bloody urine, rectal bleeding, nosebleed, and traumatic bleeding. Externally the root is poulticed to treat carbuncles, swellings, external ulcers, and chapped hands and feet. It has also been used for the treatment of burns, scalds, and chilblains.

Traditionally, the root has primarily been used for lung related afflictions, as well as a hemostatic to arrest bleeding. A prescription for stomach and intestinal bleeding, for example, calls for 6 g of the powdered root taken three times per day to stop the bleeding. If blood is being expectorated from the lungs (hemoptysis) or if there is bleeding from the rectum, another prescription combines 1 part of dried *Bletilla* root, 1 of *Sanguisorba officinalis* (salad burnet) and 5 parts of *Agrimonia pilosa* (agrimony). The latter two herbs are also used to stop bleeding in western herbal traditions. The powder of the three herbs is combined and then made into a paste, which is shaped into tablets to be taken to treat the conditions.

A clinical study in the Chinese literature reports on the use of these tablets for the treatment of silicosis (a lung disease resulting from inhaling quartz dust). Five of the tablets were taken three times a day. In 44 cases that were treated from 3 to 12 weeks, symptoms were reduced in most of the patients, and the functional energy of the lungs was reported to be somewhat improved.

Animal experiments have confirmed that the root has the ability to stop bleeding. The root also has experimental antibacterial activity against gram-positive bacteria and *Mycobacterium tuberculosis*.

Additional Chinese clinical and pharmacological reports have focused on the use of *bai-ji* for bleeding ulcers, gastric and duodenal ulcers, and for the treatment of pulmonary tuberculosis.

In Western terms, the root is considered bechic (cough relieving), astringent, expectorant, and demulcent (due to its mucilage content). Early Western observers noted the use of the root for dyspepsia, dysentery, and fevers; it was used externally for malignant ulcerations. The root is seldom seen on the American herb market outside of Chinatown herb shops in major cities.

CONTRAINDICATIONS

Bletilla is not used with aconite root preparations or in chronic lung diseases. Large or frequent doses are potentially toxic. The root should be used only under the supervision of a TCM practitioner.

DOSE

3–9 (16) g of the dried root; 5–10 g of the dried powdered root in decoction. In a poultice, fresh or dried as required.

DESCRIPTION

Bletilla is a terrestrial perennial orchid growing to about two feet tall in clumps up to 12 inches across. The base of the stem enlarges into a distinct semiround, compressed corm (pseudobulb). Three to five pleated leaves surround the stem with folded sheaths. They are oblong lance shaped, with a sharp pointed tip. The terminal flower stalks yield 6 to 12 beautiful violet-purple to rose-pink blooms. The flowers are about an inch across. It blooms from April to June, depending upon climate. A rare white-flowered form is available from some orchid sellers.

DISTRIBUTION

This orchid grows in fields, thin forests, and mountain valleys, in moist situations in Hebei, Henan, Shanxi, Shaanxi, Gansu, Shandong, Jiangsu, Anhui, Zhejiang, Jiangxi, Fujian, Hubei, Hunan, Guangdong, Guangxi, Sichuan, Guizhou, and Yunnan provinces. In short, it occurs throughout the southern and eastern two thirds of China. Guizhou province is the major commercial producer of the root and produces the best quality. Bletilla is also recorded in Japan, Hong Kong, and other Pacific islands, where it is also valued as an ornamental. It is grown as a showy hardy orchid, both in gardens and as a houseplant, in Europe and the United States.

CULTIVATION

Bletilla is once of the easiest orchids to grow. The plant likes a warm situation with about 50 percent shade and moist, rich, well-drained, sandy soil, high in organic matter. In mountainous areas of China it is grown on north-facing slopes. The tubers are divided to propagate the plant. In north China, the roots are divided in April or May. In south China, plants are divided in February. The tubers can be sliced to divide them. Each section should have a bud or "eye" to further increase the planting. Plants are spaced at about 8 inches in rows about a foot apart. The tubers are planted about 2 to 3 inches deep. Water every 3 to 4 days to keep the plants moist. When the young plants are about two inches high they are side-dressed with compost or well-rotted manure. A second side-dressing is applied later in the season. In northern areas, plants are mulched with straw during the winter to prevent winter kill.

S. Foster has grown the plant outdoors in Arkansas, where without mulch, they survived temperature of –12° F. Keep one plant in a pot, bring it indoors in the late fall, forcing the plant in late November or early December. You will then enjoy flowering bletillas to brighten Christmas and the New Year.

HARVESTING

In some areas of China, first-year roots are chosen for harvesting. In other regions, roots are not harvested until after plants are three years old. The roots are harvested in early winter. Stems and lateral rootlets are removed, and young lateral tubers are divided off for replanting. The white-colored roots must be processed at once or else they oxidize and turn an undesirable black color. Before processing, the roots are sorted according to size.

PROCESSING

Soon after harvesting, the roots are blanched in boiling water for 3 to 5 minutes or steamed until the interior of the root becomes greenish-white or yellowish white, without whitish coloration. The roots are then dried in the sun until about half dry. At this point the outer covering (cortex) of the root is removed, either by "pushing" the interior of the root out of the cortex or by putting the roots in burlap sacks along with sharp stones and broken shards of glass. The ends of the sack are tied together to make handles, and two people take hold of the ends and shake the bag back and forth, allowing the broken glass and stones to wear off the cortex. Once the cortex is removed, the root is dried under sun until it is 100 percent dry. Metal tools should not be used to process the root.

ADDITIONAL SPECIES

Bletilla yunnanensis Schultr. and *B. ochracea* Schultr. ("little *bai-ji*") are used as substitutes in Yunnan and Sichuan. *Bletilla ochracea* has white or light yellow flowers and is found in mountains, fields, and thin forests in Shaanxi, Gansu, Sichuan, and Yunnan.

OTHER USES

The dried juice of the stem has been used as a binder for making tablets. In Guizhou, the plant is cultivated for the stem gum. At one point in history, Chinese alchemists attempted to make artificial blood from the stem juice. The root is reportedly insecticidal.

Cockscomb
Ji-guan-hua and *Qing-xiang-zi*

Botanical Names: *Celosia cristata* L. (*C. argentea* var. *cristata* (L.). Kuntze) and *Celosia argentea* L.
Chinese Names: Pinyin: *Ji-guan-hua* (flowers of *C. cristata*); *Qing-xiang-zi* (seeds of *C. argentea*). Wade-Giles: *Chi-kuan-hua* (flowers of *C. cristata*); *Ch'ing-hsiang-tsu* (seeds of *C. argentea*).
English Names: Cockscomb is the best-known name for *Celosia cristata*. The genus name *Celosia* is also used as a common name for *C. argentea* and *C. cristata*. Woolflower is applied to all species of the genus.
Pharmaceutical Names: Flos Celosiae Cristatae; Semen Celosiae.
Family: Amaranthaceae—amaranth family.

HISTORY

The flaming red, orange, or yellow broad-triangular flowerheads of cockscomb (*C. cristata*) are a familiar sight in gardens throughout the world. Increasingly they are being planted to add colorful array to back borders of American herb gardens. However, its herbal use is buried in obscurity in the West. The cockscombs are a plant group that has been used for parallel purposes by Asian, American, and European cultures for many centuries.

The genus *Celosia* has about fifty species native to warm temperate climates of Asia, the Americas, and Africa. *Celosia argentea* is now a widespread tropical weed. *Celosia cristata* is not known from the wild but is a cultigen (a form that has evolved under cultivation), best known as an ornamental for its white, yellow, purple, violet, red, or crimson broadplumed flower heads. Numerous cultivars (cultivated varieties) are available.

Celosia cristata was known in European gardens as early as 1570. A number of seventeenth- and eighteenth-century botanical explorers from Europe observed the plant in the gardens of Japan, China, and India. European colonists brought the plant to North American gardens at a relatively early date; *Celosia argentea* was known in American gardens by 1737.

The name *Celosia* derives from the Greek *kelos*, meaning burnt, referring to the burnt appearance of the flowers of several species. Both species were named by Linnaeus in *Species Plantarum* (1753).

The plant is briefly described with other amaranth family members in both the 1597 and 1633 editions of Gerard's *Herball*. A "gentle binding faculty" (astringency), plus "cold and dry" qualities are attributed to the plant group. Uses included allaying all types of bleeding and bloody flux (diarrhea with bleeding). The same uses for amaranth species had been recorded by Greek authors 1,500 years earlier.

The first popular American herbal, Samuel Stearn's *The American Herbal or Materia Medica* published in Walpole, New Hampshire, in 1801, treated the amaranths generically as well. He writes, "The flowers of the common, large garden kind, dried, and powdered, have been recommended for incontinence of urine, diarrheas, dysenteries, and hemorrhages of all kinds."

Celosia argentea is also common in India, where it has been used as food and medicine. According to William Dymock in *Pharmacographia Indica* (1893), the young shoots were eaten as a vegetable, but are considered very heating. It was generally eaten only during famine. The seed was used as a treatment in diarrhea. One early Indian work noted that 180 grains of the seed, with an equal quantity of sugar, were taken daily in a cup of milk as an aphrodisiac. The seeds have also been used in the treatment of blood diseases, mouth sores, and eye diseases.

The astringent flowers of *C. cristata* have been used in India for diarrhea. The seeds have been employed as a demulcent and astringent for painful urination, cough, and dysentery.

The first mention of the use of cockscomb seed comes in the third class of drugs in *Shen Nong Ben Cao Jing*. As in India, the seeds were used to stop bleeding and for the treatment of eye disease. Celosia flowers are mentioned in the Tang Dynasty herbal, *Ben Cao Shi Yi*, (Omissions from the Materia Medica), 720 A.D. attributed to the physician Chen Cang-qi. The flowers of *C. cristata* have a history of use for blood diseases, bleeding, hemorrhoids, diarrhea, and dysentery. Li Shi-zhen first lists uses of the young stems and leaves of cockscomb in the 1596 *Ben Cao Gang Mu*. In Chinese tradition, fresh *C. argentea* stalks and leaves were used in folk medicine as a poultice on wounds, infected sores, and skin eruptions.

Taste and Character

Celosia cristata is slightly sweet and cool. *Celosia argentea* is somewhat bitter and cool.

Functions

Cools the blood, stops bleeding, clears up heat in the liver.

Uses

The seeds of *C. argentea* and the flowers of *C. cristata* are official drugs of the 1985 Chinese *Pharmacopeia*. The seeds of *C. cristata* are essentially treated as a substitute for *C. argentea*, as they are very similar and virtually impossible to distinguish from one another. If pieces of the flower head are present, the species can be identified from the style; the flower style of *C. cristata* is 2 to 3 mm long, while that of *C. argentea* is 4 to 6 mm long.

The dried flowers of *C. cristata* are used in prescriptions to treat leukorrhea, dysentery, hemorrhoids, expectoration or coughing of blood (hemoptysis), vomiting with blood (hematemesis), nose bleed (epistaxis), urine with blood (hematuria), urinary tract infections, and uterine bleeding. A traditional prescription for profuse menstruation, for example, called for powdered red cockscomb flowers dried in the sun to be taken before meals with alcohol. This prescription was contraindicated with fish, seafood, and pork.

The seeds are used for similar purposes and for treatment of cloudy urine, dizziness, and hypertension. In modern China they are primarily used in prescriptions for eye ailments, such as inflammation of the cornea, iris, and ciliary body, and acute conjunctivitis. Seed preparations have been shown to dilate the pupils and have an antiphlogistic effect. A recent pharmacological study shows that the seeds may have promise in reducing blood pressure. Extracts of *C. celosia* flowers have an antiprotozoic effect against *Trichomonas vaginalis*.

The young stems and leaves, considered a folk remedy, are used in decocted prescriptions for diarrhea with blood, vomiting with blood, nosebleeds, and uterine bleeding. A decoction of the whole plant is used as a wash for urticaria (skin eruptions associated with severe itching). A poultice of the fresh leaves is used for the bite of centipedes.

DOSE

Flowers 4.5–15 g; seeds 3–15 g in decoction.

DESCRIPTION

Celosia argentea is an erect annual herb growing up to 3 feet tall, with linear to oval lance-shaped leaves, about 2 inches long. Flowers range from silvery-white to pink-red in drooping or erect spikes.

Celosia cristata, is a branching, erect annual, 2 to 3 feet high, with oval to lance-shaped, alternate leaves, 2 to 5 inches long. The inflorescence (flower head) is terminal or in leaf axils, in short spikes, or more commonly broad, showy, fan-shaped heads. They come in white, purple, violet, pink, yellow, salmon, orange, red, and crimson forms. The tiny seeds of both species are shiny and black.

DISTRIBUTION

Celosia argentea is a weedy plant widely distributed in warmer climates throughout the world. *Celosia cristata*, thought to originate under cultivation in East Asia, is commonly grown as a garden ornamental throughout the world.

CULTIVATION

Both species like warm conditions. Celosias are easily cultivated in a half-rich sandy loam with well-rotted stable manure. In China, seeds are planted in March or April at a very shallow depth. Seeds from the middle part of the seed head are used for propagation. Germination takes about a week at temperatures of 65 to 70°F. When seedlings are 3 to 4 inches high they are thinned to a spacing of 6 to 12 inches. The plants like a fair amount of water, though established plants can be forced to flower if allowed to dry out for short periods of time. Seedlings, however, may lose their leaves if allowed to dry out. *Celosia argentea* thrives well in dry exposed areas. *Celosia cristata* prefers a richer, moist soil. Numerous cultivated varieties (cultivars) are available.

HARVESTING

From July to October, the flowers are harvested and dried in the sun. When the seed is ripe, from September through October, the whole plant is cut, dried in the sun, and the seedheads are rubbed to remove the seeds. They are sifted or winnowed to separate the chaff.

OTHER USES

In East Africa, the leaves of *C. argentea* (known as mfungu) are used as a type of spinach. In the seventeenth century, European explorers found *C. argentea* cultivated in the Moluccas, where the leaves were also eaten like spinach. The flowering spikes have been used in China as an ornament on cakes, using the colorful flowers to form written characters on the top of cakes. Historically it was considered a troublesome weed in Chinese flax fields, and was gathered for use as a potherb. The Toba-Bataks of central Sumatra in Indonesia used the plant as a ceremonial protective offering to spirits. In India the leaves of *C. cristata* have been eaten as a potherb, and the strong fiber from the stems has been used for making rope. When the seedlings are still quite young they are considered an acceptable spinach substitute in Malaysia.

Daylilies
Xuan-cao

> **Botanical names:** *Hemerocallis fulva* (L.) L.; *H. citrina* Baroni, *H. minor* Mill. Also *H. middendorffi* Trautv. et C. A. Mey.; *H. lilioasphodelus* L.
>
> **Chinese Names:** Pinyin: *Xuan cao* (*H. fulva*); *Xuan cao-gen* (*H. lilioasphodelus, H. citrina, H. minor*); Wade-Giles: *Hsüan-ts'ao* (*H. fulva*); *Huang-hua-ts'ai-kên, Hsüan-ts'ao-kên* (*H. lilioasphodelus, H. citrina, H. minor*).
>
> **English Names:** Orange Daylily, Tawny Daylily, Fulvous Daylily (*H. fulva*); Dwarf Yellow Daylily (*H. minor*).
>
> **Pharmaceutical Name:** Radix Hemerocallis.
>
> **Family:** Liliaceae—lily family.

HISTORY

Few Asian plants have become as integral a part of American gardens—and roadsides, for that matter—as the common daylily *Hemerocallis fulva*. Daylily hybrids for gardens are now available in sizes from 6 inches to 6 feet in height, numerous color patterns, and every color except for the elusive blue daylily. The American Hemerocallis Society, a horticultural society of devoted daylily enthusiasts, has been active since 1946. Currently there are over 275 registered daylily breeders, hundreds of amateur breeders, and nearly 30,000 named cultivars (cultivated varieties). In the past thirty years, Americans have gone mad for daylilies.

In 1753, Linnaeus adopted the Latin name *Hemerocallis* to refer to daylilies. In 1544 the name *Hemerocallis* was first used by the Venetian physician, Peitro Andrea Mattioli, in references to Mediterranean species of lilies (*Lilium*). Hemerocallis is a transliteration of the "*emerokallis*" of the first century Greek physician Dioscorides. Dioscorides' name actually applied to another plant, not daylilies, and his comments have been erroneously ascribed to daylilies by some authors.

Prior to the sixteenth century, Asian daylilies were unknown to European authors. The first European authors to write of daylilies were three contemporaries, the Belgians Rembert Dodoens (1517–1585) and Charles de l'Ecluse or Clusius (1526–1609), and the Frenchman Mathias de l'Obel or Lobel (1538–1616). The three were good friends and colleagues. All shared their observations and notes and the woodcut illustrations that were used interchangeably in their publications. The first illustration of *H. lilioasphodelus* (*H. flava*) appeared in 1554 in Dodoens' herbal *Cruÿdeboeck*. A 1570 work coauthored by de Lobel and Pierre Pena described the plant and mentioned that they had seen the plant used as medicine in Venice and Antwerp. *Hemerocallis lilioasphodelus* was figured in de Lobel's 1576 work, *Plantarum Stirpium Historia* (History of Plants), as was the common daylily *H. fulva*. This was the first European illustration of our common daylily.

A 1583 work of Clusius mentions the occurrence of the daylily in Hungary. Clusius is credited with introducing daylilies from eastern to western Europe in the late sixteenth century. How and exactly when daylilies arrived from East Asia to eastern Europe is unknown. What is known is the daylilies were rare in castle gardens of eastern Europe in 1554 and they were not known in the gardens of western Europe until the 1580s. After the 1580s, daylilies are mentioned in numerous western European herbals.

The first Englishman to write about the plant was Henry Lyte in his 1578 *A Niewe Herball*. This work was basically an annotated English edition of a French edition of Dodoens' *Cruÿdeboeck*. In the 1597 edition of *Gerard's Herball*, Gerard becomes the first English author to use the English name daylily which has remained with us ever since. Daylily is subsequently mentioned in European herbals of the seventeenth and eighteenth centuries. By the nineteenth century, it is rarely mentioned as a medicinal plant in the European literature.

Hemerocallis fulva was introduced into America at an early, but unknown, date. The famous naturalist Thomas Nuttall observed naturalized specimens of the common daylily near Philadelphia in 1812.

In Chinese literature, the daylily appears to be first mentioned in a collection of ancient folk songs, odes, and hymns attributed to Confucius. Confucius lived from 551–479 B.C. A treatise called *An Introduction to the Daylily* by Chi Han was published in 304 A.D. He describes the use of the flower as a vegetable.

In Chinese herbals it first appears in an annotated revision of *Shen Nong Ben Cao Jing* published around the year 656 A.D. in the Tang dynasty. An herbal published about 1059 A.D. in the Song dynasty attributed diuretic qualities to the root and mentioned its use in jaundice. This work also contained the first published illustration of *xuan-cao* in China, and presumably the first in the world. In *Ben Cao Gang Mu* (1596), published about the same time as the first edition of *Gerard's Herball*, Li Shi-zhen quoted all earlier publications on the plant and added his own observation on its habitat, growth habits, distribution, and recorded medicinal uses. He mentions use of a root poultice for abscesses of the breast, as well as other ailments it is still used for in modern China. Li Shi-zhen notes that the flavor of the cooked shoots is like creamed onions. The juice of the root was used to counteract arsenic poisoning.

Xuan-cao is also mentioned as a food plant in various emergency food guides published in China from 1409 A.D. on. From Chinese records it is clear that the same source plant(s) is used today for the same purposes as in ancient times.

According to Dr. Shiu Ying Hu (1968), one meaning for the Chinese word *xuan* is to "push aside" or "forget worry." "*Cao*" means herb. The Chinese name, translated to "forget-worry herb" may refer to the alleged hallucinogenic effect of eating large doses of the tender young leaf shoots. See S. Y. Hu (1968) for a fascinating and complete account of the history, botany, and uses of daylilies.

TASTE AND CHARACTER

A little sweet, cool.

FUNCTIONS

Good for urination, cools the blood, somewhat toxic.

USES

Daylily is not often used as a remedy in China. It is primarily considered a folk medicine and is not listed in the Chinese *Pharmacopeia*. Three species (*H. fulva*, *H. citrina*, and *H. minor*) are used as primary source plants of the herb.

The root is used in the treatment of edema, poor or difficult urination, turbid urine, leukorrhea, jaundice, hepatitis, cystitis, hematuria, nosebleeds, toothache, cervical lymphadentitis, bloody stool, uterine bleeding, and mastitis. Cooked with pork, it has also been used in preparations to promote growth of blood cells and to provide strength for feverish conditions. The fresh root was traditionally ground into a mudlike consistency and used as a poultice for the pain and swelling of mastitis. As a diuretic for edema, the dried roots and leaves were decocted in water that had previously been used to rinse rice. Decocted with fresh ginger and taken with a little wine, the root decoction is recorded as a folk treatment for bloody stool. For jaundice the fresh root of *xuan-cao* was washed, stuffed inside a female chicken, roasted for three hours, and then eaten once a day or once every two days.

Modern Chinese studies indicate that *H. citrina* root is antibacterial and kills blood flukes. It is has been used clinically in China to treat blood flukes and tuberculosis. Recent studies confirm some diuretic activity against edema. However, the plant is too toxic for self-medicated use.

In Western terms, the flowers are described as anodyne, antiemetic, antispasmodic, depurative, febrifugal, and sedative. The root is considered to be diuretic, anti-inflammatory, depurative, and hemostatic, and has been used to treat dropsy, gout, jaundice, and, as a poultice, mastitis. A poultice of the root has been used as a folk remedy for breast cancers.

WARNING

While the flower buds are considered edible, the roots of daylilies are generally considered toxic and should not be ingested. Overdoses may cause urinary incontinence, respiratory arrest, dilated pupils, and even blindness. Traditional Chinese works warn that the root should never be taken in 30 g doses, since they may damage the eyesight. Several hospital reports confirm that the use of the root can adversely affect eyesight, even cause blindness. However the 206th hospital in Jilin province used the root of *H. minor* in over 60 cases without reporting eye-affecting side effects. It may be surmised that *H. minor* is the preferred species for medicinal use.

A number of compounds in the root, including colchicine and rhein, have helped reduce tumors in laboratory experiments, but this activity is due to their high toxicity. Hemerocallin, another component, is also considered highly toxic. The poisonous components of the root are said to accumulate in the system with repeated or prolonged use. In traditional prescriptions, *Coptis* and *Phellodendron amurense* have been used to counteract the root's toxicity. Daylily root is *not* an herb for self-medication. It should only be used under qualified medical supervision—and for a prescription involving daylily root, you will probably have to travel to China to find a qualified medical practitioner.

DOSE

4.5–6 g, in decoction. Poultice of fresh or dried root; fresh root juice used externally.

DESCRIPTION

Hemerocallis fulva is a perennial growing to 6 feet tall, forming clumps from the spreading rhizomes. The basal, linear leaves are about two feet long and about 1½ inch wide, keeled, two-ranked, somewhat flattish, and grass-like in appearance. The root is spindle-shaped, thickened, and fibrous. Flowers are on erect scapes (stalks arising from the base of the plant). The flower tubes are funnel-shaped opening to bell-shaped at the ends, orange or rusty-orange. They are up to 5 inches long, and 3½ inches wide, and bloom from May to July.

Hemerocallis citrina is a perennial to four feet in height with leaves up to 3½ feet long, and more than 1 inch wide. The fragrant lemon-yellow flowers, up to 6 inches long, bloom at night, June through July.

Hemerocallis minor, grows to about 18 inches high, has slender leaves to about 20 inches long (¼ inch wide), and yellow fragrant blooms to 4 inches long. It blooms in spring.

Hemerocallis lilioasphodelus grows to about three feet. The leaves are about 2 feet long and ¾ inch wide. The fragrant yellow flowers are about 4 inches long, on a drooping scape, and bloom in spring.

Hemerocallis middendorffi is a foot or more tall, with leaves up to 2 feet long, drooping at the tips. The fragrant orange blooms are nearly 3 inches long. It blooms in late spring. The flowers of this species are in mostly sessile head-like clusters, with short, broad bracts beneath.

DISTRIBUTION

Hemerocallis fulva (tawny daylily) grows wild in mountain valleys or near water, moist forest openings, and under shade in grassy fields on west-facing slopes. It is cultivated throughout China. It is also common in Japan. Tawny daylily has become so widely naturalized in the eastern United States that, according to Dr. Shiu Ying Hu, it is actually more common in the United States than it is in China. In China, major production regions include Shaanxi, Hunan, Jiangxi, Zhejiang, and Fujian.

Hemerocallis citrina grows in mountainsides and rice fields in Hebei, Shanxi, Shandong, Jiangsu, Anhui, Zhejiang, Jiangxi, Hubei, Henan, Shaanxi, Gansu and Sichuan. It, too, is cultivated throughout China. It is grown commercially in Jiangsu, Zhejiang, Anhui, and Shandong, with lesser production in Hebei, Henan, Shaanxi, Gansu, Hubei, and Sichuan.

Hemerocallis minor grows wild in moist soils on mountainsides, grass-lands, hillsides, and forest margins. It is cultivated throughout China. It is also native to Japan and eastern Siberia. In China *H. minor* is mainly produced in Heilongjiang, Jilin, Liaoning, and Nei Mongol, as well as in in Hebei, Shandong, Shanxi, Shaanxi, and Gansu. The major sales are to the northeast and north central regions.

Hemerocallis lilioasphodelus (*H. flava*) grows primarily in the northern Yangtze River valley, in mountain meadows and fields. It is distributed in Jilin, Liaoning, Hebei, Henan, Gansu, Xinjiang, Jiangsu, Zhejiang, Anhui, Hubei, Guizhou, Yunnan, and Sichuan. This species is also cultivated throughout China. It is very closely related to *H. minor*, and some Chinese botanists combine the two species.

H. middendorffi occurs in high mountain meadows in northern China, Korea, adjacent Russia, and Japan.

CULTIVATION

According to Dr. Shiu Ying Hu, a leading authority on the history and botany of daylilies, their attractive foliage and exquisite flowers, together with their ability to withstand drought, compete with weeds, and flourish in the face of neglect, have endeared them to gardeners. Anyone can grow daylilies. It is a hardy perennial. Requirements are relatively simple given any good average garden soil with adequate moisture. Propagation is by division of the rootstocks, in early spring or fall. They are sometimes grown from seed. Since thousands of hybrid varieties are available, only a few of the original species are actually cultivated in gardens, mostly by collectors or breeders. By far, *H. fulva* is the most commonly grown species. Daylilies are cultivated throughout China, often in raised beds, on the levees between rice paddies.

HARVESTING

·The root is harvested in July to September after flowering. After digging, the above-ground portions of the plant and lateral rootlets are removed; the root is cleaned and then dried in the sun.

PROCESSING

The base of the stem and foreign matter are removed, and the roots are covered with a wet cloth until the center is moist and soft. Roots are then cut into sections and dried in the sun.

ADDITIONAL SPECIES

Hemerocallis thunbergii Hort. ex Bak. is also used in China.

OTHER USES

The dried or fresh unopened flower buds are sold as a vegetable in China, primarily used in soups and as a condiment in meat dishes. They are called *jin-zhen-cai*, and have a mucilaginous, somewhat sweet taste. The flower buds are found in the stockrooms of every good Chinese restaurant. Virtually every edible plant guide for North America mentions cooked daylily buds as an edible delicacy.

The leaves of *H. lilioasphodelus* have traditionally been used by peasants and the Tartars of the Upper Obi region to weave small mats to place underneath saddles.

The young shoots of *H. fulva*, considered potentially hallucinogenic in large doses, are used in Chinese folk medicine. They are considered a little sweet and cool and are used to promote diuresis, eliminate wetness heat, remove oppression and a hot feeling in the chest, alleviate problems with digesting food (over a two- to three-day period), and for jaundice and bloody urine. Prescriptions call for doses of up to 15–30 g of the fresh herb in decoction.

The flower buds of *Hemerocallis* are also used in folk medicine. They are considered a little sweet and cool and are used in prescriptions to promote diuresis, eliminate wetness heat, and remove oppression and hotness in the chest. Prescriptions use 15–30 g doses to treat bloody astringent urine, jaundice, piles, bloody stool, sleeplessness, and lung ailments.

Dianthus
Qu-mai

Botanical names: *Dianthus chinensis* L. and *Dianthus superbus* L.
Chinese Names: Pinyin: *Qu-mai* (herb). Wade-Giles: *Ch'ü-Mai* (herb).
English Names: Fringed pink (*D. superbus*), Chinese pink, rainbow pink (*D. chinensis*).
Pharmaceutical Name: Herba Dianthi.
Family: Caryophyllaceae—pink family.

HISTORY

The *Dianthus* genus is most famous for the fragrant, prized carnation (*D. caryophyllus* and its hybrids). It also includes dozens of less well known plants widely grown as ornamentals for their mat-forming, mounding, or other characteristics suitable for specialty gardens. There are more than 300 species in the genus *Dianthus*, members of the pink family. Most occur in Eurasia. In the United States pinks are often grown in rock gardens. Two species grown in American gardens, fringed pink (*D. superbus*) and Chinese or rainbow pink (*D. chinensis*), are source plants of a Chinese herb known as *qu-mai*.

Also known as Jove's flower, *Dianthus* is derived from the Greek *Dios*, referring to Jupiter (Jove), and *anthos*, flower. Linnaeus named both *Dian-*

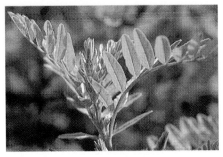

Astragalus
Astragalus membranaceus

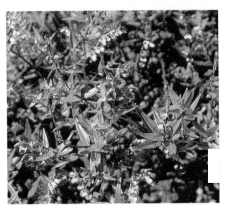

Baikal Scullcap
Scutellaria baicalensis

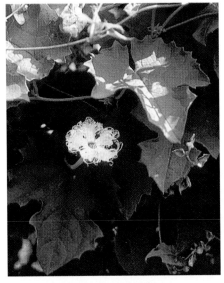

Chinese Cucumber
Trichosanthes kirilowii

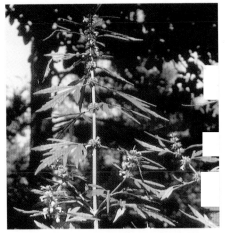

Chinese Motherwort
Leonurus artemisia

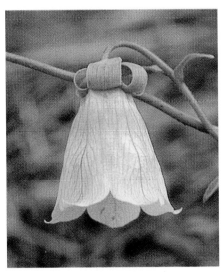

Codonopsis
Codonopsis spp.

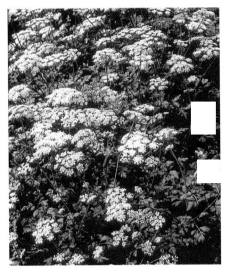

Dang-gui
Angelica sinensis

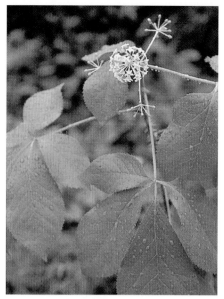

Eleuthero
Eleutherococcus senticosus

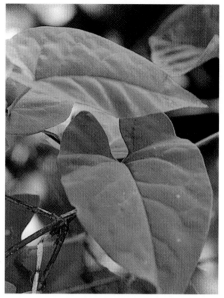

Fo-ti
Polygonum multiflorum

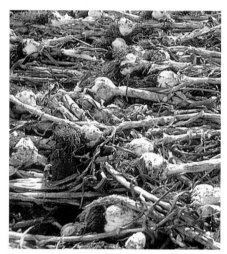

Garlic
Allium sativum

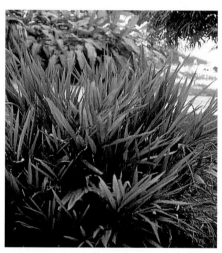

Ginger
Zingiber officinale

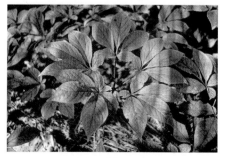

Asian Ginseng
Panax ginseng

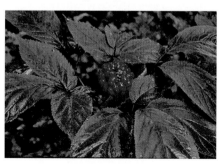

American Ginseng
Panax quinquefolius

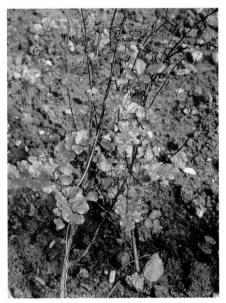

Licorice
Glycyrrhiza uralensis

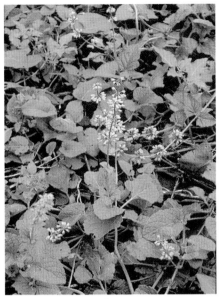

Red Sage
Salvia miltiorrhiza

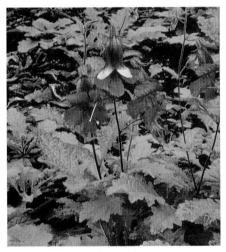

Rehmannia
Rehmannia spp.

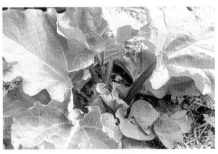

Common Rhubarb
Rheum x *cultorum*

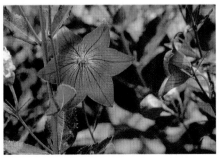

Balloonflower
Platycodon grandiflorum

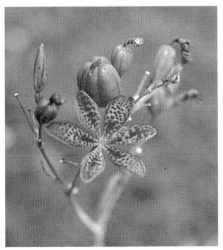

Blackberry Lily
Belamcanda chinensis

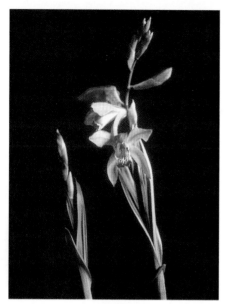

Bletilla
Bletilla striata

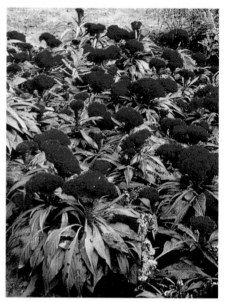

Cockscomb
Celosia cristata

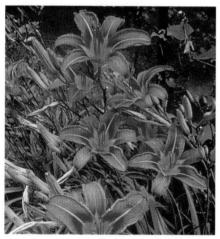

Daylilies
Hemerocallis fulva

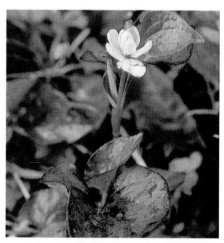

Houttuynia
Houttuynia cordata

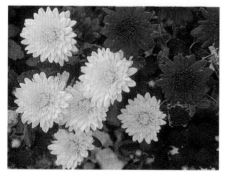

Mums
Chrysanthemum x *morifolium*

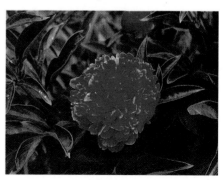

Peony
Paeonia lactiflora

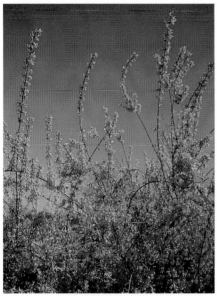

Forsythia
Forsythia suspensa

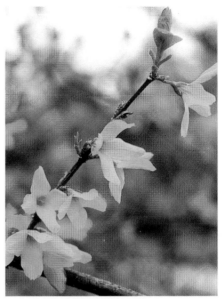

Forsythia flowers
Forsythia suspensa

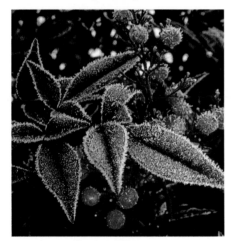

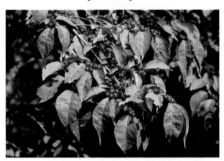

Matrimony Vine
Lycium spp.

Heavenly Bamboo
Nandina domestica

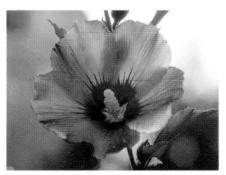

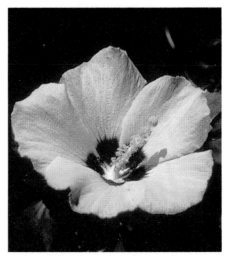

Rose-of-Sharon (pink-flowered cultivar)
Hibiscus syriacus

Rose-of-Sharon (white-flowered cultivar)
Hibiscus syriacus

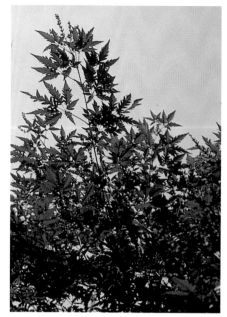

Vitex
Vitex negundo

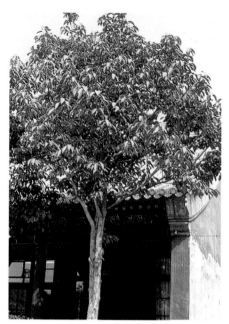

Eucommia
Eucommia ulmoides

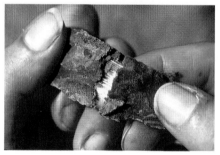

Eucommia bark
Eucommia ulmoides

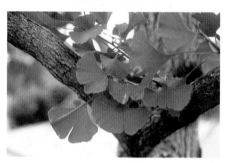

Ginkgo
Ginkgo biloba

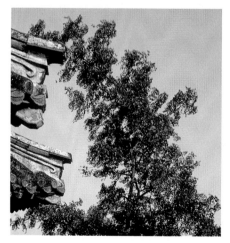

Jujube
Ziziphus jujuba var. *spinsoa*

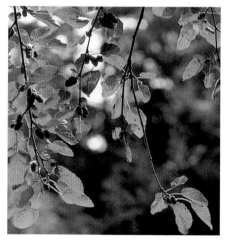

Mulberry
Morus alba

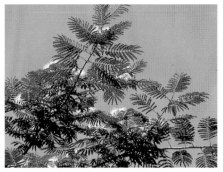

Silk Tree
Albizia julibrissin

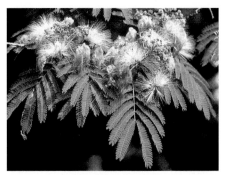

Silk Tree flowers
Albizia julibrissin

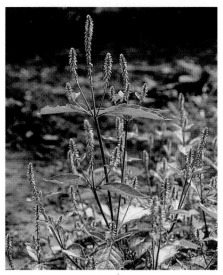

Achyranthes
Achyranthes bidentata

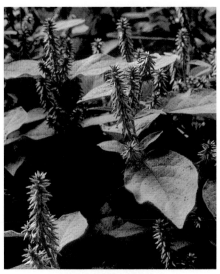

Achyranthes (detail)
Achyranthes bidentata

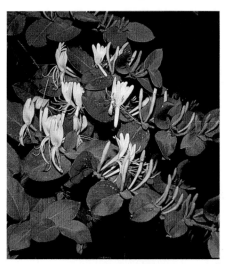

Japanese Honeysuckle
Lonicera japonica

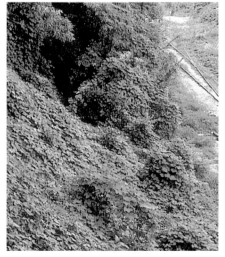

Kudzu
Pueraria lobata

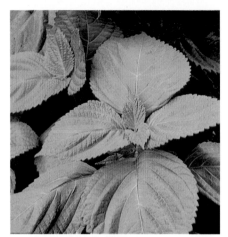

Perilla
Perilla frutescens

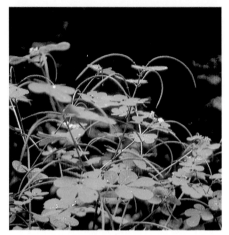

Sicklepod
Cassia obtusifolia

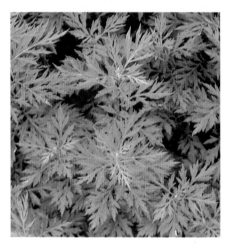

Sweet Annie
Artemisia annua

Photographs not available for:
Schisandra
Dianthus
Gardenia
Privet
Summer Cypress

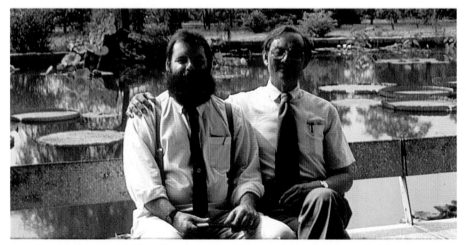

Steven Foster and Yue Chongxi at the Botanical Garden, Botanical Institute, Academy of Sciences, Beijing.

thus chinensis and *D. superbus*. He noted cultivation of *D. chinensis* in his gardens and those of his patrons at Uppsala in 1737 and 1748. Previous to that *D. chinensis* was mentioned in James Petiver's 1713 publication on rare plants found in the Physick Garden at Chelsea. Petiver (1658–1718) was apothecary to the Charterhouse, London, and a keen observer of new medicinal plants introduced into England, particularly Chinese medicinal plants. Philip Miller writes of the plant in his *Gardener's Dictionary* (1768).

Originally known as *Caryophyllus sinensis*, the first seeds of the plant to reach Europe were sent to Paris in 1705 by French missionaries. All specimens sported single flowers until 1719, when the first double-flowered forms bloomed in Paris. *Dianthus superbus* is itself native to Europe.

The whole plant, harvested when the flowerbud is swollen and about to open, is the Chinese medicinal herb. *Dianthus chinensis* and *D. superbus* are used interchangeably; however, *D. chinensis* is most often used. They are very closely related species, differing chiefly in the form of the calyx. The use of this medicinal plant is first mentioned in *Shen Nong Ben Cao Jing*. The Chinese name *qu-mai*, refers to the similarity of the seeds to wheat.

TASTE AND CHARACTER

Bitter, cold.

FUNCTIONS

Disperses heat, promotes diuresis, moves stagnant blood, stimulates menstrual flow.

USES

The dried herb of both *D. superbus* and *D. chinensis* are source plants of the traditional Chinese drug *qu-mai* in the 1985 Chinese *Pharmacopeia*. The herb is used in prescriptions to treat infrequent urination, urinary infections, stones, calculi, bloody urine, gonorrhea, edema, suppressed menstrual flow, carbuncles with swelling, eye inflammations, boils with toxic matter, and eczema. Folk uses have included mixing the powdered herb with peanut oil, stir-frying until warm, and then applying externally to treat sores with swelling. An ancient folk treatment for skin ailments (perhaps eczema) called for stir-frying the flowers until they turned yellowish in color, and then grinding them into powder. Mixed with the saliva of a goose, it was used as a poultice as necessary.

In Western terms, it is considered diuretic, antipyretic, anticoagulant, and antibacterial. In experiments, diuretic action has been confirmed, which is believed to be due to its effect on potassium salts. One experiment showed that the flowering tops had a more potent diuretic effect than the stems. Animal experiments have confirmed intestinal stimulating action, cardiovascular simulating activity, and antiparasitic activity against blood flukes. It has also been shown to impair the metabolism of hexobarbital. Clinical studies on the herb have involved urinary tract infections, cystitis, and suppressed menstrual flow. The plant is much more likely to be seen in American gardens than in herb outlets in the United States.

DOSE

4.5–9 g used in decoction, pills, powders or poultice.

WARNING

Contraindicated for kidney and spleen deficiency and during pregnancy.

DESCRIPTION

Dianthus chinensis has a solitary flower or a loose cluster of several flowers. The plant is unbranched except at the top. The flowers are 1½ to 2½ inches wide, with ovate bracts about half as long as the the flora tube (⅞ inch). *Dianthus superbus* differs from *D. chinensis* primarily in the length and shape of the calyx. The bearded lacerations of the petals of *D. superbus* are generally much longer than those of *D. chinensis*. Both flower from June to September.

Dianthus superbus is a perennial, growing to 3 feet. The leaves are linear lance-shaped. The flowers are quite fragrant, bearded as described above, with petals up to one inch long; they come in colors from pink to purplish to white.

Dianthus chinensis (sometimes called rainbow pink), is an annual, biennial, or short-lived perennial, growing from 8 to 20 inches tall. Leaves are up to 3 inches long, and linear. The flowers are ½ to 1 inch across, not fragrant as in *D. superbus*, and generally rose to lilac, with a darker purple center. Several cultivars of both species are available.

DISTRIBUTION

Dianthus chinensis grows in mountains and fields. It is often cultivated. *Dianthus superbus* grows in the countryside in open forests, forest edges, and nearby streams. Both are grown in gardens and yards throughout most of China. *Dianthus superbus* has a wide natural range occurring not only in China, but in Japan and Siberia, westward through middle Europe to Denmark.

Important provinces with commercial production include Hebei, Henan, Liaoning, Hubei, Jiangsu, besides in Hunan, Zhejiang, Shanxi, Shaanxi, Anhui, Gansu, Qinghai, Xinjiang, Fujian, Yunnan, and Guangxi.

CULTIVATION

Dianthus does best in a warm, moist climate, with a friable, well-drained, rich sandy loam. Dry sandy soils are not suitable. Before planting in China, the ground is fertilized with well-rotted barnyard manure or night soil. The soil is worked to a depth of at least a foot. Beds about 5 feet wide are carefully prepared and raked, making the soil surface very fine.

Propagation is by seeds, planted in late March to early April. In South China, seeds are planted in September or October. The tiny seeds are mixed with sand or thin soil before sowing. They are very lightly covered with soil and kept moist until seedlings emerge in about 15 days. Individual plants are thinned to about 10-inch spacings.

The plants can also be propagated by division in late March or early April. The entire plant is dug up and separated into 3 to 4 divisions. The divisions are replanted with a spacing of about 10 inches. When plants are 3 to 5 inches high, the soil is cultivated and weeded. This is repeated every 2 to 3 weeks. Plants are watered often and side-dressed with manure 3 times per year.

In North China plants are mulched for the winter after October 20, an important farm day in China that recognizes and celebrates the coming of the frost. It also marks the time that traditional doctors start watching for cases of frostbite and stocking medicines to treat winter diseases.

On April 20, the day that marks the coming of the spring rain, burned earth fertilizer (charcoaled grass) is added to the soil. The first spring shoots are cut back after April 20. The leaves to follow will grow more vigorously. At this time plants are side-dressed with night soil. Care is taken to ensure that the soil is well drained.

HARVESTING

The plant is collected in summer or autumn when the flower bud is very full and swollen, just before the flower opens. Two to three cuttings can be made a year on cultivated crops. The whole plant is dried in the sun, or the fresh plant can be is cut into small pieces before drying.

PROCESSING

Considered optional. Foreign matter is removed, including root pieces; the plant is washed, covered with a moist cloth and allowed to sit until uniformly moist, and then cut in sections before drying under sun.

ADDITIONAL SPECIES

In the northeast (Liaoning, Jilin, Heilongjiang) *Dianthus amurensis*, *D. versicolor*, and *D. subulifolius* are used as substitutes. In Ningxia, *D. orientalis* is used. *Dianthus amtifolia* Fisch. has also been used as a substitute. In Guizhou *Aletris spicata* has been recorded as an adulterant. In Yunnan, adulterants have included *Melandrium rubicundum* (Franch) Hand-Mazz., *Jasminum beesianum*, Forst. et Diels. *Avena fatua* L. and *Polygonum aviculare* L.

Dianthus caryophyllus the familiar and common carnation, is the source of carnation absolute, the aromatic oil used in sophisticated perfumes. The absolute is extracted using solvents. The flowers have been used in India as a cardiotonic and diaphoretic. The whole plant was once used as a vermifuge.

OTHER USES

The root has also been used as a folk remedy for the treatment of rectal or esophagal cancer. Both the fresh and dried herb were used, primarily in the form of a poultice. For esophagal cancer, the powder was traditionally blown onto the back of the throat.

Gardenia
Zhi-zi

Botanical Names: *Gardenia jasminoides* Ellis, *G. jasminoides* Ellis
var. *radicans* Thunb.
Botanical Synonyms: *Gardenia florida* L., *G. augusta* (L.) Merrill.
Chinese Names: Pinyin: *Zhi-zi* (fruits). Wade-Giles: *Chih-tzu,*
Huang-chi-tzu.
English Names: Gardenia, Cape jasmine.
Pharmaceutical Name: Fructus Gardeniae.
Family: Rubiaceae—madder family

HISTORY

Gardenia has long been grown under glass by American florists for its
delightfully scented flowers used in table arrangements, corsages, and
boutonnieres, though its popularity is not what it once was—through no
fault of the beauty and fragrance of the flowers! The name *gardenia* serves
as both the common English name of the plant as well as the generic part
of the Latin name. Of the nearly 200 species of the genus *Gardenia* native
to subtropical regions of Asia and Africa, only *Gardenia jasminoides*, the
Cape jasmine, is commonly cultivated in America.

The Cape jasmine arrived in England in the 1750s, but it was found
difficult to propagate. John Ellis, an English botanist who published the
first western account of the plant in 1761, suggested that the plant be given
to James Gordon, a gardener at Mile-end.

Gordon, described by Ellis as "a man who seems to be possessed of a
knowledge peculiar to himself," was successful in propagating many rare
plants after other growers had failed. After receiving two cuttings of the
plant in August 1757, Gordon was able to propagate it and sold it with
great success. The name *jasmine* as applied to this plant comes from a
painting by one of the most famous of natural-history illustrators, George
Dionysius Ehret. Ehret, unsure of the plant's identity, labeled his plate
"jasminum" with a question mark next to the caption. Since gardenia
flowers superficially resemble those of jasmines (trailing plants of the olive
family), it was given the species name *jasminoides*. The name Cape jasmine
arises from Ellis's 1761 account, which attributed the origin of a double-

flowered gardenia to the Cape of Good Hope. The name has stuck since.

Gardenia is named for a correspondent of both John Ellis and Linnaeus, Alexander Garden (1730–1791), a physician and naturalist from South Carolina. The genus name *Gardenia* has since become the best-known English name for the plant. In China, the drug composed of the fruits is called *zhi-zi*, which refers to a wine vessel with a shape similar to dried gardenia fruits.

Zhi-zi is first mentioned in the oldest Chinese herbal, *Shen Nong Ben Cao Jing*, attributed to Shen Nong, who placed it in the second of his three classes of drugs. In Chang Chung-ching's great classics, *Shang Han Lun* and *Chin Kuei Yao Lueh* (*Essentials of the Golden Chest*), written in the late second or early third centuries A.D., *zhi-zi* was the main ingredient in three of ten prescriptions for jaundice. Chang Chung-ching stated that "a good doctor treats a disease before it aggravates." He noted that liver disease could result in spleen disease and that it was therefore important to enhance spleen function to treat liver disease. According to Chinese medicine theory, jaundice is a disease of the spleen. The liver stores blood, while the spleen governs blood. Modern understanding of the role of the spleen and liver show that these concepts have a scientific basis (Kong 1977).

TASTE AND CHARACTER

Bitter, cold.

FUNCTIONS

Disperses heat, purges fire, cools the blood, removes toxins.

USES

Today the fruits are used in Chinese prescriptions for jaundice, high fever, fidgets, insomnia, and vomiting with blood. Externally, the fruits are used in prescriptions for sprains, swellings, and pain of bruises. Teas are also made from the roots and the fruits to treat canker sores, dysentery, and fevers. The fruits are considered useful against fevers, for dispersing the blood accumulated in bruises, and to stop bleeding; they are purgative and sedative. It is officially listed in the Chinese *Pharmacopeia*.

Various Japanese and Chinese studies confirm a rational scientific basis for the traditional use of gardenia fruits in jaundice. Many Western studies on traditional herb remedies are being undertaken to discover the active chemical constituents and their mode of action, with the goal of eventually synthesizing and manufacturing a drug from the compound.

Tests with gardenia fruits indicate such a simplistic approach does not recognize or acknowledge the full potential of the crude herb itself. While the glycoside, geniposide, is recognized as the key active chemical component of gardenia fruits, taken alone it does not produce as much benefit to the liver as the whole fruits themselves. One or several of the fourteen or more additional chemical components, acting alone or together, contribute to gardenia's fever-reducing, purgative, and tranquilizing actions.

Several studies of treating obstructive jaundice have indicated that extracts of gardenia fruit can reduce plasma bilirubin levels without any side effects such as damage to liver tissue and other systems (Kong *et al.* 1977).

Studies have shown that the seeds can lower systemic arterial blood pressure (Chow *et al.* 1976, Koo and Li 1977). Extracts have also been shown to possess antibacterial and antifungal qualities.

Clinical studies in China using a decoction or powder of gardenia fruits have reported positive results in icteric hepatitis, sprains, and contusions; when sterilized, the drug can be used to stop bleeding in the gastrointestinal tract as well as local bleeding.

Dose

6–12 g of the dried fruits, used in tea, powder, or pill form.

Warning

In traditional Chinese medicine, patients with weak spleens or diarrhea are not given the fruits.

Description

Gardenia is a bushy evergreen shrub growing up to 6 feet in height. The glossy, thick, leathery leaves are opposite or in whorls of three. They are lance shaped to oblong lance shaped, 2½ to 5½ inches long and 1½ to 2½ inches wide. The fragrant, tubular, often double white flowers are borne singly atop a branch or are clustered in the upper leaf axils. The calyx has five long teeth, which persist with the dried fruits. The elliptical or oval-shaped capsule, 1 to 2 inches long, is orange, fleshy, and marked by 6 to 8 winged grooves.

DISTRIBUTION

Gardenia occurs in low mountains, thin forests, stream banks, and road-sides in central and southern China, growing in Zhejiang, Jiangxi, Fujian, Hubei, Hunan, Sichuan, and Guizhou provinces, and is cultivated in most other provinces. The eastern coastal province of Zhejiang produces the highest quality drug, although production is most abundant in Hunan. Gardenia is scattered in Japan, Taiwan, the Ryukyu Islands, and Vietnam as well. In the United States it has long been popular as a greenhouse plant and today is grown indoors for cut flowers and, in mild climates, outdoors as an ornamental.

CULTIVATION

Gardenia enjoys warm weather and will usually not survive a freeze below 20°F. As a house plant, the key to success lies in keeping its environment sufficiently moist, misting the plant twice a day, and giving it plenty of water, without overwatering. It must be protected from cold drafts and extreme temperature fluctuations. It thrives in a warm house closed to drafts with even temperatures. Night temperatures should be above 65°F. A south-facing window will provide the full sun necessary for healthy plants. Outdoors, mature plants prefer full sun, though they should be protected by dappled shade during the hottest part of the summer.

It is not particular about soils, but a light acid to neutral sandy soil is best. A pH of 5 to 6 is optimum. An alkaline soil will adversely affect the plant's growth. The soil should contain enough organic matter to retain a good supply of moisture. Add peat if necessary. A saline-alkaline or heavy clay soil is not suitable.

To encourage blooming, plants can be side-dressed with manure or blood meal, or fed every three to four weeks with fish emulsion. To control competitive weeds, mulching is preferred over cultivating to avoid damage to the shallow lateral root systems.

Gardenia is propagated by both seeds and cuttings. Seeds can be plant-ed in spring to a depth of 1½ inch, in rows spaced at about 1 foot. Young seedlings can be protected from harsh sun by planting under lath sheds for the first four to six months. Thin seedlings to spacings of about 3½ inches. Once they reach about a foot in height they can be transplanted to their per-manent location. The plants and permanent rows should be spaced at 4 to 5 feet.

Cuttings can be made in March or April when budding begins. Choose three- to four-year old cuttings with 3 to 4 buds, and make cuttings 5 to 8 inches long. Place obliquely in a rooting medium. Give bottom heat and frequent misting to stimulate growth. An 80 percent survival rate can be expected. The cuttings can be transplanted the following spring. Plant the root crowns relatively high, as you would for azaleas and rhododendrons.

HARVESTING

The fruits are harvested in October when the surface begins to yellow, usually after a frost. They are dried in the sun or under low heat.

PROCESSING

The gardenia fruits are processed in a variety of ways before use. The crude dried fruits can be used; sometimes before drying the freshly harvested ripe fruits are boiled for a short time or steamed for a half hour in a bamboo steamer. The ends of the fruits are sliced off, or the fruits are sliced in half to remove the seeds. Another method is to stir-fry the fruits under a low heat until they turn a golden-yellow color. "Burned gardenia fruits," a separate drug, are stir-fried over a strong fire until the peel is charcoaled but the interior of the fruit retains an orange-yellow color.

Houttuynia
Yu-xing-cao

Botanical Names: *Houttuynia cordata* Thunb.
Botanical Synonyms: *Polypara cordata* (Thunb.) Kuntze; also erroneously spelled *Hottuynia cordata*, or *Houtuynia*.
Chinese Names: Pinyin: *Yu-xing-cao* (herb). Wade-Giles: *Yu-hsing-ts'ao* (herb).
English Names: Houttuynia, chameleon plant.
Pharmaceutical Name: Herba Houttuyniae.
Family: Saururaceae—lizard's tail family.

HISTORY

Increasingly, if you go into a nursery selling perennials or herb garden plants, you will find a small, low-growing herb with heart-shaped leaves. *Houttuynia* has quietly become a relatively common ornamental in American gardens. If you rub the leaves to emit their fragrance you'll be in for a surprise—and for most people an unpleasant one. The odor is unexpected, but familiar. The Chinese name, *yu-xing-cao*, means "fish-smell herb," and it does indeed smell like fish. Eating the raw leaf imparts the odor of fresh fish to one's breath. This unusual odor is attributed to components of the essential oil. In Japan the plant is called *"dokudami,"* which means detoxicant. A local Japanese name for the leaf, *"kaeruppa,"* meaning frog leaf, refers to a belief that a half-dead frog can be resuscitated by eating the leaf. After tasting the leaf yourself, you might just become a believer in this tale.

Houttuynia is monotypic, represented only by *Houttuynia cordata*. The Latin name was first published in a 1783 publication by C. P. Thunberg, predating his *Flora Japonica* by one year (1784). He named the genus in honor of a Dutch botanist and physician, Martins Houttuyn (1720–1798). In an 1891 publication, Kuntze placed the plant in the genus *Polypara*. That botanical name has slipped into obscurity. Thunberg's original Latin name is widely used today. Apparently Houttuyn, in a 1780 publication, had once named a plant of the Iris family *Houttuynia capensis* after himself, causing some obscure confusion on the application of the generic name. It is unclear when the plant was first introduced to Western horticulture. The Dutch explorer Cleyer is thought to have met with the plant in Japan as early as 1680.

In China *yu-xing-cao* is first mentioned in *Ming Yi Bie Lu* by Tao Hong-jing (500 A.D.) in the lower grade of herbs. The dried whole plant (harvested when in flower) is an official drug of the 1985 Chinese *Pharmacopeia*.

TASTE AND CHARACTER

Warm, mild, cold.

FUNCTIONS

Eliminates wetness-heat, dispels abscesses, detoxifies.

USES

Yu-xing-cao is used in prescriptions for vomiting of blood with pus caused by lung abscesses, coughing of thick yellow phlegm, leukorrhea, edema, urinary infections, chronic bronchitis, hemorrhoids, rheumatism, rectal prolapse, carbuncles, and boils. Eaten fresh, the leaves are used in folk medicine as an appetite stimulant. The leaf juice has been used as an astringent for anal prolapse. The juice has been applied externally to sores and snake bite, and as a poultice is a folk remedy for cancer. The crushed leaves have been applied to promote bone growth at the site of a fracture. The distillate of the whole herb is applied topically to herpes simplex. For skin disease, the fresh or dried herb is poulticed. A famous traditional prescription for lung infections combines two parts of the herb with one part of the root of balloonflower in decoction.

Clinical studies in China have focused on the uses of the herb for infections of the upper respiratory tract, including pneumonia, lung abscesses, and chronic bronchitis. It has been used in various preparations, including a decoction and injectable forms of a steam distillate of the herb, as well as injectable chemical isolates. Other clinical studies have included the use of a tablet made from the leaves in the treatment of leptospirosis (caused by leptospira infections); its curative and preventative effects in postoperative surgical infections; and treating inflammation of the middle ear (with a 95 percent success rate), sinusitis, chronic inflammation of the cervix and other types of pelvic inflammation, and chronic nephritis. The herb is also reportedly a folk remedy for cancer and has been used externally in the treatment of psoriasis.

In one clinical study an injection of the herb was used for lobar pneumonia. Eight patients were involved. All returned to good health in one to three days. Efficacy rates in other lung-related diseases reported in clinical studies in the Chinese literature have been impressive.

In experiments the herb has a diuretic action; strengthens capillary walls; is antifungal, antibacterial, and antiviral; and lowers blood pressure. The herb may have some immunostimulant function. One study showed that a decoction of the herb significantly enhanced the phagocytic activity of human peripheral leukocytes against *Staphylococcus aureus*. In Western terms, the herb is considered refrigerant, detoxicant, anti-inflammatory, antipyretic, and diuretic.

DOSE

15–30 g in decoction, poultice, or as a wash. Before decocting, the herb is soaked in water first, and then simmered for only three minutes. When used in prescriptions with other herbs, it is added after the rest of the prescription has been decocted. It is said that eating too much of the herb will cause shortness of breath.

DESCRIPTION

Houttuynia is a creeping perennial herb with a stoloniferous rhizome up to 3 feet in length. Stems are up to 18 inches long. The fetid leaves are heart shaped at the base, broadly oval, sharp pointed at the apex, 1 to 3 inches long, and entire (without teeth). There are conspicuous sheathing stipules at the base of the leaves. The unique flower is a short clublike spike, less than an inch long, subtended by 4 to 6 white, petal-like bracts. The fruit is rounded.

A number of cultivars are available in American horticulture, notably 'Chameleon,' (also called 'Variegata'), which is variegated with green, cream, and pink-red splotches, and 'Flore Pleno,' sporting enlarged double white bracts beneath the flower head, with purple-tinged leaves.

DISTRIBUTION

Houttuynia occurs in moist, shaded lowlands and is cultivated from India to China, and on Pacific islands including Japan, Taiwan, and the Ryukyus. It grows in much of eastern China, especially in the Yangtze River valley, and in marshy places of Anhui, Zhejiang, Hunan, Jiangsu, and Jiangxi. In Japan it is very common in Honshu, Shikoku, and Kyushu. In India it is found throughout the subtropical Himalayas at heights of up to 6,000 feet. Much of the Chinese drug supply is harvested from the wild.

CULTIVATION

Houttuynia likes a cool, moist, rich, shaded situation, including ditches and swamps. In such conditions it prospers, and can become invasive if not held in check. It is easy to keep under control, however, in an average garden situation with partial shade where it is allowed to dry out occasionally. The plant is very easily propagated by dividing the rhizomes. In the United States it has become a more popular and abundant ornamental in recent years, primarily due to the introduction of the variegated form.

HARVESTING

The leaves are harvested in mid to late summer, before the leaves die back. Leaves will die back relatively early in the growing season if they are allowed to dry out. It is best harvested just as it comes into flower in June or July. The herb is cleaned, and then dried in the sun.

PROCESSING

While the fresh juice of the herb is strongly antibacterial, hot extracts of the herb have been shown to have insignificant antibacterial action, suggesting that some components may be volatilized upon heating.

ADDITIONAL SPECIES

A California plant *Anemopsis californica* is closely related to *Houttuynia*; in fact, was once classified as *Houttuynia californica*. It grows from southern Oregon down to northern Mexico, Arizona, Nevada, and western Colorado. This plant was used for remarkably similar purposes to *yu-xing-cao* by native American groups of California, Mexico, and Nevada. It was used for sores, lung afflictions, and as an antiseptic wash. The root was used for menstrual cramps (like a Chinese folk remedy utilizing houttuynia roots). Eclectic medical practitioners of the late nineteenth century used *Anemopsis* to treat rheumatism, asthma, colds, indigestion, and impure blood.

OTHER USES

Another common Chinese name for the plant *chu p'i ku*, meaning "pig thigh," is applied to the herb in Chinese markets where it is sold as a culinary herb.

The root has been eaten as a vegetable, raw or cooked. Because of their unique and unusual flavor the leaves are sometimes used sparingly in salads or as a condiment.

Mums
Ju-hua

Botanical Name: *Chrysanthemum* x *morifolium* Ramat.
Botanical Synonyms: *Dendranthema morifolium* (Ramat.) Tzvel.,
Chrysanthemum sinense Sabine, *Dendranthema sinense* (Sabine)
Des. Moul., *Pyrethrum sinense* (Sabine) DC, *Tanacetum sinense*
(Sabine) Sch.-Bip., *Tanacetum morifolium* (Ramat.) Kitam., etc.
Chinese Names: Pinyin: *Ju-hua* (flowers). Wade-Giles: *Chu-hua*
(flowers).
English Names: Florist's chrysanthemum, mum.
Pharmaceutical Name: Flos Chrysanthemi.
Family: Asteraceae (Compositae)—aster family.

HISTORY

Perhaps no plant group except the roses has been the subject of so many
books and articles as the chrysanthemums. Chrysanthemums have been
loved by gardeners for many years. The Chinese have cultivated them for
at least 3,000 years. The genus *Chrysanthemum* is a diverse group of annual
or perennial plants with as many as 200 or as few as five species, depending
upon the botanical authority cited. Differences in opinion are recognized
in current modern publications by scientists of equal authority. Our subject, *Chrysanthemum morifolium* (which is considered a complex hybrid by
many botanists), is now placed in the genus *Dendranthema*. In 1961 a
Russian botanist published the name *Dendranthema morifolium*, which is
used in some modern floristic works, including the *Flora of China*. The
name *Chrysanthemum sinense* also refers to the plant in some works on
Chinese medicinal plants. Most modern works on Chinese medicinal
plants, however, use the name *Chrysanthemum morifolium*, which we will
use here to help reduce confusion.

Jac. Breyn (1637–1716), a merchant from Danzig, frequented flower
gardens of Holland in the latter seventeenth century and described the
plants he saw in a two-part work published in 1680 and 1689. In the 1689
work we find the first Western description of the mum. Breyn mentioned
six varieties he observed in the gardens of the Dutch. The plant then fell
into obscurity. Mums were not generally known in Holland or other parts
of Europe until they were reintroduced to Europe in 1789. Now, as they

have been for over 200 years, the many varieties and cultivars of mums are valued as an ornamental of the flower garden, greenhouse, or conservatory, blooming especially in the autumn months.

The genus name *Chrysanthemum* was published by Linnaeus in 1753. The species *C. morifolium* was established in a 1792 publication by Thomas Albin Joseph d'Audibert de Ramatuelle, who lived from 1750–1794. Given the length of his name, one can see the value of the abbreviated author citation "Ramat." at the end of the scientific name. In 1823, the English botanist Joseph Sabine (1770–1837) named the plant *Chrysanthemum sinense*, a name used in many nineteenth-century works. Sabine wrote five major publications on chrysanthemums published between 1821 and 1826. The name chrysanthemum is derived from *chrysos*, gold, and *anthos*, flower, in reference to the yellow color of many chrysanthemums.

Chrysanthemum morifolium flowers are the Chinese herb *ju-hua*. There are many types of *ju-hua* with qualifying name variations, depending upon production region, processing methods, time of harvest, and other factors (see "Harvesting" and "Processing" sections). There are some slight distinctions made in the use of different forms of chrysanthemum, but the medicinal action is considered primarily identical. The flowers were first mentioned in *Shen Nong Ben Cao Jing*. The leaves were first mentioned in *Ming Yi Bie Lu* (*Miscellaneous Records of Famous Physicians*) by Tao Hong-jing, published during the North and South kingdoms, about 500 A.D.

TASTE AND CHARACTER

A little sweet, bitter, cold.

FUNCTIONS

Expels wind and heat, disperses liver fire to treat eye disease and detoxifies.

USES

Ju-hua is used in prescriptions for colds with wind and heat, headache, inflamed eyes, swelling and pain in throat, vertigo, tinnitus, sores such as boils, and tightness of the chest with anxiety. Pillows stuffed with the flowers have been used for the treatment of cold and headache. Soaked in wine, the flowers make "chrysanthemum wine," a historical restorative beverage. A traditional treatment for vertigo calls for the "very dry" powder of *ju-hua* added to rice wine and taken as needed. Even the dew gathered from the flowers has been thought to have restorative powers. White *ju-hua* flowers are also traditionally used for heart disease.

A prescription for the treatment of high blood pressure and arteriosclerosis calls for a decoction of 24 to 30 g of *ju-hua* with 24 to 30 g of Japanese honeysuckle flowers (*Lonicera japonica*). This is one day's prescription, which is divided into 4 doses and drunk instead of tea. The same herb material is decocted for two day's dosage. The dose is adjusted by a physician as necessary. After two weeks, the amount is reduced to 9 g of flowers. If the patient has serious vertigo, 12 g of mulberry leaves (*Morus alba*) are added to the prescription. If arteriosclerosis and hyperlipemia are present, 12 to 24 g of the fruits of Chinese hawthorn (*Crataegus pinnatifida*) are called for in Chinese clinical works.

A clinical report using this prescription in 46 cases, over a three- to seven-day period of administration, notes a reduction of headache, vertigo, and other symptoms in most patients. Blood pressure was reduced to normal in 35 percent of the patients. The remainder of the patients showed some improvement in blood pressure after 10 to 12 days.

A clinical report in the Chinese literature for the treatment of heart disease used a decoction of *ju-hua* in 61 cases of angina pectoris. It was found to be effective in 80 percent of the patients; very good in 43.3 percent, and in 36.7 percent of the patients, some improvement was noted. It was considered particularly useful for mild cases of angina. For patients with tight chest, palpitations, vertigo, and numbness, the decoction had a moderate effect. Forty-five percent of patients showed some changes on electrocardiograms. Obvious effects were observed in 18.8 percent of patients, and some improvement in 27.1 percent. High blood pressure was reduced in some patients. One patient experienced stomachache and diarrhea as side effects. Former ulcer patients did not have any adverse effects.

Additional clinical studies have focused on the use of the flowers in hypertension, arteriosclerosis, infections of the upper respiratory tract, bronchitis, tonsillitis, conjunctivitis, local infections, and burns.

Experimentally, the flower extract helps to stabilize the central nervous system, dilates blood capillaries, and is antibacterial and antifungal. An alcohol-precipitated decoction produced marked dilation of coronary vessels, thus increasing blood flow.

While the large number of Chinese varieties are considered to have comparable medicinal value, a wide variation in chemical composition and quantity could be predicted from the genus, necessitating more research to find the highest-quality cultivars for medicinal use. The white chrysanthemum has been reported to be higher in flavonoid glycosides, and contain additional components such as coumarins and alkaloids.

DOSE

4.5–12 g.

CONTRAINDICATION

The roots of *Atractylodes macrocephala* and *A. lancea*, the root of *Lycium chinensis*, and the inner bark of *Morus alba* are not used with *ju-hua*.

DESCRIPTION

Considered hybrids of several other chrysanthemums, the ancestry of modern-day mums may involve as many as six *Chrysanthemum* species. The highly variable common mum is a stout, near-woody, hardy perennial growing up to 3 to 5 feet in height, with erect or spreading stems. The alternate leaves are about 3 inches long, highly aromatic, thick, and gray-hairy beneath. They are variously lobed, entire, or coarsely toothed. The daisylike flower heads are highly variable in size, shape, and color. The disk florets are yellow, but ray flowers range from yellow, white, pink, bronze, reddish, or purple.

Two basic types of the common florist's chrysanthemum are generally available, including those with large flower heads grown in containers, or more bushy, hardier types grown as border plants in the perennial garden. The flower head-size of the container-type mums is determined by selection, as well as by attention to cultivation and the skill of the grower. Factors such as pruning, disbudding, propagation, and soil types affect the size of the flower heads. If left to grow on their own, they produce bushy plants with smaller heads.

The hundreds of mum cultivars are further classified by flower shape into several basic types. The double-flowered compact types are known as "cushions." The single daisylike, yellow-centered forms are known as "daisies." "Decoratives," which are generally taller and larger than the cushions, have double or semidouble flowers. "Pompons" are compact forms with ball-shaped flowers. "Buttons" represent plants with small double flowers, generally less than an inch in diameter.

DISTRIBUTION

Cultivated throughout China. Major production areas include Anhui, Henan, and Zhejiang. A famous production region for white *ju-hua* is Hangzhou in Zhejiang province. Mums are widely grown in European and American horticulture.

CULTIVATION

According to Chinese works, the plant is not particular about soil; however, saline-alkaline, poorly drained soils are unsuitable. It does best in high dry areas with full sun, little wind, and a rich, sandy, well-drained soil. In an early twentieth century English work, G. Nicholson's *An Encyclopedia of Horticulture*, the author has a different opinion:

> [The soil] can scarcely be too rich when the plants are strong and placed in the flowering pots. Good loam, heavy rather than light, should be used in about equal proportions with rotten manure, including some cow dung. A little soot intermixed with this tends to give the leaves a dark green colour, and materially assists them. Crushed bones are sometimes used for drainage, with a large crock over the hole (1886, p. 321).

Propagation is by seed, stem cuttings, or by dividing the roots in autumn or spring. Seed can be sown in February or March, lightly covered with soil, and placed in a warm area. Seeds germinate readily. Young seedlings should be pinched back after they are about three inches high to encourage bushy growth. In April to May, cuttings 4 to 6 inches long are made. Place in a rooting medium and maintain temperatures of 55 to 60°F. They root in about 20 days. Transplant when strong. Roots can be divided in fall or spring, toward the end of April. When the young plant is 5 or 6 inches high, dig up plants, choosing seedlings with "white" roots. These are considered best for medicinal plantings. Over the long term, mums do better if divided at least every three years.

Rows should be spaced at about 18 inches; individual plants are spaced at 12 inches. When about 1 foot high, pinch back the tops to encourage branching and better flower development. Side-dress plantings with horse manure.

Additional cultivation information can be found in any good gardening book. Chrysanthemum culture has been raised to the level of an art. There are as many ways of growing mums as there are artists to perform the task.

HARVESTING

The flowers are harvested around the third week of October. They bloom very well at this time in China's important production regions. After harvest, they are baked over light heat until dry, or steamed and then dried in full sun. Another method its to dry in shade in a well-ventilated room.

For "white" *ju-hua* (*bai-ju*), the whole plant is cut, tied in bundles, and hung to dry. Flowers are removed once dry.

To produce "*chu-ju*" (from Anhui), when most of the flowers are blooming the whole plant is harvested and hung in a dark attic to dry. Sulphur is used to fumigate the plants until the flowers and leaves become soft (about 60 percent dry). The plants are sifted or shaken until the flowers are rounded in form, and they are then completely dried. The sulphur fumigation process causes the flowers to have a light color and kills insects.

In another form, *gung-ju* (from southern Anhui province), the flowers are harvested and then baked until dry.

PROCESSING

White *ju-hua* is produced by steaming the flowers and then drying them in the sun. "Yellow" *ju-hua* (*hang-ju*) is produced by baking over a light fire until dry. Both are produced in the Hangzhou area and throughout Zhejiang province. Chrysanthemum flowers produced in the Hangzhou area are sometimes called *hang ju-hua*.

For charcoaled *ju-hua*, the flowers are stir-fried until dark brownish-yellow, so that they retain their character (not burned). Clean water is sprinkled clean on the herb to cool it, and it is then dried.

ADDITIONAL SPECIES

Chrysanthemum indicum, ye-ju-hua, is used for similar purposes. Actually native to China and Japan, it is widely grown in India as an ornamental, where it is also used as a stomachic and aperient. In Indochina the leaves have been prescribed for migraine headaches, a similar use to the leaves of

Tanacetum parthenium (feverfew), now popularly sold in Western herb markets for the treatment of migraine. Other Chinese chrysanthemum species have been used as folk cancer remedies.

OTHER USES

The root, young stem, and old leaves are used as folk medicines.

The leaves, *ju-hua-ye*, are considered a little hot, a little sweet, and neutral. They have been used for boils, sores, vertigo, and blurred vision. A decoction of the dried leaves, juice from the fresh leaves, or a poultice of the fresh leaves are used.

For boils the fresh leaves (or the root in winter) are juiced. A small amount (unspecified) of the juice is then taken.

For boils, with toxic material, general soreness, pain, and swelling, the leaves and the roots are juiced. The juice is added to a small teacupful of hot wine. Another method is to soak the leaves in warm alcohol or eat the fresh leaves.

The young stems, *ju-hua-miao*, are collected in early summer and then dried in shade. They are considered a little sweet, a little bitter, and cool. They are used to clear away liver fire in order to treat eye disease, vertigo, and vaginitis. The dried stems are used in decoction or as a powder.

For the treatment of vertigo and a heavy feeling in the chest, a traditional treatment uses a moxa of the powdered young stems placed on the temples. Then, while fasting, a five-finger pinch of the dried stems are taken with a little wine. The next day two five-finger pinches are taken. The third day, three five-finger pinches are taken.

To make the eyes clear and calm the patient, the stem is cut into small pieces and then eaten with rice porridge, flavored with salt.

For the treatment of vaginitis, a decoction of the stem is used as a wash.

Peony
Bai-shao and *Chi-shao*

Botanical Names: *Paeonia lactiflora* Pallas is the source of *bai-shao*. *Paeonia veitchii* Lynch is the official source of *chi-shao* in the Chinese *Pharmacopeia*.

Botanical Synonyms: *Paeonia albiflora* Pallas., *P. edulis* Salib.

Chinese Names: Pinyin: *Bai-shao* (white or cultivated peony roots), *Chi-shao* (red or wild peony roots). Wade-Giles: *Pai-shao* (white or cultivated roots) *Ch'ih-shao* or *Ching-shao* (red or wild roots).

English Names: Peony, Chinese peony, common garden peony.

Pharmaceutical Names: Radix Paeoniae Alba (*bai-shao*), Radix Paeoniae Rubra (*chi-shao*).

Family: Peoniaceae—peony family; or Ranunculaceae—buttercup family.

HISTORY

Peonies have been cultivated as ornamentals in China since about 900 B.C. There are two well-known ornamentals in the genus *Paeonia*. The roots of both species are famous medicines in Chinese tradition. One is *Paeonia suffruticosa*, the moutan or tree peony, which produces an official drug of the Chinese *Pharmacopeia*, *mu-dan-pi* (the bark of the root). The other is *Paeonia lactiflora*, the herbaceous peony so common in American gardens. It produces two distinct herbal drugs, *bai-shao* (cultivated root), and *chi-shao* (wild-harvested root). The plant, itself, is known as *shao-yao*. The common garden peony, or *shao-yao*, sporting white, red, or pink flowers, is among the most popular and widely grown of garden perennials throughout the northern hemisphere. Blooming peonies can be seen in every city, town, and tiny hamlet in the United States from May through June. *Paeonia lactiflora* is the primary subject of this article, but a few words on the tree peony are necessary first. It is commonly grown as an ornamental in China, but is less commonly seen in the United States.

The Chinese call the tree peony *mu-dan*. Two or three weeks after the arrival of spring, its blooms celebrate the lush explosion of vegetation. Another name for it is "rich flower." Perhaps this name refers to the size of the flower. The Chinese believe that the plant is a symbol of richness.

There are many stories about the flowers of *mu-dan* in China. One of them is known to all. During the Tang dynasty, the empress Wu Ze-tien ordered all flowers to bloom on the following day. It was deep winter. The next day all of the flowers blossomed except *mu-dan*. This made the empress very angry. She was in a rage and drove the plant from the capital of Cheng'an to Luoyang. So Luoyang flower is another name for *mu-dan*.

In Zhung-Shan Park in Beijing, there are many famous and precious breeds of *mu-dan*, such as *bai-yu* (white-flowered), *wei-zi* (purple-flowered), and *yao-huang* (light yellow-flowered). Every spring many people flock to Zhung-Shan Park to enjoy the *mu-dan*. Two or three weeks following the blooming of *mu-dan*, the flowering of *shao-yao* (*P. lactiflora*, source of the Chinese drug *bai-shao*) begins. Most people in China prefer the flowers of *mu-dan* because its flowers are much larger, fuller, delicate but strong, and do not lose their petals as easily as *P. lactiflora* does. Perhaps some day the Chinese peoples' appreciation of the *mu-dan* peony will be adopted by Americans.

Ten species of peony are found in Europe. *Paeonia* is named after the mythical physician Paeon. Apollo, god of healing and son of Zeus and Leto, was the father of Aesculapius, god of medicine. Paeon, a pupil of Aesculapius, served as physician to the Greek gods. Leto gave the peony plant to Paeon on Mount Olympus. He used it to cure Pluto of a wound, the first mythical use of peony for medicinal purposes. This aroused the jealousy of Aesculapius, who plotted to kill Paeon. When Pluto heard of the plot he changed Paeon into the plant that has since borne his name.

The genus *Paeonia* was established in Linnaeus's *Species Plantarum* (1753). *Paeonia*, historically placed by botanists in the buttercup family, is now placed in the separate peony family, which contains 33 species of temperate-climate herbs or shrubs. The German-born Peter Simon Pallas (1741–1811), who made extensive botanical explorations of the Russian Empire, first named *P. lactiflora* in a 1776 publication. He also authored the synonym *P. albiflora* in 1788, but the previously published, *P. lactiflora*, is the earliest valid name for the plant in question.

The plant is thought to have been introduced to European gardens from Siberia as early as 1558. By 1805 *Paeonia lactiflora* was known in English gardens, introduced by Sir Joseph Banks (1743–1820). When numerous varieties were imported from the East in the mid nineteenth-century, their popularity as garden plants grew immensely. Peonies were undoubtedly introduced to American gardens at an early date. They were grown in Virginia as early as 1771.

The root, produced from cultivated *P. lactiflora* (with bark removed), is known as *bai-shao*. Wild-harvested roots of *P. lactiflora* and *P. veitchii* (generally with bark intact) are known as *chi-shao*. They are treated as distinct herbal products and are very commonly used in Chinese medicine. Both are listed as official drugs in the Chinese *Pharmacopeia*. The earliest mention comes in the second or middle class of drugs in *Shen Nong Ben Cao Jing*. In *Ben Cao Gang Mu*, Li Shi-zhen noted that there were two kinds, *bai-shao*, or white peony, and *chi-shao*, red peony. He stated that the color of the root follows the flower color, though this is not necessarily true. In fact the *bai shao* or white peony is the root drug prepared from cultivated peonies. It is described as strong, rich, and straight. *Chi-shao*, the red peony, is the root derived from wild harvested plants. The root is white, small, thin, and crooked. Other major distinctions between the two types of peony root have to do with processing methods.

Taste and Character

Bai-shao is bitter, sour, and slightly cold. *Chi-shao* is sour, bitter, and cool.

Functions

Bai-shao nourishes the blood, nourishes and balances the liver, reduces acute pains, soothes liver *qi*, and is astringent to yin (stops sweating). *Chi-shao* expels blood stasis, allays pain, cools blood, disperses heat, and subsides swelling.

Uses

Bai-shao is used in prescriptions for hypertensive headache, vertigo due to blood deficiency with liver heat, pain in the chest and sides, spastic pains in the stomach and intestines, abdominal pains due to diarrhea or dysentery, appendicitis pain, feet and hands stiff with pain, painful systremma (charley horse of the calf), abnormal menstruation, painful or difficult menstruation (dysmenorrhea), uterine bleeding, leukorrhea, spontaneous perspiration, night sweats, and fever due to yin deficiency.

    Chi-shao is used in presciptions for amenorrhea, abdominal mass, abdominal pain due to blood stasis, pains of the chest and side, heat in blood, vomiting with blood, nosebleeds, dysentery bleeding, uterine bleeding, dysmenorrhea, red eyes, carbuncles with swelling, furuncles, sores, and traumatic injury.

    Bai-shao and *chi-shao* have been used for thousands of years in China, both in TCM and folk medicine. For example, to treat a knife wound with much bleeding and pain, a folk treatment calls for 30 g of *bai-shao*, fried until yellow, powdered and taken in a 6 g dose with either wine or water that was previously used to rinse rice. At the onset of the injury the prescription was given 3 times per day, and then the dose would be increased to 4 or 5 times per day. Combined with licorice root, *bai-shao* is used both as a decocted tea and external wash for the treatment of ring-worm of the feet with swelling and pain.

Experimentally, *bai-shao* has an antispasmodic and analgesic action in animal experiments. The herb has been shown to prevent gastric secretions and may help to prevent gastric ulcers resulting from nervousness. It is also antibacterial and antiviral. In experiments with mice, it prolonged sleeping time, acted as an anticonvulsive, lowered blood pressure, and was anti-inflammatory. The major active component, paeoniflorin, has tranquilizing, analgesic, anti-inflammatory, and antispasmodic activity.

In Western terms, *bai-shao* is considered to promote circulation and to be analgesic, spasmolytic, diuretic, antibiotic, emmenagogic, sedative, and expectorant. It is primarily used in the United States by TCM practitioners.

DOSE

Bai-shao is used in doses of 4.5 to 12 g in decoction, pills, or powder. *Chi-shao* is used in doses of 3 to 9 g.

WARNING

Bai-shao is contraindicated in prescriptions with *Veratrum nigrum*, which is itself poisonous, and during pregnancy. It is also contraindicated for persons with diarrhea accompanied by abdominal coldness. *Chi-shao* is contraindicated with *Veratrum nigrum* and during pregnancy. Peony-derived medicines should only be administered in prescriptions by TCM practitioners.

DESCRIPTION

The common garden peony is a perennial growing from 1½ to 3 feet in height. The stems are glabrous (smooth), each bearing two or more flowers. The leaves are alternate, lower leaves are often 2- to 3-parted, shining above, and dull green beneath. Individual leaflets are elliptical to lanceolate in shape. They are entire (without teeth) or may have lobed margins. The large fragrant flowers from 2¾ to 4 inches in diameter are usually white, although they come in various shades of pink, red, and red-purple. Many cultivated forms have double flowers. Literally hundreds of cultivated varieties (cultivars) have been developed from this single species.

There are several books on peonies and their cultivation, plus an American Peony Society.

DISTRIBUTION

Paeonia lactiflora occurs on mountainsides, and in grassy fields and shrub thickets in both valleys and high mountain fields. The wild plant occurs in Heilongjiang, Jilin, Liaoning, Hebei, Shanxi, Nei Mongol, Shaanxi, Gansu, Ningxia, Qinghai, and Xinjiang. It also occurs in Siberia.

Major cultivated supplies are produced in Henan, Shandong, Anhui, Zhejiang, Sichuan, and Guizhou provinces. Hunan and Shaanxi also have commercial production. The root produced in Anhui is called *bo bai-shao*. Its surface is smooth. That produced in Sichuan is called *chuan bai-shao*. The root grown in Zhejiang is called *hang bai-shao*, and is distinguished by its noticeably wrinkled surface.

The best quality has a large strong root, without white color in the center of the root and without cracks.

Paeonia lactiflora, wild-harvested for *chi-shao*, is produced in Heilongjiang, Liaoning, Jilin, and Hebei, as well as in Shanxi, Nei Mongol, Shaanxi, Gansu, and Ningxia. The supply is sold throughout China.

Paeonia veitchii, growing in elevations of up to 8,100 to 11,000 feet, is found along forest margins, in dark shaded forests, and on mountainsides in Shanxi, Shaanxi, Gansu, Qinghai, Sichuan, and Xizang. The root is primarily produced in Sichuan, as well as in Shanxi, Gansu, Shaanxi, and Qinghai, where it is consumed locally.

Paeonia obovata, found in deciduous forests, forest margins, and mountain valleys in Heilongjiang, Jilin, Liaoning, Hebei, Shanxi, Nei Mongol, Shaanxi, Gansu, Xinjiang, Henan, Anhui, Jiangxi, Hubei, Hunan, Sichuan, Guizhou, and Yunnan, as well as in Sakhalin and Japan, has also been used as a source plant of *chi-shao*. However, it is reported to be used only as a local source in Shaanxi.

Paeonia lactiflora, and its hundreds of cultivars, are very commonly grown in Western horticulture. *Paeonia veitchii* and *P. obovata* are also found in American gardens, primarily those of peony collectors.

CULTIVATION

The common garden peony prefers warm, moist climates, but is tolerant of cold weather. The soil should be well-drained, loose, rich in organic matter, and somewhat sandy. Clay soil or poorly drained lowlands are not suitable for cultivation. Propagation is by division of roots. A bud with a 2 inch piece of root attached is selected. Sections are separated into several parts with one or two buds, and planted in rows spaced at 2 to 3 feet, with individual plants spaced at about 1½ feet. Soil is hilled up over the clumps in winter to provide protection. In China, the flower buds are pinched backed before opening to send more energy to the roots. In Zhejiang, to make large roots, the lateral rootlets are cut off the live plants during the winter when they are dormant. This makes the root grow very large. The method is performed from the second year on.

HARVESTING

Roots of the cultivated *bai-shao* are harvested after 4 to 5 years of growth, in August through October. The roots are then graded according to size, placed in hot water, and boiled until the interior of the root in cross section is no longer white, or until sticky and fragrant. Once it reaches this stage, it is immediately immersed in cold water. The root bark is removed after this point, although in some production regions, the root bark is removed before boiling. A bamboo knife or broken piece of porcelain, rather than a metal instrument, is used to scrape off the bark. Next, it is dried in the sun for one day, and then piled into pyramid-shaped heaps to make the root "sweat." This procedure is repeated several times until the internal part of the root is completely dry. The dry roots are cut into slices before use.

A less elaborate process is to scrape away the outer bark, boil for 5 to 15 minutes (until the interior is soft), and then dry in the sun. Slice as needed.

The wild harvested *chi-shao* (*P. lactiflora, P. veitchii,* and *P. obovata*) is collected in spring or autumn, although autumn is preferred. The rhizome and lateral rootlets are removed, and the root is cleaned and dried until half dry. Curved roots are straightened by hand to improve appearance, uniformity, and market value. Then, the roots are graded according to size, tied up into small bundles, and placed in the sun to dry to 100 percent. In Sichuan, the root bark is removed before drying.

PROCESSING

For stir-fried *bai-shao,* slices are placed in a pan and stir-fried over a light fire until the exterior has a yellow color.

To make alcohol-processed *bai-shao*, slices are sprinkled with yellow wine, covered with a moist cloth for a short period of time, and stir-fried until the surface has a yellow color. For every 100 lbs. of *bai-shao*, 10 lbs. of yellow wine is used.

To produce black-surface *bai-shao*, slices of the root are stir-fried until the surface is blackish-yellow in color, and are then cooled.

"Roasted" or fried *chi-shao* is stir-fried for a short time until the roots are mostly yellow and have a few charred points on raised areas of the root.

ADDITIONAL SPECIES

Paeonia lactiflora var. *trichocarpa* (Bunge) Stern. is found in Jilin, Liaoning, Hebei, Shanxi, and Nei Mongol. The root is used as *chi-shao*.

The root of *Paeonia anomala* L., distributed in Gansu and Xinjiang, is used in these regions as a type of *chi-shao*.

Paeonia suffruticosa, the moutan (*mu-dan*) or tree peony, also produces an official drug of the Chinese *Pharmacopeia*, *mu-dan-pi*, which is the bark of the root. It is used in prescriptions to eliminate heat from the blood, disperse blood stasis, in the treatment of feverish diseases, vomiting of blood, amenorrhea, and external inflammation. It too is grown in American gardens.

The European peony (*P. officinalis*) was mentioned in the texts of Dioscorides, Pliny, and other classical *materia medica*. Like the Chinese peony, the European species has traditionally been used for the treatment of female ailments, as well as a sedative or antispasmodic. It is also used as a tonic, alterative, depurative, and antiepileptic.

The root of the western North America species, *Paeonia brownii*, was used by the Costanoans of central California for stomachache, indigestion, pneumonia, and as a laxative. Other native American groups in the West used it for a wide range of purposes, including coughs, kidney ailments, diarrhea, sore throat, externally as a wash for sore eyes, or as a poultice for cuts, wounds, sores, and burns.

OTHER USES

In fourteenth- and fifteenth-century England, the roots of *P. officinalis* were used to flavor roast pork. Peony seed was also used as flavoring. The root of *P. lactiflora* have been used as a food by nomadic groups in Mongolia.

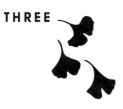

THREE

Ornamental Shrubs

Forsythia
Lian-qiao

Botanical name: *Forsythia suspensa* (Thunb.) Vahl.
Chinese Names: Pinyin: *Lian-qiao* (fruits). Wade-Giles: *Lien-ch'iao* (fruits).
English Names: Forsythia, golden-bells.
Pharmaceutical Name: Fructus Forsythiae.
Family: Oleaceae—olive family.

HISTORY

In every town in America, spring is marked by the bright yellow blooms of forsythias, which appear before the leaves emerge. Forsythia is one of the best-known spring flowering shrubs grown as an ornamental in North America. Forsythias are adaptable to many soil types, grow with ease, thrive on neglect, grow in city environs where other plants will not survive, and are virtually free from insect and disease pests. They are such a common part of the American landscape that they are taken for granted by most, and few people ever consider the plant's origins. Many people fail to realize that forsythia originates in East Asia, and fewer still know that the fruit of *Forsythia suspensa* is an important herbal product in traditional Chinese medicine.

The genus *Forsythia* of the olive family includes seven species, six of which are native to East Asia, with one species from Albania in southwestern Europe. *Forsythia suspensa* (Thunb.) Vahl was first classified in Western terms as *Ligustrum suspensum* by Carl Peter Thunberg, in his 1784 classic *Flora Japonica*. In 1804, the Danish botanist Martin Vahl (1749–1804) named the plant *Forsythia suspensa*, the Latin name by which it is known today. The generic name also serves as the English common name. Forsythia is named in honor of William Forsyth (1737–1804), a prominent Scottish horticulturist and botanist.

The famous Scottish botanical explorer, Robert Fortune, is credited with bringing forsythias from Asia to Europe in 1844. In those days, trips from China to England had to go around "the Horn," and the trip took four to five months. It was extremely difficult to transport seeds, and especially plants, under the adverse, unrefrigerated storage conditions of sailing vessels of the day. Fortune used Wardian cases (solariums) to transport the plants. Before setting sail, scions (or plants) were placed in soil inside the case, and they were then sealed in glass and put in a protected hold in the ship, where they would not be subject to salt spray. In his writings Fortune stated that "large vessels with poops" were the best means of transportation from the Orient. The "poop," or deep hold, helped to protect the plants from the elements.

The use of the fruits is first mentioned in the third class of herbs in the first-century A.D. *Shen Nong Ben Cao Jing*. The stems and the leaves, *lian-qiao-jing-ye*, are first mentioned in the 1596 *Ben Cao Gang Mu*. The use of the root, *lian-qiao-gen*, is first recorded in the 1670 Qing dynasty work by Zhang Lu, *Ben Jing Feng Yuan*.

TASTE AND CHARACTER

Bitter, a little cold.

FUNCTIONS

Forsythia capsules dispel heat, detoxify, disperse swelling, disperse accumulations resulting from blockage of vital energy (*qi/ch'i*), and disperse accumulations from blocked blood energy circulation.

USES

The seed capsules are used for febrile diseases, "hot" disease, carbuncles with swelling, sores with toxic matter, swollen lymph nodes, urinary infections, infection of the urethra, colds due to wind and heat, sore throat with swelling, inflammatory disease with redness of skin, scrofula, and boils.

The crude drug of forsythia is derived from the dried ripe fruits. It has primarily been used for its pus-eliminating and anti-inflammatory effect, both internally and externally. For example, for the treatment of inflamed sores a decoction of the fruit is used.

Clinical reports in the Chinese literature have focused on, among other ailments, the treatment of acute nephritis. A decoction of the capsules, taken before meals three times a day, was used for 5–10 days, depending upon the condition of the patient. Patients were not allowed to have hot (pungent) or salty food during this time. Eight cases were treated in this manner. Before treatment, all patients had edema and high blood pressure. After treatment, six of the patients had a complete reduction of edema, and two patients were much improved. The blood pressure had an obvious reduction in all cases.

For the treatment of lung abscesses, an intramuscular injection of *lian-qiao* was used (1 ml is equivalent to 1 g of crude drug). One dose was administered twice per week. Twenty-five cases were treated. Fourteen were cured, 10 were much improved, and one patient died. The mean success of treatment was 12 days in 18 patients.

Other clinical studies in China have focused on the successful use of *lian-qiao* in acute infectious disease, pulmonary tuberculosis, cervical lymph node tuberculosis, skin infections, acute viral hepatitis, hemorrhage of the retina, and purpureal skin lesions.

In laboratory experiments, *lian-qiao* is a broad spectrum antibiotic against numerous gram-positive and gram-negative bacteria. Forsythiaside is considered the strongest bacteriostatic compound in the fruits. The fruits have also been shown to have antifungal, anti-inflammatory, antipyretic, antinauseant, and diuretic action, and also have a slight tonic effect on the heart, show liver-protectant action, and may slightly lower blood pressure.

In Western terms, the fruits are considered antiphlogistic, laxative, diuretic, antifebrile, antitussive, tonic, and emmenagogic. They are primarily prescribed in the United States by TCM practitioners.

DOSE

Fruits: 6–15 g, in decoction, pills, powder, poultice, or as a wash.

DESCRIPTION

Forsythia is a glabrous (smooth), somewhat sprawling shrub growing from 3–9 feet in height. The internodes of the stems are hollow, but the nodes themselves (where leaves attach) have a solid pith. The opposite, simple leaves, often three-divided, are ovate or elliptical-ovate, up to 4 inches long, and toothed, except at the base. The tubular yellow flowers, appearing in spring before the leaves, are deeply four-parted giving the appearance of four petals. It is commonly planted in the United States, and numerous cultivars (cultivated varieties) are available. In addition, a hybrid between *F. suspensa* and *F. viridissima*, known as *F.* x *intermedia*, is also widely planted.

DISTRIBUTION

Wild plants grow in low mountain thickets and forest margins in Liaoning, Hebei, Henan, Shanxi, Shandong, Jiangsu, Jiangxi, Hubei, Shaanxi, Gansu, Ningxia, Sichuan, and Yunnan. Forsythia is commonly cultivated as an ornamental in China.

Major commercial production of the fruits is in Shanxi, Henan, Shaanxi, and Shandong. Shanxi and Henan are the two most important provinces in terms of production. "Old or yellow" *lian-qiao* is the most common forsythia product, sold throughout China. "Green" or unripe capsules, known as *qing-lian-qiao* or *qing-qiao*, are sold to Sichuan, Zhejiang, and the three largest cities in China, Beijing, Tianjin, and Shanghai.

Forsythia is widely planted and naturalized in Japan, Europe, and the United States.

CULTIVATION

Forsythia likes full sun or dappled shade, a warm, relatively moist situation, and is hardy throughout the United States. It is best grown in a sunny situation, sheltered from the wind. This shrub is tolerant of a wide variety of soils, growing well in a sandy or somewhat silty loam. In China, it is grown in gardens, along roadsides, or in idle fields with good drainage.

Seeds, divisions, cuttings, or layering are used for propagation. The seeds can be sown in spring. In China, before sowing, seeds are mixed with white sand and stratified underground for about 60 days. Once planted, they are covered with about ⅛ inch of soil. The soil is kept moist until emergence. In China ashes are used as a fertilizer on seed beds. When seedlings are about 1 foot high, they are transplanted to permanent locations. Individual plants are spaced at 5 to 7 feet apart.

If cuttings are used for propagation, the best time to take scions is spring or summer. Cut on the node itself, which will quickly develop roots. Divide the plants in spring to increase the size of planting. Old dead branches are trimmed off to stimulate new growth.

Normal forsythia plantings yield relatively few fruits. Recent studies at the Nanchuan Institute of Medicinal Plant Cultivation in Sichuan province have focused on the biological basis for low-yielding forsythia plantings. Fruit production can be increased through management by training the plants, proper timing of harvest, and prevention or elimination of disease and pest problems.

HARVESTING

"Green" *forsythia* or *qing-lian-qiao* (unripe seed capsules) is harvested in late August or early September (before September 10th), when the fruits are not very ripe and still have a greenish color. They are par boiled for a short time or steamed until "ripe." Then they are dried in the sun.

To produce "yellow, or old" *lian-qiao*, the ripened, yellowish seed capsules are harvested in late September or early October (before October 10). According to ancient tradition, the seeds themselves are removed and discarded, and the capsule is dried in the sun. The boat-shaped valve sections of the dried fruit, usually with the seeds removed, is the traditional form of the herbal product. However, during production of the 1977 edition of the *Pharmacopeia of the People's Republic of China*, researchers discovered that the seeds were rich in the active chemical components of the plant. Based on this modern discovery, the seeds are now retained as part of the herbal product. Applying modern science to traditional methods has helped to further refine and develop Chinese herbal remedies.

PROCESSING

Processing involves sifting away foreign matter, rubbing the capsules open, and removing stems or branches.

ADDITIONAL SPECIES

Forsythia europaea Degen & Bald. is from Albania. *Forsythia giraldiana* Lingelsh., *F. viridissima* Lindl., *F. ovata* Nakai, and *F. japonica* Mak., all from East Asia, are grown in American gardens. *Forsythia viridissima* is also used as a source plant for *lian-qiao*. In addition to *Forsythia suspensa*, *F. viridissima* and *F. ovata* have reportedly become locally naturalized in North America.

OTHER USES

The root of forsythia, *lian-qiao-gen*, is considered bitter, cold, and slightly poisonous. It has been used for high fever and jaundice. The root decoction has also been used as a wash on cancerous sores.

The stem and leaves of forsythia, *lian-qiao-jing-ye*, have traditionally been used in decoction as a folk remedy to treat accumulation of heat in the heart and lungs at a dose of 6–9 g.

Heavenly Bamboo
Nan-tian-zhu

Botanical names: *Nandina domestica* Thunb.
Chinese Names: Pinyin: *Nan-tian-zhu-zi* (fruits); *Tian-zhu-zi* (fruits); *Nan-tian-zhu* (plant); *Nan-tian-zhu-ye* (leaves); *Nan-tian-zhu-gen* (root). Wade-Giles: *Nan-t'ien-chu-tzu* (fruits); *T'ien-chu-tzu* (fruits); *Nan-t'ien-chu* (plant); *T'ien-chu-tzu-yeh* (leaves); *T'ien-chu-tzu-kên* (root).
English Names: heavenly bamboo, sacred bamboo, nandina.
Pharmaceutical Name: Fructus Nandinae.
Family: Berberidaceae—barberry family.

HISTORY

Heavenly bamboo is not a bamboo at all, but a semi-evergreen member of the barberry family, with dark green shiny stems that superficially resemble bamboo stalks. In China it is well known as a house plant. In Japan it has been grown as an ornamental for at least 1,200 years. In the United States, it is primarily planted as an ornamental in the south for the rich autumn color of the fruits, which persist late into the winter. The fruits are the source of a traditional Chinese Medicine, *tian-zhu-zi*.

Only one species in this genus, *Nandina domestica*, has long been cultivated in Asia as an ornamental. The genus *Nandina* was named by Thunberg in 1781. He named the species *Nandina domestica* in his *Flora Japonica* (1784). *Nandina* comes from the Japanese name of the plant, *nanten*, which is derived from the Chinese name "*nan tian-zhu*," meaning "southern heavenly bamboo." The specific epithet, *domestica*, refers to the fact that the plant is widely cultivated. The plant was introduced into English gardens in 1804 by William Kerr, who was appointed botanical collector in Canton for the Royal Botanical Garden at Kew in 1803.

Writing about heavenly bamboo in January 1849, the famous nineteenth-century Scottish botanical explorer, Robert Fortune, said:

> In the winter season at Shang hai a plant with red berries is seen in the gardens, which takes the place of our English

Holly. It is the N. domestica. The Chinese call it *tein chok* [t'ien chu] or "Sacred [Heavenly] Bamboo." Large quantities of its branches are brought at this time from the country and hawked about the streets. Each of these branches is crowned with a large bunch of red berries, not very unlike those of the common holly, and, contrasted with the dark, shining leaves, are singularly ornamental. It is used chiefly in the decoration of altars, not only in temples, but also in private dwellings and in boats—for here every house and boat has its altar. The Nandina is found in English gardens, but from these specimens no idea can be formed of its beauty. It does not appear to produce its fruit so freely in England as it does in China. (quoted in Bretschneider, 1898, Vol. 1)

The fruits are first mentioned in *Kai Bao Ben Cao* (*Materia Medica* of the Kai Bao Era), attributed to Ma Zhi, and published during the Song dynasty in 973 A.D. The use of the leaves is first noted in *Ben Cao Gang Mu Shi Yi* (Omissions from the Grand Materia Medica), authored by Zhao Xue-min, published in 1765 during the Qing dynasty.

Traditionally, a gourd-shaped charm of the wood was made and hung around the neck of a child to ward off whooping cough. Ancient herbals mention the planting of heavenly bamboo in gardens to prevent fire. Historically, it has also been planted next to washbasins in Japanese gardens to protect against evil.

TASTE AND CHARACTER

Fruit: sour, a little sweet, neutral, somewhat toxic. Leaves: bitter, cold, without poison. Root: bitter, cold.

FUNCTIONS

The fruit is astringent for lung, stops cough, disperses liver heat, tonifies tendons, benefits vital energy (*qi/ch'i*), and clears eyes. The leaves allay colds, stop cough, and reduce swelling. The root expels wind, disperses heat, expels wetness, and eliminates phlegm. The root and stems disperse heat, clear wetness, stimulate menstrual flow by removing blockage of menstrual-controlling meridians.

Uses

The fruit is used for chronic cough, asthma, whooping cough, malaria, and ulcer of the penis. It is also said to be useful in restoring the nervous system and quieting drunkards, and has been used as an antidote to fish poisoning. Folk tradition holds that the seeds increase virility.

The leaves are used for the common cold, whooping cough, red eyes, swellings with pain, scrofula, bloody urine, and infantile malnutrition.

The root is used for headache due to wind and heat, cough due to lung heat, jaundice with wetness and heat, rheumatism with pain, red eyes, carbuncle and furuncles, and scrofula.

The root and stem are used for fevers, the common cold, conjunctivitis, coughs due to lung heat, jaundice with wetness and heat, acute gastro-enteritis, infection of the urinary tract, and traumatic injuries.

The fruits, leaves, roots, and roots with stems of heavenly bamboo are traditional remedies that are not official in the current Chinese *Pharmacopeia*, and are seldom used in modern practice. Basically, the fruits are considered astringent to the lungs, strengthening to tendons, and beneficial to vital energy (*qi/ch'i*). As a folk remedy for whooping cough, the fruits are decocted with raw sugar added. For the treatment of malaria, one ancient remedy called for the "old fruits" of heavenly bamboo, (at least one year old). They were steamed until well done, and then a dose equal to one fruit for each year of the patient's age was given in the morning with boiled, hot water. The fruits were also once used as an antidote to arsenic poisoning. About 5 ounces of the fresh fruits or 1 to 2 ounces of the dried fruits were pulverized, and then taken with water. If the fresh fruits were used, they were simply soaked in water, but the dried fruits were decocted for the antidote. Fresh fruits were preferred. Given the potential toxicity of the fruits, the cure might have been worse than the poison.

A decoction of the leaves was used as a folk eyewash for heat and swelling of the eyes. For malnutrition in babies, the leaves were decocted and given instead of tea. The whole plant has been used as a poultice to treat inflammation of sores. For jaundice, a traditional prescription called for the fresh roots of the plant in decoction. For rheumatism, the fresh root was decocted with one or two pig's feet in red wine and water. This "soup" was simmered for several hours then taken in two to three doses. For the treatment of sciatica, one folk remedy called for a decoction of the root taken with alcohol. A folk cure for the treatment of traumatic injuries with shock called for a section of the root to be made into a paste with strong alcohol and hot water, which was then rubbed onto the affected area.

In laboratory experiments the fruits have proven antibacterial. The alkaloids domesticine and nandinine have an effect similar to that of morphine in cold-blooded animals, but have caused paralysis in experiments with warm-blooded animals. These alkaloids also have a cardiovascular inhibitory effect. In Western terms, the fruits are considered antitussive, and tonic. While the plant is widely grown as an ornamental in the southern United States, the herbal derivatives are not seen in markets outside of Chinatown herb shops.

DOSE

Fruit: 6–15 g in decoction, or burned into charcoal, retaining character; externally used as a poultice or ash powder mixed with oil for external application. Leaves: 9–15 g in decoction, poultice, or wash. Root: 30–60 g in decoction, tincture, poultice, decoction, wash, or applied to the eye.

WARNING

At least ten different alkaloids have been identified from the fruits. They are considered potentially toxic and should be used only by qualified TCM practitioners. Cases of respiratory paralysis have been reported from the use of the fruit in cases of pertussis in children.

DESCRIPTION

Heavenly bamboo is a semievergreen, smooth, spare branched shrub, somewhat resembling bamboo in appearance. It grows to a height of 8 feet. The stems are about as thick as a finger, somewhat jointed and cane-like, as in bamboos, although it is not related to bamboos. The alternate leaves are two- or three-divided, with leaflets narrowly ovate to broadly lance shaped, to 2 inches long; they turn red in autumn. The small, six-petaled, white (rarely purple) flowers are in terminal panicles. The bright scarlet fruits, up to ⅜ inches across, appear in late autumn, often persisting until the following spring. One cultivar has white berries. Many cultivars are known in Asia.

DISTRIBUTION

Heavenly bamboo grows in mixed forests, on mountain sides, and in shrub thickets. It is very commonly grown as a yard and garden ornamental in China, but is best known as a houseplant. It is sometimes cultivated for production of various plant parts for medicinal use. Heavenly bamboo is found in the middle and lower Yangtze River valley including Hebei, Shandong, Hubei, Jiangsu, Zhejiang, Anhui, Jiangxi, Guangdong, Guangxi, Yunnan, and Sichuan. It ranges from central China to India, and has been cultivated in Japan for many centuries (since at least 850 A.D.), where it is now naturalized in ravines and mountain valleys on the warmer parts of Honshu, Shikoku, and Kyushu. It is widely cultivated in the southern United States and is reportedly naturalized in some areas.

CULTIVATION

Heavenly bamboo prefers a warm, moist climate, and cannot bear extreme cold. It is root hardy where temperatures dip to –20°F., but attains full growth only where temperatures do not go below 0°F. It tends to be more hardy if well established. Good drainage is essential, and a neutral to slightly alkaline pH is preferable. It is propagated by seeds or root division. Plant the seeds after the last spring frost and keep them moist until emergence, about 30 days later. After two to three years' growth, seedlings can be transplanted. Divide roots in spring or late autumn. Give full sun.

HARVESTING

The root and stem are harvested at any time. The root is harvested from three- to four-year old plants, then cut into sections and dried in the sun. In autumn, winter, or the following spring, the persistent fruits are harvested and then dried in the sun. Seeds are produced after two or three years of growth. The fruits are subject to insect infestations and must be stored in tightly closed containers.

PROCESSING

None noted.

ADDITIONAL SPECIES

Nandina domestica is monotypic.

OTHER USES

The stem and branches, *nan-tian-zhu*, are used as a separate remedy in folk medicine. They are used to stop cough and to treat asthma. They may also act as a stimulant.

According to *The Wealth of India* (1948–1985), the wood has been used for chopsticks in China.

Matrimony Vine
Gou-qi-zi and *Di-gu-pi*

> **Botanical names:** Lycium barbarum L., (*L. halimifolium* Mill.);
> *Lycium chinense* Mill.
> **Chinese Names:** Pinyin: *Gou-qi-zi* (fruits); *Di-gu-pi* (root bark).
> Wade-Giles: *Kou-ch'i-tzu* (fruits); *Ti-ku-p'i* (root bark).
> **English Names:** Chinese matrimony vine (*L. chinense*), Duke of
> Argyll's tea tree (*L. barbarum*), boxthorn, wolfberry, etc.
> **Pharmaceutical Names:** Fructus Lycii, (fruit of *L. barbarum* and
> *L. chinense*); Cortex Lycii (root bark of *L. chinense* and *L. barbarum*).
> **Family:** Solanaceae—nightshade family.

HISTORY

According to an old myth, European species of matrimony vine were considered a curse to matrimonial bliss. If the plant grew next to a home, it meant misfortune for the marriage within. Perhaps this tale results from the thorny nature of the plant. Given its common name, however, in modern times, matrimony vine is associated more with marital bliss, rather than its demise.

The genus *Lycium* of the nightshade family includes about 100 species of warm temperate shrubs, especially abundant in the western United States as well as in South America. There are two centers of distribution in the Americas: Arizona, where 10 of the 14 native North American species are endemic, and Argentina, where 22 of the 30 South American species occur. Three species occur in Europe. There are at least six species in China.

In 1768 *Lycium chinensis* was first described and named by Phillip Miller (1691–1771) in his celebrated *Dictionary of Gardening*. *Lycium barbarum* was named by Linnaeus in his 1753 classic, *Species Plantarum*. The fruit of *L. barbarum* is an official drug listed in the 1985 Chinese *Pharmacopeia*, while the root bark of *L. chinense* and *L. barbarum* are official listings. *Lycium barbarum* has been cultivated in Europe for many centuries. *Lycium chinense* was cultivated in European botanical gardens as early as 1696.

The genus name *Lycium* derives from the Greek *lykion*, an ancient name of a species of *Rhamnus* (buckthorn) from Lycia. Linnaeus transferred that name to the genus of the nightshade family now referred to as *Lycium*. Pliny noted that *Lycium* was good for sore eyes, inflammation, and other ailments. Dioscorides also noted medicinal uses of *Lycium*, stating that preparations of various plant parts relieved inflammation and related ailments. *Lycium* was also mentioned by other writers, including Celsus and Galen.

The *Lycium* of the ancient Western world, however, is probably not the same plant group we refer to today. *Lycium* was imported from India, and is mentioned in listings of Indian drugs by the Roman custom house at Alexandria about 176–180 A.D. In the ancient world, *Lycium* was held in high esteem and was kept in vases or jars that were reserved expressly for the storage of this one drug. In 1833 the British botanist John Forbes Royle wrote "On the *Lycium* of Dioscorides," published in the *Transactions of the Linnean Society of London* in 1837, noting that the Indian *Lycium* of the ancients was identical to an extract known as rasaut (*rusot* or *rasot*), a high alkaloid extract of *Berberis* (barberry) species. The names *rusot* or *rasot* (*rasaut*) seem to have been used in a thirteenth-century Arab work by Ibn Baytar to refer to the ancient *Lycium*. Then, as now, *rasaut* is sold in bazaars in India and is used for the treatment of eye diseases. It should be noted that both North American and European *Berberis* species are used for the same purpose. The Indian *Lycium* so highly esteemed by the ancient Greek and Romans was probably *Berberis lycium*.

The bark of the root of *L. chinensis*, and *L. barbarum*, known in modern China as *di-gu-pi*, is initially mentioned in the first class of drugs in *Shen Nong Ben Cao Jing*. The fruit, *gou-qi-zi*, is first mentioned in the 500 A.D. work *Ming Yi Bei Lu* by Tao Hong-jing.

TASTE AND CHARACTER

Fruit: sweet, neutral. Bark: a little sweet, cold.

FUNCTIONS

The fruit invigorates the liver and kidney and supplements vital energy (*qi/ ch'i*). The bark dispels heat, reduces fever, cools the blood, and reduces blood pressure.

USES

The fruits are used in prescriptions for vertigo and dizziness, tinnitus, poor eyesight, cough due to deficiency, lower back pain, kidney deficiency, impotence, headache, seminal emission, and diabetes.

The root bark is used in prescriptions for low fever from tuberculosis, coughs and asthma due to lungs with heat, diabetes, vomiting with blood, nosebleed, bloody urine, high blood pressure, and bad sores.

The fruit of both *L. chinense* and *L. barbarum* is the Chinese traditional drug *guo-qi-zi*, which has long been a famous tonic in TCM. It is said to nourish the vital essence, serve as a general tonic, and improve the vision. In traditional applications it is used to tonify deficiency of the liver and "kidney." Many traditional prescriptions refer to the herb's "tonic" effects. A general tonic to improve skin color and impart strength called for two cups of the fruit to be macerated in 50 percent alcohol and left to stand for one week. The tincture was then strained, and the patient was given a nip every day. A tincture of the bruised fruits of matrimony vine was also prescribed for deficiency of the liver, or as a wash if the eyes had become "burned" by a strong, dry wind. In the summer time, weak patients were given a tea made by soaking matrimony vine fruits and schisandra fruits for three days, which they would drink instead of tea. In the 1985 Chinese *Pharmacopeia*, only the fruits of *L. barbarum* are listed as official drugs.

Lycium fruits are suggested for the enhancement of nonspecific immunity. The fruit extract has an experimental atropinelike effect for eye ailments. Fruit extracts experimentally reduce blood sugar, have a hypotensive effect, promote regeneration of liver cells, and prolong the time it takes for blood to coagulate. In rats, long-term ingestion resulted in increased serum and liver phospholids. The fruits contain betaine (about 1 percent), which is considered by some researchers to be its primary active component. The fruits are considered to be of low toxicity.

The root bark of both *L. barbarum* and *L. chinense* is official in the Chinese *Pharmacopeia*. The bark is primarily used to help reduce fever, reduce blood pressure, and act as a hemostatic. A decoction of the bark and a few tea leaves was used as a traditional folk remedy for malaria. Two or three hours before the anticipated return of the fever, the decoction was drunk. A traditional treatment for vomiting with blood, bloody urine, or bloody stool was simply to drink a decoction of the fruits and root bark of *Lycium*. Decocted with the leaves of mallow (*Malva neglecta*), the tea, with a little sugar added, was used as a treatment for boils. To relieve the pain of toothache, one folk cure called for the decoction of the root to be used as a mouthwash.

Confirming the traditional use of the root bark for treating toothache, a clinical report assessed its use for abscessed teeth. An extract of the root bark was made using 30 g of the root bark in 500 ml. of water, reduced to 50 ml. It was then filtered, and applied directly to the infected tooth with a cotton swab. Of 11 patients treated, all experienced a mitigation of pain. The average time it took to mitigate pain was one minute.

Studies in recent years have focused on the hypotensive, antibacterial, hypoglycemic, and fever-reducing activity of the root bark. A water extract of the root bark is considered to have a blood pressure-lowering effect due to a dilating effect on the blood vessels. A clinical report for the treatment of high blood pressure utilized 60 g of fresh root bark or whole root, or 30 g of the dried root bark. Two doses of the decoction were given per day. The course of treatment was 30 days. In the treatment of 36 cases, after 1 to 3 courses of treatment, 20 patients were reported to be much better, 5 patients had noticeable improvement, and 11 patients did not have any reduction in blood pressure. However, all of the patients reportedly felt better.

Lycium fruits are sold in American herb markets, but the root bark is not often seen.

DOSE

Fruits: 6–12 g. Bark: Decoct 6–15 g, or use in pill or powdered form, as a poultice, gargle, wash, or macerated in oil.

DESCRIPTION

Lycium chinense is a vigorous hardy deciduous shrub with arching or prostrate branches up to 12 feet long, often without thorns. The alternate or fascicled leaves are oval to lance-shaped, bright green, and up to 1½ to 3 inches long. The purplish flowers are five-lobed and ½ inch or more across. The lobes are nearly as long the the flower tube. The bright red-orange fruit is oval to oblong in shape, nearly 1 inch long, and half as wide. Fruiting is from June to September.

Lycium barbarum is a deciduous shrub with arching or spreading branches to 10 feet long. The linear to linear-oblong leaves are about 1 inch long. The five-parted corolla is pale rose in color. The stamen filaments are smooth at the base. There is considerable confusion about differences between *L. barbarum* and *L. halimifolium* Mill. (*L. barbarum* var. *vulgare* Ait.). In his *Manual of Cultivated Trees and Shrubs* (1954), Alfred Rehder notes that *L. barbarum* is not hardy in the northern United States and is distinguished by having smooth filaments (of the stamens) and narrower, smaller leaves. However, the confusion still persists today. *L. halimifolium* is often listed as a synonym for *L. barbarum*. For practical purposes in terms of herbal use, *L. barbarum* and *L. halimifolium*, cultivated or naturalized in the United States, are generally considered synonymous.

DISTRIBUTION

Lycium barbarum L. grows at high altitudes from 6,000 to 9,000 feet in sandy soils, dry soils, or thickets near streams. It often grows in cold areas in salty, sandy soil, in Hebei, Nei Mongol, Shanxi, Shaanxi, Gansu, Ningxia, Qinghai, and Xinjiang. It occurs westward to southeastern Europe, Iran, and North Africa. The plant is widely cultivated in Ningxia, where it is considered one of the most important medicinal plants. It is also commercially grown outside of the city of Tianjin (east of Beijing) from plant material introduced from Ningxia. There is also minor commercial production in Nei Mongol, Xinjiang, and Gansu. *Lycium barbarum* (*L. halimifolium*) is widely cultivated, and has escaped from cultivation in the eastern United States.

Lycium chinense occurs along mountain streams or small rivers, along roads, and rocky clefts in mountains and foothills, to a height of about 7,500 ft. It is common in much of East Asia, including eastern China, Japan, and Korea. It is naturalized both in Europe and the United States. In the United States it occurs in waste places and along roads from Massachusetts south to Virginia and Louisiana, west to Oklahoma, and north to Michigan.

CULTIVATION

Matrimony vine prefers a relatively cool climate and a sandy soil. It likes an alkaline soil, and thrives with a side-dressing of manure. It prefers a relatively moist but well-drained situation.

Seeds are used for propagation. In China, the dry fruits are soaked in water for one or two days, and then the seeds are washed out and dried in the sun. Sow the seeds in rows, and cover with less than a half inch of soil. Keep the seed moist. Emergence takes place in about ten days. Thin out weak seedlings as appropriate. The following year, seedlings are transplanted to permanent locations in early April. Rows are spaced at about 8 feet, with 6 foot spacing between individual plants.

Lycium is also propagated with cuttings. In spring before buds fully develop, choose growth from the previous year, cut into 6 inches sections, and place obliquely in a rooting bed. Keep warm until the leaves appear. Transplant once new roots are established. In China, during the second year of growth, when plants reach about four feet in height, the tops are pruned back to encourage branching. Every year, the crown is pruned two or three times to give the bushes a rounded form, making the fruit harvest easier. Plants are kept watered during the flowering and fruiting period. In spring and summer, dead or dense branches are pruned.

HARVESTING

The fruits are harvested when ripe in late summer or autumn. They are spread thinly on a bamboo mat to dry and are dried in a shaded, well-ventilated area, or baked under light heat. The fruits are not turned while drying since this may bruise them, causing them to turn black.

The bark of the root is harvested in spring or autumn. The best time is considered from November to the spring of the following year. The root is cleaned and dried in the sun.

PROCESSING

The calyx are removed from the fruits, along with any extraneous branchlets or leaflets. No special processing noted.

The root bark is washed, although not too vigorously, dried in the sun, and then cut into sections.

ADDITIONAL SPECIES

Several additional species of *Lycium* are used as substitutes in various parts of China. *Lycium turcomanicum* and *L. potaninii* (*L. chinensis* var. *potaninii*) are produced in Gansu. *Lycium dasystemum* is used in Xinjiang.

In Fujian the bark of *Clerodendron cyrtophyllum* has been used as an adulterant to *Lycium* root bark.

OTHER USES

The leaves are also used in Chinese medicine, and the young shoots, like those of *L. europeum*, are eaten in spring. A folk belief holds that using the leaves year-round instead of tea will promote excellent health. The leaves have been used as a tonic in degenerative diseases and to allay symptoms of pulmonary consumption.

Thorny matrimony vines such as *L. barbarum* are sometimes grown as hedge plants. The fruits of some species are eaten.

In India the leaves of *L. barbarum* are considered poisonous to livestock and camels. Severe digestive tract lesions have been reported in cases of poisoning among sheep and calves in the United States.

Privet
Nu-zhen-zi

Botanical names: *Ligustrum lucidum* Ait.
Chinese Names: Pinyin: *Nu-zhen-zi* (fruits). Wade-Giles: *Nu-chen-tzu* (fruits).
English Names: Chinese privet, Glossy privet, Nepal privet, wax-leaf privet, white wax tree.
Pharmaceutical Name: Fructus Ligustri Lucidi.
Family: Oleaceae—olive family.

HISTORY

In the United States, the word *privet* is associated with hedges. The privets, especially European privet, *Ligustrum vulgare*, which is native to Europe and North Africa, has been a favorite and one of the most widely grown hedges for many decades. In *More Aristocrats of the Garden* (1928, p. 71), E. H. Wilson describes privets as "greedy feeders unmerciful to flower-border and lawn. They grow freely and quickly and need clipping three or four times a year to keep within proper shape and bounds."

Our subject, the glossy or Chinese privet (*L. lucidum*) is grown in the southern United States as an evergreen hedge shrub. It is not hardy where temperatures dip below 0°F. However, it is found in another form in American herb markets, especially Chinatown herb shops. The dried fruits are the Chinese herb product *nu-zhen-zi*. In Chinese tradition the evergreen leaves of *L. lucidum* have been regarded as a symbol of chastity, hence the Chinese name, *nu-zhen*, meaning "female chastity." "*Zi*" means "fruits."

The genus *Ligustrum* of the olive family has about 50 species native to Europe, East and Southeast Asia, and Australia. The group includes both deciduous and evergreen shrubs and small trees, generally known as privets. *Ligustrum vulgare*, the common or European privet, has been grown as a hedge plant in Europe since the end of the sixteenth century. It is widely naturalized in North America. The Japanese species *L. ovalifolium* is commonly grown as a hedge plant in Europe today. The Chinese privet, *Ligustrum lucidum*, was introduced to England from China in 1794 by Sir Joseph Banks.

The genus *Ligustrum* was established by Linnaeus in 1753. It derives from the Latin *ligare*, meaning to tie, referring to the use of the flexible branches for lashing. *Ligustrum lucidum* is the name given to the Chinese privet in 1810 by the British botanist William Aiton (1731–1793).

The fruits first appear in the primary class of drugs in *Shen Nong Ben Cao Jing*, and are mentioned in all of the ancient *ben cao*. The plant used today is the same as identified in the ancient *ben cao*. The use of the bark of *L. lucidum* is first mentioned in Su Song's 1061 classic, *Tu Jing Ben Cao*. The use of the leaves is first noted in *Ben Cao Gang Mu*.

TASTE AND CHARACTER

A little sweet, bitter, neutral.

FUNCTIONS

Invigorates the liver and kidney, strengthens the waist and knees, clears the ears and eyes, darkens hair.

USES

For yin deficiency of the liver and kidneys, vertigo, tinnitus, premature gray hair, habitual constipation of older persons, and benzene poisoning.

The fruits of *L. lucidum* (*nu-zhen-zi*) are official in the 1985 Chinese *Pharmacopeia*. In traditional Chinese medicine it has primarily served as a tonic for the liver and kidney. Primary uses have focused on "yin" deficiencies associated with these organs or body symptoms, which includes tinnitus, dizziness, blurred vision, premature graying, and low back pain. For example, a traditional treatment to invigorate the liver and kidney, strengthen the waist and knees, and stop premature graying uses *nu-zhen-zi* harvested in late December. The fruits are dried indoors, mixed with a little honey and wine, and steamed. After steaming they are allowed to sit overnight, and then are dried in the sun the next day. The fruits are then powdered, stored in an earthen container, and a little bit of the powder is taken every day.

Like *astragalus* (*huang-qi*), the fruits of Chinese privet, or *nu-zhen-zi*, have been the subject of recent studies both in China and the United States for enhancing white blood cells counts after chemotherapy or radiotherapy treatments, primarily for cancer. These treatments reduce white blood cell counts; *nu-zhen-zi* helps to raise them to normal levels. Extracts of the fruit seem to enhance immunological function. An alcohol-precipitated decoction of the fruits has experimentally increased coronary flow while inhibiting myocardial contractility, but without a marked change in heart rate. In experiments water extracts have been shown to inhibit cervical cancers in mice. Extracts of the fruits are also antibacterial.

Clinical trials in China have used *nu-zhen-zi* for leukopenia (reduction in white blood cell count from chemotherapy or radiotherapy), infections of the respiratory tract, hypertension, acute icteric hepatitis, early cataracts, and Parkinson's disease. Positive results were reported. Use of the fruits to help enhance immune function following chemotherapy has real therapeutic potential for Western medicine.

In Western terms, *nu-zhen-zi* is considered a mild cardiac stimulant, diuretic, immunostimulant, anodyne, nutritive, and mildly laxative. The fruits are found increasingly in herb products sold in the United States.

DOSE

Dose 4.5–15 g, in decoction, pills, powder, extract, etc. Toxicity is considered very low.

DESCRIPTION

Chinese privet is a large shrub or small tree growing to 30 feet tall. The evergreen leaves are ovate or elliptical lance-shaped, papery, glossy, and 3 to 4½ inches long. The creamy white, fragrant flowers are in panicles to 8 inches long. It blooms in July and August. The oblong blue-black fruits are about ½ inch long. Numerous cultivated varieties (cultivars) are available in American horticulture.

DISTRIBUTION

Chinese privet occurs in warm, moist soils, on sunny mountainsides, and is often cultivated in gardens or along the edges of farm fields. In China it grows in Hebei, Henan, Shanxi, Shandong, Jiangsu, Anhui, Zhejiang, Jiangxi, Fujian, Taiwan, Hubei, Hunan, Guangxi, Guangdong, Shaanxi, Gansu, Yunnan, Guizhou, and Sichuan.

Major commercial production of the fruits is in Zhejiang, Jiangsu, Hunan, Fujian, Guangxi, Jiangxi, and Sichuan. Most is sold to distribution centers in Beijing, Tanjing, and Shanghai. The provinces of Guizhou, Guangdong, Hubei, Henan, Anhui, and Shanxi all have minor production, which is usually consumed locally.

Chinese privet is grown in the southern United States, where it has escaped locally from cultivation. It is not hardy in the north. Chinese privet is commonly planted as a small street tree in southern Europe.

CULTIVATION

Chinese privet is not particular about soil and climate, though it is not tolerant of extreme cold. In China it is generally grown on plains or in low mountain hills. It is propagated by seed. The fruits are harvested in December. Just after harvest, the seeds are drilled in seedbeds with rows spaced at 2 feet. Seeds are covered with ½ to 1 inch of soil. In early spring two years later, the young seedlings are transplanted to permanent locations. Individual plants are spaced at 12 to 14 feet. The plantings are cultivated and weeded one or two times a year, and side-dressed with manure once or twice a year for 2 to 3 years. When plantings are well-established, they are side-dressed with manure once a year.

HARVESTING

The fruits of wild or cultivated plants are harvested when ripe, in late fall or early winter. Cultivated plants usually begin producing fruit in 4 to 5 years. After harvest, they are washed and dried in the sun or steamed before drying in the sun (see below). Another method involves smoking the fruits over a fire of the branches for a short time, after which the fruit is dried under sun.

PROCESSING

Alcohol-processed *nu-zhen-zi* is made by mixing 20 pounds of yellow wine with 100 pounds of the fresh fruits. They are placed in a crock and sealed up until the fruit has absorbed the wine. The fruits are then removed and dried in the sun.

Steamed *nu-zhen-zi* is made simply by placing the fruits in a double boiler and steaming them until "ripe." They are then cooled and dried in the sun. This is a new technique based on modern Chinese research on traditional processing methods, which found no difference in *nu-zhen-zi* processed with or without alcohol.

ADDITIONAL SPECIES

There are two kinds of fruit on the market. One is plump and strong, while the other is thin, shriveled and not of very good quality. Most of the fruit found in commerce are the lower-quality fruits. Both plump and shriveled fruits are found on the same plants. The plump fruits are found on branches in full sun, and have two seeds. The shriveled fruits have only one seed.

Ligustrum thibeticum is used as a substitute for *nu-zhen-zi* in Xizang (Tibet).

OTHER USES

The branches, leaves, and bark are used to expel phlegm, stop coughs, and treat bronchitis. The dose is 30–60 g.

The leaves, collected throughout the year, are considered a little bitter and neutral. They expel wind, clear the eyes, reduce pain, and reduce swelling. The leaves have traditionally been used in prescriptions for headache, vertigo, red eye, sores, swelling, ulcers, burns, and inflammation of the oral cavity. A decoction of 9–15 g of the leaves is used, or they are used as a poultice. A thin extract of the leaves is used for eye ailments, or the leaf juice is gargled for oral inflammation or peritonitis.

The bark of Chinese privet, tinctured in alcohol, is traditionally used to strengthen the kidneys. The powdered bark has also been used in prescriptions for burns, and chronic bronchitis. Either 60 g of the bark or 90 g of the branches with leaves can be decocted with a little sugar to treat bronchitis. The course of treatment is 10 days. Two courses of treatment are often administered.

The root of Chinese privet, collected in September and October, is a relatively new herbal medicine in China. It is considered bitter and neutral. It disperses blood stasis, and stops pain moving about the body due to excessive vital energy (qi/ch'i), coughs, and leukorrhea.

The wood of Chinese privet is yellowish-brown, elastic, even-grained and hard. In India it is used for making small agricultural implements. In China the wood has been used for walking sticks, hay forks, and umbrella handles.

The shrub also produces an exudation of the branches—a white wax caused by an insect. The Chinese white wax was once widely used, and is considered superior to ordinary waxes because it is less sticky and burns with a brighter flame when used in candles.

Rose-of-Sharon
Mu-jin-hua

Botanical Name: *Hibiscus syriacus* L.

Chinese Names: Pinyin: *Mu-jin-hua, Da-jin-hua* (flowers); *Mu-jin-pi* (bark); *Mu-jin-zi* (seeds); *Mu-jin-gen* (root). Wade-Giles: *Mu-chin-hua, Ta-chin-hua* (flowers); *Ch'uan-chin-p'i, Mu-chin-pi* (bark); *Mu-chin-tzu* (seeds); *Mu-chin-kên* (root).

English Names: Rose-of-Sharon, shrubby althaea, Syrian rose, Syrian ketmie.
Pharmaceutical Names: Flos Hibisci; Cortex Hibisci.
Family: Malvaceae—mallow family.

HISTORY

Native to China, the name Syrian rose is a misnomer. It does not occur naturally in the Middle East, but was brought to Europe via western Asian trade routes at some point prior to 1600. The genus *Hibiscus* contains about 200 species native to warm temperate and tropical regions. *Hibiscus syriacus* is the most commonly cultivated hardy flowering hibiscus in American and European gardens. The plant was named by Linnaeus in 1753. *Hibiscus* is an old Greek name for a large-flowered mallow.

While rose-of-Sharon had been known in European flower gardens for at least three centuries, it was not until the end of the nineteenth century that the native home of the plant was determined by European explorers. The Irish-born physician Augustine Henry and the Scot Robert Fortune observed it growing both wild and cultivated in China during the nineteenth century. It arrived in the United States at an early date, brought by European colonists. The medicinal use of the plant was described in the 1588 *Hortus Medicus et Philosophicus* by the German physician and botanist, Joachim Camerarius the Younger (1534–1598). The shrub is also mentioned in the 1633 Thomas Johnson edition of *Gerard's Herball*. While noted in sixteenth–century herbals, it is virtually unknown as a medicinal plant in the West.

The Chinese name for the flowers *mu-jin-hua* refers to the fact that the flower lasts for a short time, blooming in morning, then withering in evening. The flowers were first mentioned in the *Ri Hua Zi Ben Cao*, a work published in the Tang dynasty around 915 A.D. The medicinal use of the fruit and bark are first mentioned by Li Shi-zhen in *Ben Cao Gang Mu*. The dried flower is the main traditional drug produced from the plant, but the trunk and root bark, fruits, root and leaves are also used.

TASTE AND CHARACTER

Flowers: bitter, a little sweet, neutral. Bark of tree and root: a little sweet, bitter, cool. Root: a little sweet, neutral. Fruit: a little sweet, neutral, without poison.

FUNCTIONS

The flowers dispel heat, cool blood, detoxify, reduce swelling, and promote diuresis.

The bark of tree and root dispels heat, promotes diuresis to eliminate wetness, detoxifies, stops itching, and kills worms.

The root is considered to be without poison and clears away heat and toxic matter, promotes diuresis to eliminate wetness, and subsides swelling.

The fruit clears away lung heat, is an expectorant, dispels toxic matter and stops pain.

USES

The flowers are used in prescriptions for dysentery, mucous vaginal discharges, diarrhea, bloody stool, and dysentery. Externally, they are poulticed for sores, boils, hemorrhoids, carbuncles with swelling, and burns.

The bark of tree and root is used in prescriptions for bloody stool, diarrhea with blood, dysentery, prolapsed anus, and mucous vaginal discharges. Externally it is used for ringworm, hemorrhoids, scrotum itch, eczema, and athletes foot.

The root is used in prescriptions for cough, lung abscesses, acute appendicitis, bloody stool, swelling and pain of hemorrhoids, mucous vaginal discharges, and ringworm.

The fruit is traditionally used for asthma with phlegm and cough, headache due to nervousness, and migraine.

The flowers, bark of the stem and root, root, and fruit are relatively minor articles of *material medica* in traditional Chinese medicine and are not official in the 1985 Chinese *Pharmacopeia*. In laboratory testing the flowers have been shown to have weak antibacterial activity. The flowers are considered nontoxic. The root has some antibacterial and antifungal activity. Water extracts of the fruits been used as a folk cancer remedy.

The flowers have been used as a traditional treatment for dysentery, hemorrhoids, and patients "with confused mind due to wind and heat." Traditional prescriptions using the flower sometimes call for a particular flower color. For example, for dysentery, a decoction of 30 g of white rose-of-Sharon flowers with 30 g of lump sugar is used. One dose is taken per day. For severe dysentery, accompanied by shivering and an inability to eat food, one prescription calls for the red-flowered form of rose-of-Sharon. The calyx of the flower is removed; the flower is then dried in the shade and added to biscuit batter. The biscuits are eaten to give the patient some nutrition, as well as to be as a delivery method for the herb. An old prescription to treat a patient with "confused mind due to wind and phlegm," calls for the powder of the sun-dried flowers to be baked, and then one or two spoonfuls of the powder to be taken before meals in very hot water. In this case, the white-flowered forms of rose-of-Sharon are preferred. In treating vaginal mucous discharge, 6 g of the powdered flower is mixed with human milk and taken. The dried flowers have been used in decoction for the treatment of hemorrhoids. The fresh flowers, mixed with a little "sweet vine," have been applied externally as a folk treatment for boils.

A clinical report for the treatment of bacterial dysentery used 2 g doses of the dried flowers in powder. One dose was administered every two hours for three days. In the treatment of 300 patients, temperature was reduced and stools returned to normal in two to three days in 96.3 percent of those treated.

The powdered bark, considered to have an antifungal affect, is traditionally mixed with vinegar, decocted for hours until it becomes thick and sticky, and then applied to ringworm. A solution of the bark in salt water has been used as another folk remedy for ringworm. The bark is also used in prescriptions as an external folk treatment for neurodermatitis. Internally, a decoction of the bark, drunk instead of tea, has been used as a folk treatment for diabetes.

A decoction of the root used as a steam bath or wash is a folk remedy for the treatment of hemorrhoids.

An ancient prescription for impetigo used the fruit that has been stir-fried until browned on the outside, without destroying the character, and then mixed with the bone marrow of a pig and used as a poultice on the affected area.

Several clinical reports have focused on using the bark to treat chronic cases of bronchitis. The bark is decocted two times. The two decoctions are combined and boiled down to an thin extract. A doses is given once in the morning and once at night. The reported course of treatment was 10 days. In the treatment of 177 cases, only 2 patients were cured (1.3 percent). Twenty-five patients experienced marked improvement (14.13 percent) of symptoms, while there was some improvement in 72 cases. No serious side effects were reported, but some patients experienced light vertigo, with some stomach swelling.

In Western terms, the flowers are considered astringent, antidiarrheal, and expectorant. The bark and root are considered mucilaginous, demulcent, antifungal, and febrifugal. Herb products derived from the plant are seldom seen in American herb markets outside of Chinatowns in major cities. The plant is commonly grown as an ornamental, especially in the southern United States.

DOSE

Dried flowers are used in doses of 3–9 g. The fresh flowers are used in doses of 30–60 g. They are used decocted, poulticed, in powder, or in ointment made by mixing the powdered fried flowers into sesame oil. The dried bark of shrub and root is used in 3–9 g doses in decoction, externally as a wash, steamed or as a fumigant (smoke), poulticed after soaking in wine, or powdered and mixed with vinegar for a poultice. A tincture of the bark in 50 percent alcohol is used externally. The fresh root is used in doses of 30–60 g in decoction or as a poultice or wash. The fruit is used in doses of 9–15 g, poulticed (for impetigo) or charcoaled and mixed with sesame oil and applied as necessary. The burning fruit is used as a smoke fumigant, with the smoke directed at the affected area.

DESCRIPTION

Rose-of-Sharon is a deciduous shrub of about 9 feet, or occasionally a small tree of 15–18 feet. Leaves are alternate, palmately veined or lobed, ovate or rhombic-ovate, 2 to 4 inches long, usually three-lobed, and coarsely toothed with rounded teeth. They are smooth above, with a few hairs on the veins beneath. The attractive, solitary, broad bell-shaped, five-lobed flowers are white, pink, red, or purple-violet, and 3 to 4 inches across. Stamens are numerous, surrounding the five-lobed style. Double-flowered or semi-double varieties are available. The oblong, short, beaked, densely hairy seed capsule holds dark-brown, hairy seeds. Numerous cultivated varieties are available in American horticulture, including cultivars with variegated leaves. It flowers from July to September. Rose-of-Sharon is widely cultivated for its showy, late-blooming flowers.

DISTRIBUTION

Rose-of-Sharon grows wild in South China and is cultivated throughout most of China. It is grown in Liaoning, Hebei, Shaanxi, Gansu, Ningxia, Shandong, Jiangsu, Zhejiang, Jiangxi, Fujian, Henan, Hubei, Hunan, Guangxi, Guangdong, Sichuan, Yunnan, Guizhou, and Xizang (Tibet).

Major production is in Jiangsu, Hubei, Sichuan, Henan, Hebei, and Shaanxi. Sichuan is the major producer of the dried flowers. Major production of the dried fruits is in Jiangsu and Guangxi.

The shrub has escaped from cultivation in the United States and is naturalized along roadsides and in thickets from Connecticut and New York south to Florida, and west to Texas.

It is widely cultivated as an ornamental in Europe, the Middle East, India, and Japan as well.

CULTIVATION

The tree is not particular about its surroundings; it is generally considered very adaptable. It is a frost-hardy plant if not grown in too dry a location. It does best in a rich, somewhat sandy, well-drained soil in a sunny situation. Rose-of-Sharon will tolerate heavy pruning. Usually propagated by cuttings, it can also be increased through layering or grafting. In Sichuan, from February to March, strong branches about ¼ inch thick are selected, cut into sections 6 to 8 inches long, and placed in beds to root.

HARVESTING

The flowers are collected on a sunny day in full bloom during the peak flowering season. They are dried in either sun or shade in well-ventilated conditions. Large white-colored flowers are considered the best quality. The root is harvested in autumn, and then dried in the sun. The bark is harvested in April or May and dried in the sun. The ripe fruits are harvested when they have turned a yellowish-green color in September to October, and dried in the sun.

PROCESSING

The bark is processed after harvesting by soaking it in water for a short time, then covering it with a wet cloth until uniformly moist. It is then cut into sections before being dried.

ADDITIONAL SPECIES

Some species, such as *H. cannabinus* L., known as kenaf, are cultivated for fiber. It is currently being grown in the southern United States as a possible paper pulp source. Other species are grown for their wood, or for the use of the fleshy calyx in beverages, jellies, and other foods. The leaves of some species are eaten like spinach.

OTHER USES

The fresh leaves (*mu-jin-ye*) have been used as a folk remedy to treat bloody stool, as well as heat and thirst from dysentery. From 30 to 60 g of the fresh leaves are used in decoction or poulticed for the treatment of boils. The leaves are crushed, mixed with salt, and applied to boils. The leaves are also considered stomachic and have been used as a tea substitute in China. In Western terms the leaf is considered stomachic, diuretic, and expectorant.

The stems yield a strong fiber. It has been used as a fiber plant. The flowers are considered edible.

Vitex
Huang-jing-zi

Botanical Names: *Vitex negundo* L., *Vitex negundo* L. var. *heterophylla* (Franch.) Rehd. In Chinese tradition *Vitex negundo* L. var. *cannabifolia* (Sieb. et Zucc.) Hand.-Mazz. is considered a separate drug-producing plant.

Chinese Names: Pinyin: *Huang-jing-zi* (seeds); *Huang-jing-ye* (leaves); *Huang-jing-zhi* (branches); *Huang-jing-gen* (root). Wade-Giles: *Huang-ching-tzu* (seeds); *Huang-ching-yueh* (leaves); *Huang-ching-chih* (branches); *Huang-ching-kên* (root). *Vitex negundo* var. *cannabifolia* is known as *Mu-Jing* (Pinyin) or *Mu-ching* (Wade-Giles).

English Names: Vitex, five-leaved chaste tree.

Pharmaceutical Name: Fructus Viticis negundinis.

Family: Verbeneaceae—verbena family.

HISTORY

Vitex negundo is a very common species in China. In and around Beijing, it is one of the most common wild shrubs. The seeds of the plant are wild-harvested in the mountains just outside of Beijing and throughout much of China for local markets. In China, seed preparations are widely used as a cold remedy. The shrub is grown in American gardens, primarily in the South, for the ornamental effect of the violet flower spikes.

The genus *Vitex* of the verbena family includes about 250 species in tropical and temperate regions of the world. *Vitex negundo* was named by Linnaeus in 1753. Since this species is highly variable, with at least seven varieties recognized in China, numerous botanical synonyms are found in the literature. The typical species, as well as *V. negundo* var. *heterophylla*, and *V. negundo* var. *cannibifolia*, are used in Chinese medicine. *Vitex negundo* was introduced into Parisian botanical gardens around 1697, from Jesuit missionaries stationed in China. It arrived in English botanical gardens by the 1740s. *Vitex negundo* var. *heterophylla* arrived in Europe around 1750. The date of introduction to the United States is not clear. *Vitex* is the old Latin name for this, or shrubs of similar appearance, mentioned in the writings of Pliny.

The fruit is the main part of the plant used in Chinese medicine. It is first mention in *Tu Jing Ben Cao*, attributed to Su Song and published in 1061 A.D. Some Chinese scholars believe the plant was first described in *Shen Nong Ben Cao Jing*, but modern Chinese scholars of bencaology (study of Chinese herbals), believe that Shen Nong may have referred to another species. It is also listed in *Ben Cao Gang Mu Shi Yi*, a 1765 Qing dynasty work by Zhao Xue-min. The leaves are first mentioned in *Ben Cao Gang Mu Shi Yi*. The use of the branches was first mentioned in a recent work, and is not found in the ancient *ben cao*.

TASTE AND CHARACTER

Fruits: hot, bitter, warm. Root: bitter, a little hot, neutral. Leaves: a little sweet, bitter, neutral. Branches: Hot, warm.

FUNCTIONS

Fruits are used in prescriptions to expel wind, expel phlegm, stop cough, relieve asthma, regulate vital energy, and stop pain.

The root is used to clear away heat, stop coughing, expel phlegm, and treat malaria.

The leaves are used to clear away heat, dispel pathogenic factors from the exterior of the body through diaphoresis, expel wetness, treat malaria, and are used as a detoxicant.

The branches expel wind, dispel pathogenic factors through diaphoresis, reduce swelling, and are detoxicant.

USES

The fruits are used in preparations for the common cold, chronic bronchitis, cough, asthma, stomachache, dyspepsia, enteritis, dysentery, hernias, joint pains, malaria, rheumatism, and hemorrhoids.

The root is used in prescriptions for chronic bronchitis, malaria, hepatitis, the common cold, coughs, asthma, rheumatism, stomachache due to summer heat, and malaria.

The leaves are used in prescriptions for the common cold, enteritis, dysentery, malaria, infections of the urinary system, summer fever, vomiting and diarrhea, and jaundice. Externally, poultices are used for eczema, skin diseases, skin inflammations, injuries, scabies, and ringworm. The fresh leaves are poulticed for insect and snake bites, and are insecticidal against mosquito larvae and maggots.

The branches are traditionally used for the common cold, cough, sore throat, rheumatism, pains of the bones, and toothache.

The seeds (fruits), root, and leaves of vitex have been valued in Chinese traditional medicine their for stomachic and cough suppressing value, primarily in the treatment of the common cold, coughs, asthma, and digestive disturbances. The seeds of *huang-jing* are the primary part that is used. The oil from the seeds of *Vitex negundo* var. *heterophylla*, considered a separate herbal product in Chinese tradition (*mu-jing-you*) is listed as an official drug in the 1985 Chinese *Pharmacopeia*. No plant parts of typical *Vitex negundo* are officially accepted in the Chinese *Pharmacopeia*.

Experimentally, the fruits are considered expectorant and suppress coughs. A 70 percent tincture of the fruits and the essential oil of the fruits are antibacterial against *Staphylococcus aureus* and are bronchodilators, anodyne, and sedative. Leaf extracts of *V. negundo* show experimental antitumor activity against the Ehrlich ascites tumor system. Leaf extracts have also been shown to prevent joint swelling in arthritic rats.

For pain of the stomach or liver, the seeds are powdered, made into flour, and added to food. A modern prescription for pain in the stomach and intestines or pain following an operation calls for the powdered seed. A traditional treatment for asthma calls for 6–15 g of the powdered seeds with a little white sugar mixed in to taste. Divided into two doses for one day, the powder is taken in hot water. For hiccups, sour stomach, and constipation a traditional prescription calls for 15 g of the seed decocted or infused in hot water. This is divided into two doses, one in the morning and one in the evening. For bleeding hemorrhoids, the seeds are stir-fried, powdered, and then mixed with a little raw sugar. The powder is taken before meals with wine. Traditionally, to treat dysentery, enteritis, and dyspepsia, 8 parts of the seed are taken with 1 part brewer's yeast and 8 parts white sugar. The seeds are first stir-fried until they are yellow, powdered, and mixed with the white sugar and yeast. The adult dose is placed at 4–6 g (1–2 g for children), with four doses taken per day.

The fresh root is used to treat chronic bronchitis. It is decocted into a thick syrup and taken once in the morning and once at night for a period of 10 to 20 days, as necessary.

For the treatment of ringworm, 250 g of the fresh leaves are placed in a large bowl of hot water and soaked until the water turns light green. Cold water is then added, and the feet are soaked in the water for five or six minutes before going to bed at night. A poultice of the leaves has also been used as a treatment for ringworm.

To kill mosquitos, the fresh leaves are mixed with dried grass and burned as a fumigant. The windows and doors are kept closed for two hours to fumigate the house.

A folk treatment for bites of poisonous snakes, accompanied with redness and swelling throughout the body and blisters, calls for the pulverized fresh tops of the plant. The plant is juiced, and the juice is drunk. The spent leaves are used as a poultice directly on the bite. The crushed fresh leaves have also been used as a poultice for dog or centipede bites. A decoction of the fresh leaves has been used as a folk treatment for malaria.

One clinical report for the treatment of chronic bronchitis used the powdered, roasted seeds made into large "honey pills," each containing 9 g of the powder. The treatment was given 3 times per day for 9 days, and continued for two courses of treatment. Of 46 patients treated, it controlled the symptoms in 5 patients who were relieved of all symptoms in a short time; 17 patients showed great improvement; 15 patients had some improvement. The most noticeable effect was that of an expectorant. Most of the patients experienced an expectorant effect by the second day. The remedy seemed to be most effective in mild cases with "cold deficiency." No side effects were observed.

Another clinical report in the Chinese literature on treating chronic bronchitis described the use of a root decoction. The decoction was brought to a boil, simmered under low heat for two to three hours, and separated into two doses for one day. The course of treatment lasted ten days, and two courses of treatment were administered. In the treatment of 335 cases, the total rate of efficacy was placed at 84.2 percent, with much improvement noted in 34.2 percent of the patients. It controlled asthma, cough, phlegm, inflammation, and wheezing in the chest; it helped to control asthmalike symptoms best. It was considered less effective for coughs or as an expectorant. Patients with mild cases of short duration responded much better than those with long-standing cases of bronchitis. The treatment was contraindicated in patients with high blood pressure or heart disease. Side effects reported included diarrhea, stomachache, nausea, lack of appetite, headache, and heart palpitations. These side effects were described as very light in the patients that experienced them, and according to the report, they did not interfere with the treatment.

A clinical report on acute enteritis in 40 patients used five handfuls of the fresh young leaves, which were decocted and taken in one daily dose. The condition was more or less controlled in about 70 percent of the patients. In summer, a tea made from the leaves is also drunk as a preventative for enteritis.

In Western terms, various plant parts of vitex are considered expectorant, antitussive, febrifugal, tonic, astringent, antibacterial, sedative, and anodyne. It is a little-known herb product on the American market.

Vitex negundo var. *cannabifolia* is designated as a separate drug, *mu-jing* (with qualifiers designating plant parts used, including seed, leaf, root, etc.). *Mu-jing-you* the oil of this variety, and *mu-jing-you jiao-wan* (capsules of the oil) are official entries in the 1985 Chinese *Pharmacopeia*. Various plant parts and components of this variety have experimental expectorant, antitussive, antiasthmatic, antispasmodic, sedative, and antibacterial activity. The volatile oil of the leaf or seed has been shown to have a 90 percent effective rate in over 1,000 cases of bronchitis, according to one clinical study. The oil inhibits ovule production in women and has been studied as a potential contraceptive.

DOSE

Fruits: 3–9 g, in decoction (sometimes 15–30 g in powder). Leaves: 3–9 g of dried leaves in decoction; 15–60 g fresh leaves, also used as poultice or wash. Root: 6–12 g. Branches: 3–6 g, in decoction, poulticed. The branches are also used after being forged (charcoaled), retaining character; they are powdered and applied as needed.

WARNING

Vitex negundo fruits and root contain flavonoid glycosides as well as cardiac glycosides. Because of the potential adverse effect of cardiac glycosides on heart patients, the plant must be used cautiously in patients with a history of heart disease.

DESCRIPTION

Vitex negundo is a shrub or small tree to 15 feet tall. The branches are four-angled. The leaves are palmately divided into five (or three) leaflets. The leaflets are mostly lance-shaped, ½ to 4 inches long, entire, or serrate. Lower leaves have stalks; upper leaves are mostly sessile (without stalks). The leaves have fine, dense grayish hairs underneath. The flowers are in slender spikes, up to 8 inches long, grouped in a densely white-hairy terminal panicle. The individual purple flowers are ¼ to ½ inch long and flower from June through July.

V. negundo var. *heterophylla* differs chiefly in that the leaflets are deeply incised with large serrate teeth; sometimes the teeth are so large they can be described as remote leaflet segments.

V. negundo var. *cannabifolia* has leaves that strongly resemble those of marijuana (*Cannabis sativa*). The resemblance is so great that those who grow the plant are best advised to keep a pressed sample for identification purposes, lest one be accused of growing marijuana.

DISTRIBUTION

Vitex negundo grows in fields, on mountainsides, and on wasteland in hills and roadsides, along streams, and in shrub thickets in the central coastal provinces of China, as well as in Gansu, Guangxi, Guangdong, Guizhou, Sichuan, Yunnan, and Xizang (Tibet). In short, it grows throughout the country except for the northeast and northwest areas.

Vitex negundo var. *heterophylla* grows in very poor mountainsides, wastelands, ditches, and roadsides in Liaoning, Nei Mongol, Hebei, Henan, Shandong, Shanxi, Shaanxi, Ningxia, and Gansu to northern Sichuan.

Vitex negundo var. *cannabifolia* grows on sunny mountainsides, roadsides, or valleys, primarily in provinces south of the Yangtze river, as well as in the coastal province of Shandong.

Vitex negundo also occurs in southeastern Africa, Madagascar, Southeast Asia, India, and the Philippines.

In the United States, *Vitex negundo* and *V. negundo* var. *heterophylla* have been naturalized in southern Florida.

CULTIVATION

The *Vitex* species are very common in China. They are so abundant in the wild that they are not commercially cultivated for drug production. Commercial collections are made in Jiangsu, Zhejiang, Jiangxi, Hunan, Sichuan, and Guangxi. However, in most parts of China, the plant is collected on a small scale for local use.

Vitex grows well in a wide variety of soils, thriving most luxuriantly in rich, moist, well-drained soils, but it is tolerant of poor, dry soils as well. It likes full sun. Vitex shrubs have an open spreading habit, and if they become too large and sprawling can be controlled by pruning. The *Vitex* species described above are hardy to about -10°F.

Unlike many woody plants, most *Vitex* species are easily propagated from seeds and can also be quickly propagated by layering or from softwood cuttings. Cuttings can be made from May through July, before flowering begins. A dip of 1,000 to 4,000 ppm IBA-quick dip (rooting hormone) has been suggested for optimum propagation of cuttings in a peat moss-perlite mix. Cuttings can be misted to produce more rapid rooting, but misting should be reduced or eliminated once rooting actually begins since excessive moisture may result in less healthy cuttings.

HARVESTING

The fruits (seeds) are collected by rubbing the fruiting branches by hand in autumn when the fruits are ripe. It is used fresh or dried. The fruits are dried in the sun and then winnowed to separate the seed from the chaff. The root and stem are collected in late summer or autumn. They are cleaned, cut into sections, and dried under sun. The leaves are collected in early summer before flowering. After harvesting, the leaves are pressed together into a small, firm pile. Once they turn from their dark green color to black, they are spread out to dry. Major production of the leaves is carried out in the southern provinces of Guangdong and Guangxi. The leaves are also used fresh.

PROCESSING

See above.

ADDITIONAL SPECIES

There are a number of species in the genus *Vitex* that are also used in China, including *V. quinata* A.N. Willd. and *V. canescens* Kurz., which is used as a substitute for *V. negundo* in Xizang (Tibet). The fruit of another species, *Vitex trifolia*, known is China as *man-jing-zi*, is also an official listing in the Chinese *Pharmacopeia*. The seed is used as an analgesic and sedative.

The chaste tree, *Vitex agnus-castus*, a European species naturalized in the southeastern United States, has been used in Europe for many years and is increasingly common in American herb markets. The fruits (seeds) are used. Recent German studies suggest that extracts of the seeds can regulate excessive menstrual bleeding or too frequent menstruation. One study shows that plant preparations may stimulate progesterone production and have a regulating effect on estrogen. In Germany, when women stop taking oral contraceptives chaste tree products have been used to help reestablish normal menstruation and ovulation. Comparative clinical studies confirm the ability of seed extracts to increase or stimulate milk flow. One proprietary medicine manufactured in Germany has been shown to reduce water retention before menstruation, and to allay effusions in the knee joints associated with premenstrual syndrome.

OTHER USES

All parts of *Vitex negundo* are commonly used in traditional medicine in India. In the Philippines, the seeds have been boiled and eaten.

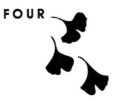

FOUR

Ornamental and Unusual Trees

Eucommia
Du-zhong

Botanical Name: *Eucommia ulmoides* Oliv.
Chinese Names: Pinyin: *Du-zhong* (bark). Wade-Giles: *Tu-chung*
(bark).
English Names: Eucommia, hardy rubber tree.
Pharmaceutical Name: Cortex Eucommiae.
Family: Eucommiaceae—eucommia family.

HISTORY

Eucommia is monotypic. It is the only member of the eucommia family.
Millions of years ago, eucommia family members existed in Europe and
North America. All are extinct except for one species. *Eucommia ulmoides*
is the only surviving member of this once widespread plant family. It has
no close living relatives. *Eu* means "well" or "good," and *kommi* means
"thread," referring to the hair- or threadlike gutta-percha (a rubbery latex)
threads found in the leaves, leaf stalks, bark, and fruits. The specific epithet
"ulmoides," means "elmlike," referring to the resemblance of the leaves to
those of elms.

The first Westerner to collect botanical specimens was Dr. Augustine
Henry, a British physician who in 1881 was attached to the Service of
Chinese Maritime Customs in Shanghai. He was transferred to Hubei
province in the following year, where he stayed until 1889. Among the
most fruitful of all European botanical explorers, he began his botanical
collections in 1885. His first collections arrived at Kew Gardens in 1886
and included a specimen of eucommia. In 1890 the first Western botanical
description of the plant appeared in a publication by the English botanist,
Daniel Oliver. Oliver, then keeper of the library and herbarium at Kew,
noted the gutta-percha threads in the bark, leaves, and seeds. His and other
publications on eucommia excited European botanists. A hardy tree of
temperate climates that produced a rubberlike substance was of great
interest!

Eucommia seed was introduced into European botanical gardens in the
1890s. In 1907 the Arnold Arboretum of Harvard University obtained
seeds from Veitch and Sons, an English nursery firm. In Europe and the

United States, the tree persists primarily as a rare specimen tree in botanical gardens and as an occasional shade tree.

Chinese knowledge of eucommia is ancient. The name *du-zhong* first appears in *Shen Nong Ben Cao Jing*. Among the 365 herbs divided into three classes, *du-zhong* is listed among the superior group of medicinal plants. According to Shiu Ying Hu (1979), *du-zhong* was described in 39 words that covered the name, synonyms, properties, distribution, and functions. Shen Nong's compilation is the first known account of the tree and its medicinal uses. It is described in all important Chinese *ben cao* since. The uses attributed to it today are the same as those listed in *Shen Nong Ben Cao Jing* (See S.Y. Hu 1979b).

In Li Shi-zhen's *Ben Cao Gang Mu*, the name *du-zhong* is interpreted as meaning that the plant was named for a Taoist who took the bark and became immortal. He happened to be the second son (*zhong*) of a family named *du*, hence the name.

CHARACTER AND TASTE

A little sweet, a little hot, warm.

FUNCTION

Invigorates the liver and kidney, strengthens bones and muscles, enhances vital essence and vital energy, and quiets a restless fetus.

USES

Eucommia bark is used in prescriptions for high blood pressure, vertigo, aching and pains of the waist and knees, weakness of the bones and muscles, frequent urination due to kidney deficiency, placental leakage, excessive fetal movement, wetness and itching of the genitals, plus placental leakage with a fetus that drops too low.

Since the 1950s, Chinese, Japanese, Russian, and American research teams have studied the pharmacology, chemistry, and clinical applications of the tree bark. In Western terms it is considered analgesic, antihypertensive, arthritic, depurative, diuretic, sedative, and tonic. Research at the department of chemistry of the University of Wisconsin, published in 1976, revealed the major antihypertensive agent, a pinoresinal diglucoside. The researchers also succeeded in synthesizing this component. However, it is still much cheaper to produce the crude bark for use as a drug than to synthesize the active component.

A clinical report in the Chinese literature on the treatment of high blood pressure uses a 10 percent tincture of eucommia. Thirty drops were administered three times per day. In 119 cases, treated for one to 23 months, the effect was considered good in 51 cases (42.8 percent), 15 cases showed some improvement (12.6 percent), and the tincture was of no use in 53 cases (44.6 percent). The average duration of treatment was nine months. No side effects were reported.

Another clinical study of high blood pressure involved the treatment of 124 patients with a 5 percent tincture of eucommia in 5 ml doses, given three times per day. The effects were reported as good at the first signs of high blood pressure. In some cases blood pressure returned to normal after 45 days of treatment. The treatment did not control serious cases of high blood pressure.

Experimental data in the Chinese literature reports reduction of blood pressure in studies with dogs, cats, and rabbits. A decoction of the roasted (processed) bark produced better results than the crude dried bark. The bark has been shown to have a stimulatory effect on the respiratory system, is diuretic, and sedative in experiments with dogs. The bark has been reported to have very low toxicity without measurable side effects.

The bark is sold at a relatively high price on world markets. Some herb products containing eucommia bark are sold in health and natural food stores in the United States. However, it is much more commonly seen in Chinatown herb shops in larger American cities.

DOSE

Dose 6–15 g, in decoction, pills, powder, or tincture.

DESCRIPTION

Eucommia is a hardy deciduous tree growing to about 70 feet in height. The elliptical to oblong-ovate leaves have an acuminate tip. They are about 3 inches long, smooth above, and slightly rough-hairy beneath. The margins are serrate. Male and female flowers are on separate trees. The oblong, somewhat compressed, one-seeded fruit has a wing, similar to those on ash species. A remarkable feature of the plant is an elastic gum or rubberlike substance, described as "silklike threads," that is abundant in the bark and seeds as well as the leaves and leaf stalks. When any of these parts are broken and pulled apart, the numerous threads are evident.

DISTRIBUTION

Wild stands of the tree are rare in China, though eucommia is widely cultivated. It grows in mountains in forests in the middle Yangtze River valley. Its native range is the Tsinling Mountains in the border area of Gansu, Shaanxi, and Sichuan in Central China. This area is famous for its large number of unique species or endemics, all remnants of an ancient flora. This flora's most famous member is *Metasequoia*, or dawn redwood, the closest living relative of the California redwoods.

Eucommia is grown commercially in every province of South China. It is grown in Shaanxi, Gansu, Zhejiang, Jiangxi, Henan, Hunan, Guangxi, Guangdong, Sichuan, Guizhou, and Yunnan. The major production regions are Sichuan, Shaanxi, Hubei, Henan, Guizhou, and Yunnan, with lesser amounts produced in Jiangxi, Gansu, Hunan, and Guangxi. The best-quality eucommia bark comes from northern Sichuan.

In the United States and Europe, it is a rare shade or specimen tree in botanical gardens, and is occasionally planted along streets. In Indianapolis, for example, it is planted on the west perimeter of Holiday Park on Spring Mill Road, between 63rd and 64th streets. Trees are available from nurseries specializing in the rare and unusual.

CULTIVATION

In China, hill country too steep for conventional crops is often used for commercial cultivation of eucommia. The tree is suitable for many growing conditions and is tolerant of severe cold, but likes plenty of sunshine and moist soils. A moist, rich, well-drained, deep soil, of a sandy or slightly clayey nature and high in organic matter is best. Nursery beds about 5 feet wide are deeply cultivated; the soil should be fine and level. In China, it is cultivated along roadsides and in yards, field margins, and corners of property.

Propagate by seeds. A tree 10 to 20 years old is chosen and the seeds are harvested. To germinate the seeds, they are dipped in hot water (140°F) for about five minutes, stirred until cool, and soaked in cold water for another 24 hours. Seeds are then mixed with sand and placed in a hole in the ground to stratify for about 20 days. When the seeds start to sprout, they are sown. Another method used in China is to soak the seeds in 68°F water for three days, changing the water one to two times per day, until the seeds swell. Seeds are planted in beds in rows spaced at 8 inches. Seeds are covered with ½ inch or less of soil, and a rice straw mulch is added. After planting, seedlings begin to appear in one or two weeks.

Cuttings can also be used for propagation, or lateral branches can be layered to produce new trees. Three- to five-inch-long cuttings of first-year growth are made in spring when the buds are swollen. They are placed directly in soil, rooting readily, and are then transplanted the following spring. A study conducted at the University of Illinois at Urbana indicated that the optimum time to take cuttings is late May to early June. A 30-second dip in chloromone resulted in 85 percent rooting in a North Carolina study.

Mechanical injury to the roots will result in suckering. The suckers can be transplanted. Transplant established (rooted) cuttings to permanent locations in spring or autumn. When young seedlings are transplanted, make sure the lateral roots are expanded (well spread-out instead of in a tight ball) tamp the soil, and water. Space plants at 5 inches when planted in nursery beds. Side-dress with manure as needed. Cut off lateral branches to cause the main trunk to grow straight and tall.

HARVESTING

In China, the trunk bark is harvested in spring. After the trees are 15 to 20 years old, the bark is harvested in April or May. Bark is removed from only one side of the tree (not girdled) in order to ensure the tree's survival. The tree will live if the bark is harvested in this manner. The bark strips are then placed face to face in layered piles and covered with rice straw. This makes the bark sweat. After about one week, the inner surface become blackish-brown. At this point, the bark is removed and pressed until flat. Then the rough outer bark is rossed off.

Another method used is to simply remove the bark, then ross away the rough outer bark. The inner bark is dried in the sun or in a shaded, well-ventilated room.

PROCESSING

For charcoaled bark, the bark pieces are put into a pan and stir-fried. A little salt water is added while frying, the bark is turned frequently to prevent it from scorching or smoking. It is treated in this manner until the surface is a black color and the silk threads are broken. The bark is not burned, retaining its "character." For every 100 pounds of bark, 3 pounds of salt is used to make a salt-water solution that is sprinkled on the bark during stir-frying.

Another method involves removing the outer bark, cleaning the inner bark, and covering it with a moist cloth until it absorbs enough moisture to easily cut the bark strips into square pieces. Then it is dried in the sun. Next the bark is soaked in a salt solution until it absorbs some of the salt water. It is stir-fried over a light fire until some of the bark has dark spots. Then it is removed from the pan and dried. After frying, the silk threads are broken. It then becomes easy to decoct the bark.

OTHER USES

The small young leaves are also used as a folk medicine for the treatment of ringworm of the feet, bloody stool, or hemorrhoids. The powder of the dried young leaves is decocted. Recent chemical studies have suggested that the leaves could be used as a substitute for the bark.

Li Shi-zhen noted in his 1596 classic *Ben Cao Gang Mu* that both the flowers and fruit are astringent and may be used in medicine. Other references to the use of the flowers and fruits in medicine are unknown.

Gutta-percha, abundant in many parts of the tree, has been extracted from eucommia and is used in the manufacture of insulation for submarine cables, wire rope, and dental material in both China and Russia. The wood has been used for making clogs, or wooden shoes. The fruits of eucommia produce up to 27 percent oil, which in China is used for various minor industrial purposes.

Ginkgo
Bai-guo

Botanical Name: *Ginkgo biloba* L.
Chinese Names: Pinyin: *Bai-guo* (seeds); *Bai-guo-ye* (leaves). Wade-Giles: *Pai-kuo* (seeds); *Pai-kuo-yeh* (leaves).
English Names: Ginkgo, maidenhair tree.
Pharmaceutical Name: Semen Ginkgo; Folium Ginkgo.
Family: Ginkgoaceae—ginkgo family.

HISTORY

Ginkgo was common 175 to 200 million years ago, when dinosaurs roamed the earth. This primitive tree is considered the oldest living tree species on earth. Ginkgo is monotypic—it is the only surviving member of the ancient and primitive ginkgo family.

In Western botany, the tree was first observed in 1690 and then described in 1712 by Englebert Kaempfer, a German surgeon working for the Dutch East India Company. It is in Kaempfer's notes that the name *ginkgo* first appears. Linnaeus bestowed the binomial *Ginkgo biloba* in 1771. A. C. Moule (1937) discussed the etymology of Chinese and Japanese names of the tree in the context of a critical review of Kaempfer's manuscripts. He concluded that Kaempfer's name *ginkgo* is a misprint, misspelling, or perhaps a corruption of a Japanese pronunciation of a Chinese name for the tree. However, H. L. Li (1956) notes that *ginkgo* is not a misprint, as Moule suggests, but rather an eighteenth-century phonetic pronunciation of a Japanese name for the tree, adopted from a name of Chinese origin. Whatever the origin, the tree is and will forever be known as ginkgo.

Numerous Chinese names are recorded from different regions and for various parts of the tree. The primary names cited here are Wade-Giles transliterations, those in brackets are Pinyin. Shiu Ying Hu (1957) records the following Chinese names: *pê-kuo* (given as *pai-kuo* in S. Y. Hu 1980) [*bai-guo*], the most common colloquial name in China, means "white fruit." *Yin-hsing* [*yin-xing*] denotes "silver apricot," and is the most common literary name used in Chinese works. *Kung-sun-shu* [*kong-sun-shu*], another colloquial name, means "grandfather and grandson tree." Since female trees do not bear seeds until they are quite old, a tree planted by a man will therefore be useful to his grandson. Bensky and Gamble (1986) record the name *yin guo* (silver fruit) for the seeds. The *Pharmacopeia of the People's Republic of China* (1985), in which ginkgo seed is listed as an official drug, uses *bai-guo*. One of the earliest names is *ya chio*, meaning "duck's foot," referring to the leaf shape.

Ginkgo has been cultivated in East Asia for hundreds of years. Numerous reports mention the existence of large specimens, some more than a thousand years old, at ancient temples in Japan and China. The tree was first introduced to North America in 1784 in the garden of William Hamilton at Woodlands near Philadelphia. Mature ginkgos are said to reach over 100 feet in height. Its longevity as an individual tree and a species in general can in part be attributed to its exceptional resistance to pests and resiliency to destruction by fire. It is also extremely tolerant of air pollution, thriving in the harshest urban environments.

Reports in the Asian literature speak of numerous instances in which specimens thought destroyed by fire resprouted from their charred remains. The Reverend G. H. Moule, writing in a letter of 8 April 1937, told of old ginkgos planted around the Kwannoan temple at Asakusa in Tokyo. The surrounding area was devastated by a raging fire after the earthquake of 1 September 1932. The ancient ginkgos surrounding the temple were believed to protect it from destruction. Moule reported that he saw numerous ancient ginkgos scorched by the fire. While other trees were completely destroyed, the blackened ginkgos sprouted again a few weeks after the fire (A. C. Moule 1937). One remarkable example of the tree's tenacity is the story of one ginkgo near ground zero of the 1945 Hiroshima nuclear bomb blast. A few months after the devastating explosion, the blackened remains of the tree sprouted new leaves.

According to H. L. Li (1956), the tree is not known to be cultivated by the ancient Chinese. The first records of cultivation of ginkgo in the Chinese literature come in the eleventh century during the Song dynasty. It was then known as a rare and precious "fruit" of eastern China in a region south of the Yangtze River. Ginkgo seed was originally sent to the ancient capital of China, Kaifeng, as a tribute to the emperor from an area now in the southern part of Anhui province. Cultivation subsequently commenced in the capital and gradually spread to other areas. One Song dynasty work *Chun Chu Chi Wen* (*Zhun Zhu Ji Wen*) mentioned that there were four large trees in the capital producing several bushels of "fruits" per year. The tree was called *ya chio tzu*, the earliest recorded name for ginkgo.

While ginkgo was a common subject of paintings and poetry during the Song dynasty, the seeds were not mentioned in herbals until the Yuan dynasty (1280–1368) in Li Tung-wan's *Shi Wu Ben Cao* (Edible Herbal) and the 1350 A.D. work, Wu-rui's *Ri Yong Ben Cao* (Herbal for Daily Usage). Wu's work mentions potential toxicity of the fruits, especially if eaten in excess by children (Li 1956). Ginkgo is also described in detail in Li Shi-zhen's 1596 *Ben Cao Gang Mu*.

TASTE AND CHARACTER

Seeds: a little sweet, bitter, astringent, neutral, potentially toxic. Leaves: a little bitter, neutral.

FUNCTIONS

The seed is considered astringent for the lungs, stops nocturnal emissions with an astringent nature, stops asthma, enuresis, excessive leukorrhea, benefits vital energy (*qi/ch'i*), and regulates urinary frequency.

The leaves promote blood circulation, stop pain, benefit the brain, are astringent to the lungs, and eliminates wetness from the upper warmer.

USES

The dried, processed seed, with the external seed coat and fleshy pulp removed, is used in prescriptions for asthma, coughs with phlegm, enuresis, mucous vaginal discharges, bronchitis with asthma, chronic bronchitis, tuberculosis, frequent urination, seminal emissions, strangury, turbid urine, and frequent urination. Externally, the seed is poulticed for scabies and sores.

The leaves are used in prescriptions for arteriosclerosis, angina pectoris, high serum cholesterol levels, dysentery, and filariasis. An infusion of the boiled leaves is also used against chilblains.

Ginkgo seeds have primarily been used in TCM for the treatment of lung-related ailments. For example, a traditional prescription for the treatment of tuberculosis calls for collecting the seeds in autumn. Once cleaned and processed, they are soaked in vegetable oil for 100 days. One seed (with the hard outer shell removed) is eaten three times per day, for 30 to 100 days. To stop nocturnal seminal emissions, a traditional prescription calls for 3 ginkgo seeds. They are decocted, then taken with a little alcohol once a day. The treatment was continued for four to five days. For the treatment of dental caries, one processed seed was eaten with each meal. For the treatment of ringworm or other fungal sores about the face or head, according to one ancient method, the fresh seeds were cut in two, and the cross section of the seed was rubbed on the affected area. A poultice of the powdered seeds has been used for the treatment of genital sores (disease not specified).

While only the seeds are official in the 1985 Chinese *Pharmacopeia*, the leaves *bai-guo-ye* or *yin-xing-ye* are widely used in clinical practice in China, as well as Europe. A modern treatment for angina pectoris uses 4.5 g of ginkgo leaves with 4.5 g of the root of *Polygonum multiflorum* (fo-ti), and

4.5 g of the bark of *Uncaria rhynchophylla*, a shrub in the madder family. The three ingredients are made into tablets. The prescription is said to be enough for one day's dosage. In Beijing an injectable preparation of this prescription has been used in hospitals. The course of treatment generally lasts six to ten weeks. In China, an extract of ginkgo leaves has also been used in the treatment of high serum cholesterol levels.

Ginkgo leaf has certainly not gone unnoticed by Western researchers. In fact, ginkgo leaf extracts are now more commonly associated with phytomedicine in Europe than they are with TCM. Based on historical reports of using the leaf tea in China to improve brain function, dozens of studies on the chemistry, pharmacology, and clinical effects of gingko leaf have been conducted by European researchers.

As one of the most widely prescribed medicinal plant products in Europe, gingko leaf extracts are used clinically for heart disease, eye ailments, ringing in the ears, vertigo, cerebral and peripheral vascular insufficiency, injuries involving brain trauma, dementias, short-term memory improvement, cognitive disorders secondary to depression, and various conditions associated with senility.

Researchers have shown that a total extract from ginkgo leaves is active, not just a single isolated component. A standardized leaf extract has been found to be beneficial in diseases involving vascular, rheological, metabolic, and immunological functions. More than 250 pharmacological and clinical studies have been published in the last two decades, the vast majority using a complex standardized extract of the dried leaves, known as EGb 761. Produced by a German-French consortium, the extract is standardized to 24 percent flavone glycosides.

The ginkgolides, bitter principles of the leaves and roots, discovered by Japanese researchers in 1932, are also being studied on a worldwide basis. These complex molecules unique to ginkgo were first synthesized in 1988. Using a highly intricate multistep procedure, a team of organic chemists at Harvard University, headed by Dr. E. Corey, synthesized ginkgolide B, considered the most active of several ginkgolides. Dr. Corey won the 1991 Nobel Prize in Chemistry for his work in synthesizing organic molecules. Ginkgolide B is a selective antagonist of platelet aggregation induced by platelet-activating factor (PAF). PAF is believed to be involved in various inflammatory, cardiovascular, and respiratory disorders. It is an inflammatory autacoid. Autacoids mediate local tissue response, such as pain perception, blood coagulation, and smooth muscle contraction. Ginkgolides have been shown to counteract the effects of PAF. Successful clinical use and the safety of the standardized extract of ginkgo leaf (EGb 761) has warranted further research on ginkgolides in a broad range of disease conditions. At present ginkgolides are being studied by a handful of research groups, while the *Ginkgo biloba* standardized extract (EGb 761) is in wide clinical usage, especially in Germany and France.

In the United States various ginkgo leaf preparations are sold as dietary supplements in the form of tablets, capsules, tincture, and standardized extracts in health and natural food stores.

DOSE

Seeds and leaves: 4.5–9 g in decoction, pills, powder, and poultice.

WARNING

The fresh fruit pulp and the processed seeds of ginkgo are considered potentially poisonous. A standardized extract of the leaf, on the other hand, is considered to have very low toxicity.

Studies have shown that seed constituents have some antibacterial and antifungal activity. In large doses (eating more than ten seeds) they can have a toxic effect, leading to skin disorders or mucous membrane irritations, or in larger doses, serious side effects. Fatalities are reported from overdoses of ginkgo seeds. Eating fresh seeds may cause stomachache, nausea, diarrhea, convulsions, weak pulse, restlessness, difficult breathing, and shock. Induced vomiting and activated charcoal with egg whites have been used as antidotes to ginkgo seed poisoning, along with the administration of a diuretic and, if necessary, oxygen.

Fresh fruits may cause contact dermatitis similar to poison ivy rash. They should be handled with rubber gloves.

DESCRIPTION

Ginkgo is a deciduous tree growing to 130 feet in height. The parallel-veined, broad, fan-shaped leaves, up to three inches across, have a notch at the apex, forming two distinct lobes, hence the species name *biloba*. They are alternate or borne on spurs in clusters of three to five. Ginkgos are dioecious (producing male and female flowers on separate plants). The male flowers are on pendulous catkins with numerous loosely arranged anthers in stalked pairs on a slender axis. In 1895 a Japanese botanist, Hirase, discovered that the pollen cells are motile (having the power to move spontaneously), and travel to the ovule of the female flowers via pollen tubes. Hirase's discovery was hailed as one of the great botanical finds of the nineteenth century. Female flowers are in pairs on long footstalks. One female flower usually aborts. The drupelike fruits have an acrid, foul-smelling pulp (likened to baby vomit or dog droppings) surrounding a single smooth, oval, thin-shelled edible nut (seeds).

In the American nursery trade most ginkgos sold represent branches of male trees grafted to seedlings. Available cultivars include "Autumn Gold," "Fairmount," "Mayfield," and others. Disadvantages of ornamental plantings of the female trees include the unpleasant scent of the fruits and the mess they make when they drop to the ground—they can cause pedestrians to slip, and their juice can stain clothing.

DISTRIBUTION

Ginkgo is known only from cultivation. The tree is not definitively confirmed in the wild in China. It has been found growing in remote forests in Zhejiang province over a ten-square-mile area, but it is impossible to determine whether these are spontaneous specimens or result from planted specimens. The occurrence of ginkgo as a wild as opposed to cultivated tree or escape has been much disputed over the past few centuries. However, H. L. Li (1956) has provided a convincing argument for its natural occurrence in the mountains of the southern border area of Anhui, Jiangsu, and northern Zhejiang, an area well known for monotypic, primitive, endemic conifers and taxads.

In modern China, ginkgo is widely planted from Liaoning, Hebei, Henan, Shandong, Jiangsu, Anhui, Zhejiang, Jiangxi, Fujian, Taiwan, Hubei, Hunan, Guangxi, Guangdong, Shaanxi, Sichuan, Guizhou, and Yunnan. The most important commercial production regions of the seeds for medicinal use include Guangxi, Sichuan, Henan, Shandong, Hubei, and Liaoning (in order of importance). It is also commonly planted in Japan and Korea as well as North America and Europe. A large ginkgo plantation, covering more than 1,200 acres, has been established in South Carolina for the production of ginkgo leaf for export to the European market. Trees are maintained at a height of about six feet, and the leaves are harvested with a modified cotton-picker.

CULTIVATION

Ginkgo trees enjoy abundant sunshine and can bear cold and dry conditions. They are exceptionally resilient, drought tolerant, resistant to pests and disease, and are tolerant of air pollution, fire, and other adversities. These factors add up to its survival on earth for up to 200 million years. The best growing condition is a deep, rich, sandy soil.

Ginkgo can be propagated from seeds, cuttings, or grafting. If seeds are planted in autumn, good germination will usually take place the following spring. The embryo is immature. After seeds are cleaned, germination is best achieved with one to two months of warm stratification, followed by one to two months of cold stratification. Cuttings can be taken in June or July. Four- to six-foot long cuttings will root in seven to eight weeks in a mix of peat and perlite that is misted frequently. Application of a rooting hormone (8,000 ppm IBA-solution) has been reported to enhance rooting.

Seeds or grafting are commonly used for propagation in China. Seeds are planted in spring or autumn. If sown in spring, seeds are mixed with white sand and stored underground for several months to stratify the seeds. During this period, care is taken to make sure that the sand is not too wet, which could possibly cause mildew. The stratified seeds are sown in rows and covered with about 2 inches of soil. Young seedlings do not like too much water, and should be protected from harsh sunlight by providing shade for the first two or three years. After growing seven to eight years, the Chinese transplant dormant seedlings to a permanent location, spaced at 10 to 15 feet.

In Sichuan, when the seeds have ripened in September, they are sown soon after dropping from the tree. Ginkgo is also propagated by grafting and cuttings. A female tree that has fruited for at least three years is chosen as propagation material. Branches with at least three to five or even six to seven short branches are chosen as scions. For grafting purposes, planting stock that was grown from seed is chosen. Grafting is performed in spring. Two or three years after grafting, the young trees are transplanted to permanent locations. In China, the young seedlings, one to four years old, are kept well weeded and are side-dressed with night soil or other nitrogen fertilizer sources. In July and October, soil around the trees is cultivated to help aerate the soil and control weeds. A second side-dressing of manure is applied in October. In autumn, every four to five years after transplanting, the soil is cultivated around the tree, a circular shallow ditch is dug, and the seedlings are side-dressed with manure.

HARVESTING

In autumn, just as they begin to turn yellow, the leaves are harvested and dried in the sun. In China the fruits are harvested in deep autumn, when the fruits are very ripe. The fleshy external seed coat is removed, and the seeds are cleaned and dried in the sun. When handling and cleaning the whole fruits, rubber gloves are recommended since the fruit pulp can cause contact dermatitis. Another harvest method calls for gathering the fruits in October and November. The whole fruits are then stacked in a pyramidal pile, which allow them to heat up, resulting in easier removal of the flesh. The fruits can also be soaked to make the fleshy external coat soft for easier removal.

PROCESSING

The inner seed is the part used. The clean seeds are fried or steamed until "ripe," and the outer shell then is removed. The thin hard shell of the seed is removed before a prescription is made, but the drug is supplied to shops with the shell intact. After the seed shell is removed, the seeds are crushed into coarse pieces.

The seeds are processed before use by steaming, stir-frying, or roasting. The seeds (with shells intact) are steamed until "ripe." Another method is to stir-fry the seeds until "ripe." They are also sometimes roasted with a simple dough made with wheat flour and water. The dough is spread over a cookie sheet before roasting, placing the seeds on top of the dough. This method is used to heat the seeds evenly without discoloring them with burn marks, or actually burning them, as may happen with stir-frying.

OTHER USES

The root and inner bark are used as folk medicines in China. The root or tree bark is collected in September and October. The bark of ginkgo was first mentioned in a twentieth-century Chinese herbal, but not in the ancient *ben cao*. Its character and taste is described as a little sweet, warm, neutral, and without poison. Functions include benefiting the heart and the brain and being useful for weak patients. The bark is used in prescriptions for mucous vaginal discharges, seminal emission, or weak, convalescing patients. The dried bark is burned to ash, mixed with vegetable oil, and used as a poultice for neurodermatitis.

The seeds, considered a delicacy in Japan and China, are edible after the acrid, foul-odored pulp is removed and the seeds are boiled or roasted. The flavor is said to be like that of mild Swiss cheese. The fresh seeds are considered toxic, and have reportedly caused death in children if eaten raw. The English botanist Robert Fortune, while traveling in China in the

1840s, observed ginkgo seeds sold widely in local markets. He likened their appearance to dried almonds. Dyed red, the nuts were traditionally eaten at weddings.

According to Dr. Shiu Ying Hu of Harvard University's Arnold Arboretum, a leading expert on Chinese food and medicinal plants in the United States, the roasted seeds are sold on streets in Shanghai. Before eating, the seeds are roasted over a medium-high heat, stirring occasionally, until the whitish seeds have browned on the exterior. They are broken open to see if they are done, which is indicated by a transparent greenish color within. Roasted ginkgo seeds are not eaten like peanuts. Only eight or ten are eaten in one day. Eating too many roasted ginkgo seeds can cause a number of unpleasant effects (see "Warning" above). Avoid standing over roasting ginko seeds—the rising steam can cause dermatitis of the face and severe eye irritation.

Jujube
Da-zao

Botanical Names: *Ziziphus jujuba* Mill., *Z. jujuba* var. *inermis* (Bunge) Rehd. (*Z. vulgaris* Lamarck var. *inermis* Bunge). Sometimes also spelled Zizyphus.
Chinese Names: Pinyin: *Da-zao* (fruits). Wade-Giles: *Ta-ts'ao* (fruits).
English Names: Common jujube, Chinese date.
Pharmaceutical Name: Fructus Jujubae.
Family: Rhamnaceae—buckthorn family.

HISTORY

Jujube is to the Chinese what apples are to Americans. The large-fruited common jujube, or Chinese date, has hundreds of cultivated varieties in China. They are grown throughout the country and are available virtually everywhere. Jujube is an excellent example of how the Chinese use food as medicine. The fruit has an ancient history of use as a Chinese herb. This small deciduous tree (sometimes a large bush) is believed to have been introduced from China into West Asia 2,500 to 3,000 years ago. The fruit was known to the Greeks and Romans, who introduced it to North Africa and Spain, where it became naturalized.

The genus *Ziziphus* consists of about 40 species of shrubs and trees native to subtropical and tropical regions. The species *Z. jujuba* was established in 1768 by Philip Miller in the eighth edition of his *Gardener's Dictionary*. The genus name, created in the fourth edition of Miller's work (1754), comes from the Greek *ziziphon*, itself derived from an ancient vernacular name of the Ziziphus tree from North Africa or southern Europe. The species name *jujube* may be derived from a Malaysian word used to denote the fruit. The varietal epithet *inermis*, means unarmed or without spines. *Ziziphus jujuba* var. *inermis* was originally named *Z. vulgaris* var. *inermis* in an 1833 publication by the Russian botanist Alexander von Bunge. In 1922 Alfred Rehder placed this variety under the species *Z. jujuba*.

Large numbers of jujube varieties were collected for introduction to the United States around the turn of the century by the Dutch-born American plant explorer, Frank N. Meyer (1875–1918). Meyer, employed by the USDA's Plant Introduction Office, was charged by David Fairchild, the first director of the Plant Introduction Office, with sending as many jujube varieties to the United States as he could. Fairchild was a champion of the jujube. He believed it would become a popular fruit tree in America because it could be grown in barren regions that would not support other agricultural crops.

However, despite his personal interest, Fairchild was never successful in the widespread introduction of this fruit tree. The Plant Introduction Office lacked funds to promote it as a commercial product. Fairchild was married to the daughter of Alexander Graham Bell, and he attempted to popularize the candied datelike fruit at social functions at the Bell home in South Florida, as well as at annual meetings of the National Geographic Society.

By 1915, experimental plantations of jujube had been established at the USDA Experiment Station in Chico, California. They were also tested in Texas and Oklahoma, but never caught on. A new intensive jujube breeding program was initiated at the USDA station at Chico in 1952, but the project was abandoned in 1959. The remaining Chico jujube planting was finally bulldozed in July of 1983. Numerous cultivars have survived, both at old plantings in the United States and in the possession of specialty fruit growers and collectors in various parts of the country.

The ripe fruit of jujube is a very commonly used traditional Chinese herbal remedy, as it has been for several millennia. It was first mentioned in the first class of herbs in *Shen Nong Ben Cao Jing*. From the old herbals we can see that the same source plant has been used for hundreds of years. Since ancient times the major jujube-producing province has been Shandong. The fruits are listed an an official drug in the 1985 edition of the Chinese *Pharmacopeia*.

One of the uses of jujube fruit is to regulate imbalances between "ying" (not to be confused with yin) and "wei" energy. It is difficult to explain in Western terms the concepts of ying and wei. In oversimplified terms, a "ying" condition means that the disease is "near the surface of the skin," not progressed very far, or a mild, acute condition. "Wei," refers to "deep-seated" disease conditions, denoting an ailment that has progressed from an acute to a chronic condition, "deep in the bones." The following story helps explain the concept:

> Two thousand years ago a famous doctor named Bian Que went to visit the Emperor.
>
> "Oh, my Emperor," he said, "You are ill."
>
> "I feel fine. I'm in very good health," the Emperor retorted.
>
> After Bian Que left, the Emperor told one of his servants that Bian Que just wanted business, so he tried to tell the Emperor that he was sick.
>
> Five days later Bian Que returned.
>
> "My Emperor, you are becoming quite ill."
>
> Again the surprised Emperor expressed that he felt fine.
>
> Five days later Bian Que returned. He looked at the Emperor, then turned around and left. The Emperor sent a servant to summon Bian Que.
>
> "Why do you leave when you see me?" asked the Emperor.
>
> "Some days ago your condition was at the surface. If you had a decoction at that point, the condition would be cured," said Bian Que, "I returned five days later. At this point the disease had become deeper. Acupuncture and herbs tinctured in alcohol could have cured you then. And now, five days later, the disease is as deep as your bones. Nobody can cure you now."
>
> Bian Que left. Several days later, the Emperor fell ill. He sent for the doctor. Bian Que arrived, but knew he could do no good. The disease was no longer "under the surface" but had manifested itself as a chronic condition.

TASTE AND CHARACTER

Sweet, warm.

FUNCTIONS

Da-zao invigorates the spleen, regulates the stomach, reinforces or invigorates vital energy (*qi/ch'i*), promotes production of body fluids, detoxifies, and balances ying (not to be confused with yin) and wei energy. Because of this function, jujube, like licorice root (*Glycyrrhiza uralensis*), is used in many Chinese prescriptions to help balance the way in which other herbs in the prescription act.

USES

Da-zao is used in prescriptions for lack of appetite and diarrhea due to spleen deficiency, loss of vital energy, blood loss, lack of strength, palpitations, purpurea due to reduction of blood platelets, insomnia, and night sweat.

Jujube crosses the line between food and medicine. On the one hand, the lustrous, dark-reddish, wrinkled fruits are relished for their sweetish-sour taste. Large, fleshy fruits are most valued for medicinal uses. They are frequently used in Chinese prescriptions as a general tonic, diuretic, and balancer of prescriptions. It helps to supplement and tonify the "spleen" and stomach, is considered moistening to the heart and lungs, and helps to nourish and pacify the spirit. It is a harmonizer in prescriptions. In experiments it has been shown to have an antiallergic effect and can prevent stress ulcers. The ethanol extract of the fruits is considered to have antiulcer activity.

Numerous prescriptions since ancient times have called for use of the fruit in a wide variety of conditions. Many of the prescriptions use the fruits as a kind of nutritional food, in combination with other "food herbs," as in the following prescriptions.

One traditional treatment for hives calls for a decoction of two ounces of the fruits. The decoction is drunk and the boiled fruits are eaten as well. The treatment is continued once a day for a week.

For spontaneous perspiration due to "imbalance of ying and wei" energy, 10 jujube fruits are combined with 9 g of *Prunus mume* fruits, 12 g of mulberry (*Morus alba*) leaves, and 15 g of wheat berries (of very poor quality, with thin shells, that float on the surface of water—basically aborted fruits). This mixture was decocted and drunk.

To invigorate and balance vital energy, one prescription calls for 10 large jujube fruits with the skin removed, and 3 g of ginseng (*Panax ginseng*) root. The fruit and roots are placed in a cloth bag and cooked in rice until they are very soft. Pills were then made.

A traditional treatment for apolexy with palpitation and a heavy feeling of the extremities involved cooking 7 large jujube fruits with 2 cups of half-ripe millet seeds. The fruits were first decocted in 1½ cups of water. Then the fruits were strained and added to the millet to make porridge.

For insomnia with anxiety, one prescription called for 20 fruits and 7 onion stems (white interior section of an onion at the base of bulb), which were boiled down to one third of its original volume in 3 cups of water, strained, and then drunk.

An external treatment for an old sore that will not heal called for 3 cups of smashed jujube fruits boiled in twice their volume of water to half of the original volume. The affected area was then washed with the decoction to help hasten the healing process.

In Western terms, the fruit of the jujube is considered stomachic, diuretic, fever-reducing, somewhat laxative, and mildly sedative. The dried fruits are sold in American herb markets as a dietary supplement. The fruits are also commonly available in Asian groceries in the United States.

Dose

Dose: 6–15 g in decoction, pills, poultice, wash, powder, paste, or ointment.

Contraindication

If the patient has fullness in the middle abdomen with much phlegm, jujube is contraindicated.

Description

Jujube is a shrub or small deciduous tree to 30 feet, with zigzagging branches, armed usually with two slender spines, one of them recurved, about an inch long, or unarmed in *Z. jujuba* var. *inermis* (Bunge.) Rehd. It is the unarmed variety that is generally used as the source plant for *da-zao*. The alternate, short-stalked leaves are oblong-ovate or ovate-lance shaped.

Margins are mostly entire, sometimes serrulate. Leaves are smooth and firm. The yellow flowers are in clusters of two to three in axils. The oblong or oval fruits, about an inch long, are brownish-red at first and then become dark red. Flowers appear from April to June; fruiting takes place from September to October. The red fruits are used in medicine. Large, red, thick-fleshed, moist, somewhat oily fruits are considered to be of the best quality. Both thorny and thornless forms are available in American horticulture.

DISTRIBUTION

The tree has been cultivated in China since time immemorial. It is found in a variety of habitats, from dry soils of plains and hillsides to plantations on river banks. Jujube is planted throughout China, except Jilin, Heilongjiang, Xinjiang, Qinghai, and Xizang (Tibet). Major production provinces include Henan and Shandong. It is also commercially produced in Hebei, Shanxi, Sichuan, and Guizhou. Shandong province produces the greatest quantity. Henan (Xin-cheng) produces the best quality. The fruit is sold throughout China and exported as well. Other provinces have some production, but it is saved for their own use.

Ziziphus jujuba, native from East Asia to southeastern Europe, has been cultivated in the Mediterranean region for several centuries and is also naturalized in some parts of the United States.

CULTIVATION

This tree is highly adaptable to growing conditions. It is generally cold hardy and tolerant of dry or wet conditions. The common jujube can be grown as far north as southern New England. The root sucker is often used for propagation in China. In spring, young suckers within 2 feet of established trees are cut away and then replanted. Night soil is given to the young suckers as a fertilizer. This is considered the easiest method of propagation in China. The root suckers are also separated from the mother tree in summer; however, they are not dug up and transplanted until the following spring. The tree does best in hot dry climates. It does not fruit as well in humid areas.

Experimental plantings in the United States over the past eighty years were primarily done in warmer parts of the country. Consequently a number of horticultural works describing its cultivation have erroneously stated that it will grow only in the southern United States.

HARVESTING

The fruit is commonly harvested about mid-September after it ripens. It is beaten from the trees and then dried in the sun. Another method is to bake the fruits until the surface of the peel is soft, then drying them in the sun. Sometimes the fruits may be parboiled until the surface is soft and wrinkled. Then they are dried in the sun.

PROCESSING

None noted.

ADDITIONAL SPECIES

The seeds of *Ziziphus jujuba* var. *spinosa* (Z. *spinosa* Hu), a wild variety common in the mountains on the outskirts of Beijing, is the source of the traditional Chinese drug *suan-zao-ren*. It is widely used in China as a sedative and hypnotic. Excellent results have been reported on the use of the seed extract for insomnia. On a trip to Beijing in 1988, Foster, suffering from severe jetlag and insomia, used the extract of *suan-zao-ren* as a sleep aid with excellent results. The seeds are an official drug in the Chinese *Pharmacopeia*.

OTHER USES

The bark, root, leaves, and seed shell have also been used as traditional folk remedies.

The leaves, *zao-ye*, first mentioned in *Shen Nong Ben Cao Jing*, are considered warming and without poisonous qualities. They have been used to treat children's fevers induced by seasonal weather and for sores and boils. They are used in decoction or as a poultice or wash.

The bark, *zao-shu-pi*, was first mentioned in *Ben Cao Gang Mu*. It is collected throughout the year, though spring is preferable. Older bark is best. It is dried in the sun. The character is considered bitter, warm and astringent. The bark is used for diarrhea, as an antiphlogistic, for chronic bronchitis, as an anti-inflammatory, and for blurred vision, burns, uterine bleeding, dysentery, and traumatic bleeding. The bark is stir-fried until charcoaled (retaining character), and used in powdered form, from 1.5 to 3 g in decoction, poultice, or applied as a wash. A tablet form of the bark is used for elderly patients with chronic bronchitis.

The root, *zao-shu-gen*, was first mentioned in *Ben Cao Gang Mu*. It is considered neutral, a little sweet, and without poison. The root is said to move vital energy (*qi/ch'i*), stimulate blood circulation, and regulate the menses. Applications include use for pains of joints, stomach pains, vomiting with blood, uterine bleeding, irregular menses, urticaria, and inflammatory diseases of the skin. Dose is 15 to 30 g in decoction, poultice, or used as a wash. For urticaria, the root of jujube is decocted with the bark of the camphor tree and used as a wash twice daily. For the treatment of joint pains, 15 g of the root is traditionally decocted with 30 g of *Eleutherococcus gracilistylis*. To treat stomach pains, 60 g of the fresh root was fried with the tongue of a pig.

The flowers are very fragrant. Honey gathered from the flowers of jujube is called *zao-mu-mi* and is considered a culinary delicacy.

Mulberry
Sang-ye, etc.

Botanical Name: *Morus alba* L.
Chinese Names: Pinyin: *Sang-ren* (fruits); *Sang-bai-pi* (root bark); *Sang-ye* (leaves); *Sang-zhi* (branches). Wade-Giles: *Sang-jen* (fruits); *Sang-pai-p'i* (root bark); *Sang-yeh* (leaves); *Sang-chih* (branches).
English Names: White mulberry, mulberry.
Pharmaceutical Names: Fructus Mori (fruits), Cortex Mori (bark), Folium Mori (leaves), Ramulus Mori (branches).
Family: Moraceae—mulberry family.

HISTORY

According to legend, the Empress of Huang-di, Si-Ling, who lived around 2960 B.C., taught the Chinese people how to raise silkworms using mulberry leaves as the worms' food. The tree has been cultivated in China for millennia. Numerous cultivated forms and varieties are grown throughout China.

Morus, the ancient Latin name for the mulberry tree, was typified by Linnaeus in 1753. The name has remained stable since. *Alba*, of course, means "white." The genus includes about seven temperate and subtropical trees, members of the mulberry family. The best-known plant in the genus is our subject, the white mulberry, *Morus alba*, native to eastern and central China and naturalized both in Europe and North America.

Cuttings of white mulberry were first brought to Tuscany from the Levant in 1434. Within 100 years it had almost entirely replaced plantations of *Morus nigra* in Italy for the purpose of feeding silkworms. An edict of the Colonial Assembly resulted in commercial plantings of mulberry in Virginia by 1623. In 1773 or 1774, William Bartram observed large plantations of white mulberry grafted to the indigenous eastern North American red mulberry (*Morus rubra*) in Charleston, South Carolina.

The possibility of commercial silk production and emphasis on planting white mulberries garnered tremendous attention in the first two hundred years of European settlement of North America. In his 1950 classic, *A History of Horticulture in America*, U. P. Hedrick wrote, "No agricultural subject in America has ever had so much attention in the press. Between the years 1828 and 1844, no fewer than 18 books, some of them running through several editions, were published. . . . The country supported four monthly magazines on mulberries and silk" (p. 217). In the end, it seems that the production of publications on silk production was more successful than American production of silk itself.

Mulberry fruits are quite frequently used in Chinese medicine. They are first mentioned in an ancient work dated at 2,000 B.C. The fruits are mentioned in the world's first official pharmacopeia, *Tang Ben Cao*, attributed to Su Jing and published during the Tang dynasty in 659 A.D. Mulberry fruit was placed in the middle class of drugs. Medicinal use of the leaves is first treated in the first-century A.D. *Shen Nong Ben Cao Jing*. The use of the young branches of *Morus alba* is originally mentioned in Su Song's 1061 A.D. Song dynasty work, *Tu Jing Ben Cao*. Li Shi-zhen's *Ben Cao Gang Mu* (1596) makes first mention of medicinal uses of the juice that exudes from the ends of fresh, heated branches. The juice of the fresh leaves used for medicinal purposes is first noted in Tao Hong-jing's *Ming Yi Bie Lu*, published around the year 500 in the dynasty of the North and South kingdoms.

TASTE AND CHARACTER

Fruits: sweet, sour, warm. Root bark: sweet, a little sweet, cold. Leaves: a little sweet, bitter, cold. Branches: bitter, neutral.

FUNCTIONS

Fruits: invigorates the liver and kidneys, nourishes the blood, promotes the production of body fluids, expels wind evil.

Root bark: reduces lung heat, stops asthma, strengthens the kidneys, reduces swelling.

Leaves: expels wind evil, disperses liver heat, clears the eyes, cools the blood, reduces fever due to wind heat.

Branches: expels wind evil and wetness, strengthens the joints and the kidneys.

USES

Fruit is used in prescriptions for vertigo, tinnitus, dizziness, palpitation, blood deficiency, diabetes, premature gray hair, thirst, dry intestines with constipation, deafness, poor eye sight (dark vision), neurasthenia, constipation due to blood deficiency, rheumatism, scrofula, and weak joints.

The root bark is used in prescriptions for asthma and cough due to lung heat, bronchitis, edema of the face, difficulty in urinating, high blood pressure, diabetes, traumatic injuries, and hypertension.

The leaves are used in prescriptions for colds due to wind and heat, headache, red eyes, sore throat, cough due to lung heat, eczema, urticaria, migratory arthralgia, and premature gray hair, and are poulticed on insect and spider bites.

The branches are used in prescriptions for stagnation and pain due to cold wind and wetness, spasms of limbs, edema of legs, itch due to wind, and arthralgia.

Virtually all parts of the mulberry tree are used in one way or another, both in TCM and in Chinese folk traditions. Mulberry leaves, bark, branches, and fruits are all official medicines in the 1985 edition of the Chinese *Pharmacopeia*. In Western terms, the root bark is considered antihypertensive, antiasthmatic, diuretic, and sedative. Experimentally, studies have confirmed diuretic and cathartic effects, a hypotensive action, and sedative, tranquilizing, anticonvulsive, analgesic, and hypothermic effects. Extracts are antibacterial. Chinese clinical studies report use in edema and bronchitis, plus esophageal and gastric cancer. In folk traditions, for centipede bites a poultice or wash of the inner bark was applied to the bite. Diaper rash is not a twentieth-century problem. A traditional

Chinese treatment for diaper rash called for the root bark of mulberry to be decocted in two large cups of water. The baby's rear end was placed in the warm decoction to treat the rash. For a patient who fell from a horse and twisted or strained back muscles, 2.5 kg of the inner bark of the root of mulberry was powdered and added to about 10 large cups of water. This was decocted until reduced to an extract, and then applied as needed.

The leaves are febrifugal, diaphoretic, and antibacterial. The fresh leaves have been shown to be strongly antibacterial against *Staphylococcus aureus*, *Streptococcus hemolyticus*, and *Bacillus anthracis*. Intravenous injections have been shown to lower blood pressure. Hypoglycemic effects have been reported in a number of studies. Chinese clinical studies on various leaf preparations have reported on its effects in the treatment of the common cold, upper respiratory tract infections, whooping cough, elephantiasis, and other ailments.

The leaves have long been used in Chinese tradition. An interesting treatment for red eyes, with pain and swelling, or eyes that feel astringent and uncomfortable, called for two mature leaves of mulberry. The leaves were placed in half a cup of very hot water. The tea was covered, and once the water was dark like thick tea the leaves were removed. This was used as an eye wash. The infusion was reheated every two hours, and used as a wash, three to five times per day. A folk treatment for open sores or boils used yellow mulberry leaves (harvested in fall after frost). They were baked until charred, powdered, and then mixed with sesame oil and applied to the affected area. For sore throat or toothache, one folk remedy is a decoction of 9 to 15 g of the leaves.

The fruits, like those of jujube, cross the line between food and medicine. Traditional medicinal prescriptions calling for the fruit often use a fruit concentrate, as noted in the following prescriptions. A traditional prescription for weak body and forgetfulness with insomnia calls for the fruits of mulberry to be boiled down until they become a thick extract. One spoonful is taken three times per day. If a patient could not sleep due to weakness of the heart and kidney and had chronic constipation, a decoction of 30 to 60 g of fresh mulberry fruits was prescribed. A traditional treatment for scrofula called for two jars of the ripe fresh fruits to be placed in a cloth sack, and the juice squeezed out and decocted down to a very thick, almost dry extract. One spoonful three times per day was taken.

The branches are antibacterial and considered antirheumatic, helping to improve joint movement.

Various mulberry tree products are sold in Chinatowns in the United

States, but are little known in health and natural food store herb outlets. Southerners still enjoy jams and jellies of mulberries, as well as eating the fresh fruit.

DOSE

Fruits are used in doses of 9–15 g, in decoction, extract, poultice or as a wash. The fruit can simply be eaten fresh or made into a fresh fruit tincture. The root bark is used in doses of 6–12 g. The leaves are used in doses of 3–12 g in decoction, powder, pills, poultice, or as a wash. Branches are used in doses of 30–60 g, decocted into a thick extract, poulticed, or as a wash or steam fumigant.

TOXICITY

Side effects from the use of injectable forms of leaf preparations have included localized pain, chills, fever, and dizziness, possibly resulting from precipitates. The reactions were mild and transient. Toxic reactions could not be found in the use of the crude leaf products.

DESCRIPTION

White mulberry is a deciduous tree growing up to 80 feet in height. The leaves are alternate, ovate, up to 4 to 6 inches long, coarsely toothed, often with thumblike lobes, and glossy green above. The flowers are unisexual, appearing in drooping catkins. The fruits, resembling a thin blackberry, are variable, ranging from white or pink to purple-black, and 1 to 2 inches long. Fruits appear in May or June. A number of cultivars are available in North American horticulture. Silkworm mulberry, a form of the species used for silk worm cultivation, has sweet black fruits; the leaves are large, dull green, and rough above. Russian mulberry, another form of white mulberry, is extremely hardy but produces fruits of relatively poor quality.

DISTRIBUTION

In China, the tree grows in mountain fields and is widely planted near villages or in cities as a shade or street tree. Cultivation in China is ancient, primarily as food for silkworm production. It occurs throughout China, but is especially common in Jiangsu and Zhejiang. Most mulberry trees in China are cultivated. Commercial cultivation of mulberry trees for fruits, silkworms, or other plant parts used in TCM takes place throughout China, especially in Sichuan, Jiangsu, Zhejiang, Shandong, Anhui, Liaoning, and Shanxi. Northern production is primarily sold to the city of Tianjin, where a mulberry-syrup manufacturing industry thrives. The provinces of Xinjiang, Yunnan, Shaanxi, Hunan, and Hubei have commercial mulberry plantations for local and regional production.

In the United States, the tree is widely planted and naturalized south and west of New York. One specimen in Kalamazoo, Michigan, has been recorded to be 82 feet in height and 16 feet in circumference.

CULTIVATION

White mulberry is adaptable to conditions, grows in warm or cool sur-roundings, and is tolerant of dry conditions. In China it is planted in mountain fields or near houses. Seeds, cuttings, or layering are used for propagation. It is said that seeds excreted from fowl fed on the fruits are more likely to produce trees bearing abundant foliage rather than fruit, and therefore, are more desirable for silkworm production. When the fruits are ripe (purple-black), they are harvested; the pulp is washed away to obtain the seeds. The tiny seeds are scattered in a seed bed and covered thinly with light soil. They are kept moist until they germinate in about two weeks. When one to two feet high, the trees are transplanted to a perma-nent location.

In China, layering is performed in March. Cuttings 8 to 9 inches long are taken and placed obliquely in the soil in the spring. In October or February of the following year, the rooted cuttings are transplanted to permanent locations.

HARVESTING

The fruits are collected in May or June when they are nearly ripe. They are dried in the sun or baked dry. Some growers steam the fruits first or blanch them in hot water before drying them in the sun. The latter method is said to make drying easier and helps to increase storage duration.

The inner bark of the root is harvested in winter. The root is dug up, cleaned, and the yellowish-brown outer bark is scraped off; the root is then cut into vertical sections. The sections are beaten with a wooden mallet to separate the inner bark from the wood. The bark is then dried in the sun. Traditionally, any part of the root found above ground is considered poisonous.

The leaves are collected after frost in deep autumn and dried in the shade.

The branches are collected in late spring or early summer. The leaves are removed and, once dried, the branches are cut into sections 12 to 24 inches long.

PROCESSING

For honey-processed root bark, the bark is placed in honey that has been heated and slightly burned, and a little hot water is added. The root bark is stir-fried for a few minutes until it turns a yellowish color. At this time the root bark should no longer feel sticky. It is then cooled. For every 100 pounds of root bark, 30 pounds of honey are used.

To make honey-processed leaves, the cleaned, dried leaves are mixed with honey and a little hot water added for good consistency. They are stir-fried until no longer sticky. For every 100 pounds of dried leaves, 20 pounds of honey are used.

For stir-fried mulberry branches, take cleaned sections of the branches, stir-fry over a light fire until a very light yellow color, and cool.

Wheat-bran processed branches calls for wheat bran, mixed with the branch sections, to be stir-fried until dark yellow. The branches are sifted to remove the bran, then cooled. For every 100 pounds of branch sections, 20 pounds of wheat bran are used.

Alcohol-processed branches are made by sprinkling alcohol on branch sections and stir-frying them until they turn a light yellow color. For every 100 pounds of branches, 15 pounds of alcohol are used.

ADDITIONAL SPECIES

Four other Chinese species of *Morus* are considered acceptable substitutes for *Morus alba*. These include *Morus australis* Poir., *M. mongolica* Schnied., *M. cathayana* Hemsl., and *M. laevigata* Wall. (*M. macroura* Miq.). *Morus australis* and *M. laevigata* have been introduced into American horticulture.

OTHER USES

Sang-li is the milky exudate from the ends of burning fresh branches of the tree. It is considered "good" for the hair and eyebrows, furuncles, and skin diseases. A traditional treatment for tetanus involves mixing the juice with good wine. The patient drinks as much as possible until becoming drunk. Upon awakening, he or she will be cured.

A clinical report in the Chinese literature on treating tetanus calls for a mulberry branch about 3 feet long and an inch in diameter. It is heated over a fire, and the dripping juice from both ends of the branch is collected. Adults were given a 10 ml (children 1 to 2 ml) dose with sugar three times per day. After administration, the patient sweats. In 17 cases, 15 returned to good health and 2 were not helped. If the patient was seriously ill, Western medicines were also used.

Sang-shuang, the processed wood of *Morus alba* made into charcoal, was first mentioned by Li Shi-zhen in *Ben Cao Gang Mu* (1596). The wood is charcoaled and then filtered with water. The wood is then steamed with much water, leaving only a few crystals. This is *sang-shuang*. It is used for treating food stuck in the throat after eating too fast; externally it is poulticed on sores and carbuncles.

Juice of the fresh leaves, *sang-ye-zhi*, is considered a little cold and bitter. It is used for carbuncles, tumors, injuries, bleeding, and centipede bites, primarily as a poultice. The juice is used as a poultice on the affected area; as an eye drop, it is used for certain eye ailments. For boils, the juice is dripped onto the affected area.

The distilled water made from the leaves, *sang-ye-lu*, is used in doses of 20–60 g for the treatment of eye disease, to expel wind, and to clear away heat.

The root, *sang gen*, is used for the treatment of epilepsy induced by fright, pains of the bones and muscles, conjunctivitis, thrush, and high blood pressure. A decoction of 15 to 30 g of the root is used. For conjunctivitis, 30 g of the clean fresh root is decocted and then drunk. A piece of pig's liver may be added when making the decoction. It is taken in the morning.

If a person uses too much Sichuan pepper (*Zanthoxylum simulans*), a decoction of mulberry root is used as an antidote. This is also used as a wash on centipede bites.

The sap of the tree, *sang-pi-zhi*, is considered bitter. It is used for the treatment of thrush in infants or traumatic bleeding. It is used as a decoction or a poultice, or the sap can be taken with hot water. The sap is applied directly to thrush infections or sores on the tongue.

The charcoaled wood (ash) of *Morus alba*, *sang-chai-hui*, is considered hot, and cold, slightly toxic. The ash is decocted in water or used as a powder, a poultice, a wash, or infused in hot water. It is used in prescriptions for edema, swelling due to sores, drinking of too much water, or edema from a head injury. For a person stabbed through the heart, the ash of the wood is used to stop the bleeding. If the roots of the hair are graying, a decoction of the wood ash is used as a hair wash. For blackheads, the ash of the wood is mixed together with lime, decocted, and the decoction is applied as a wash.

Mulberries are widely planted in subtropical regions of China, India, and other countries as food for silkworm larvae. The leaves can also be eaten as a vegetable, and have been suggested as a possible cattle fodder. They are said to improve milk yield when fed to cows.

Mulberry wood is used for making sporting goods such as the handles of hockey sticks, tennis and badminton rackets, cricket bats and stumps, and other equipment. The wood is widely used in India.

Silk Tree
He-huan-pi

Botanical Name: *Albizia julibrissin* Durazz.
Botanical Synonyms: *Mimosa julibrissin* (Durazz.) Scop.; *M. speciosa* Thunb., non Jacq.; *Acacia nemu* Willd.; *Albizia nemu* (Willd.) Benth. The genus name is also erroneously spelled *Albizzia*.
Chinese Names: Pinyin: *He-huan-pi* (bark); *He-huan-hua* (flowers). Wade-Giles: *Ho-huan-p'i* (bark); *Ho-huan-hua* (flowers).
English Names: Silk tree, mimosa, Albizzia.
Pharmaceutical Name: Cortex Albiziae (bark); Flos Albiziae (flowers).
Family: Leguminosae—Pea family; or Mimosaceae—mimosa family.

HISTORY

Commonly known as mimosa in the United States, the silk tree has become a common ornamental of the southern landscape. It is a fast-growing small tree, with a broad-spreading crown and a short trunk. Because of its low, spreading branches close to the ground, it is a favorite yard tree of children, since it is easily climbed. The delicate clusters of pink flowers continue to bloom for weeks. Herbal use of the tree is practically unknown in America. Both the bark and the flowers are used in TCM.

The genus *Albizia*, a relative of the acacias, contains about 150 species of shrubs and trees native to the Old World and South America. Our subject, *Albizia julibrissin*, was known in England by 1754. It was introduced by Richard Bateman, Esq., presumably from Persian material though it was grown in France by 1745. In 1749, the Italian for whom the tree is named, Cavaliere Filippo Albizzi, brought the tree from Constantinople to Italy. Antonio Durazzini provided the first valid botanical description of the plant in the *Magazzino Toscani* in 1772. He named the plant after Albizzi, calling it *Albizia julibrissin*, the name still in use today. The species name *julibrissin* is derived from the Persian *gul-i-abrischim*, meaning a type of silky weaving, referring to the soft silky appearance of the pink flowers.

By 1814 the tree was known to be well established in Bartram's Botanical Garden, the garden of John and William Bartram, near Philadelphia. The French botanist André Michaux had brought seeds to America from France when he arrived in 1785. He gave seeds to the Bartrams as well as to William Hamilton. Thomas Jefferson obtained seeds and grew the tree at Monticello. By the mid-1800s, the tree had become established in the South. *A Flora of North America*, by John Torrey and Asa Gray, published between 1838 and 1840, lists *Albizia julibrissin*. This work, though never completed as originally envisioned, is a foundation for systematic botany of the United States.

Torrey and Gray write: "In gardens and yards . . . cultivated and somewhat naturalized.—A small and very ornamental tree; a native of Persia. Flowers white; the stamens flesh-color or purplish above. The Persian name is said to mean Silky-flower. (1838-40, vol. 1, p. 404).

The tree is now commonly naturalized south of Washington, D.C. Though the tree primarily grows in the southern United States, certain cultivars are hardy as far north as Boston. One, *A. julibrissin* 'Ernest Wilson,' was introduced from seeds collected in the garden of the Chosen Hotel, Seoul, Korea, by E. H. Wilson in 1918.

The first Chinese herbal in which the bark is mentioned is *Ben Cao Shi Yi*, ("Omissions from the Materia Medica"), published during the Tang dynasty in 720 and attributed to Chen Cang-qi. The flower is first mentioned in a work published in a 1116 Song dynasty work, *Ben Cao Yan Yi*, attributed to Kou Zong-shi. The name *he-huan* refers to the use of the plant to "enliven the spirit."

TASTE AND CHARACTER

Bark: a little sweet, neutral. Flowers: a little sweet, bitter, and neutral.

FUNCTIONS

The bark relieves uneasiness of body and mind, disperses depressed vital energy (qi/ch'i), regulates the blood, and alleviates pain. The flowers relieve uneasiness of body and mind, nourish heat, increase appetite, and regulate vital energy.

USES

The dried bark is used in decoction for insomnia, an unsteady mind, restlessness, lung abscesses, and pulmonary abscesses. Externally it is used as a poultice for carbuncles with swelling, furuncles, painful wounds, and pain due to fracture. The flowers are used for weak nerves, insomnia, poor memory, and chest discomfort.

Both the bark of the silk tree (he-huan-pi) and the flowers (he-huan-hua) are official in the 1985 Chinese *Pharmacopeia*. Primary uses for the bark are in prescriptions to relieve depression, restlessness, and insomnia due to anxiety. Externally, the bark is used for traumatic injuries to relieve pain by invigorating blood circulation. The flowers are primarily used for their sedative and tranquilizing effects on fidgets and insomnia. In recent pharmacological studies, the flower extracts stimulate uterine contractions in animal experiments. Saponins and tannins have been identified in the bark. Tonifying, stimulating, analgesic, and diuretic effects have also been indicated for the bark.

In Western terms, the bark is considered anodyne, anthelmintic, tonic, vulnerary, discutient, and sedative. The flower is considered mildly sedative, digestive, and tonic. Stuart writes that it, "promotes joy, assuaging sorrow, brightening the eye, and giving the desires of the heart" (1911, p. 23).

He-huan-pi and *he-huan-hua* are Chinese herbs that are virtually unknown on the American herb market.

DOSE

Bark: 9–30 g. Flowers: 3–9 g.

DESCRIPTION

The silk tree, often called the mimosa tree, is a small to medium-sized, short-lived deciduous tree that grows to 40 feet. The tree branches two to four feet above the base into a wide, spreading, rounded, umbrella-shaped crown. The alternate leaves are bipinnate, with 10 to 25 divisions, each with 10 to 30 pairs of leaflets. The leaflets are oblong-lance shaped, less than an inch long; the base is unequal, and the margin entire. The graceful feathery leaves are highly ornamental. A distinct cup-shaped gland is found on the upper side of the petiole (leaf stalk), near the swollen base of the stalk. The leaves are sensitive, folding up at night. The globular, pink flowers grow at the ends of branches or in leaf axils, on short flower stalks or nearly sessile. They are described as "silky" in appearance because of the dozens of slender filaments of the stamens. The stamens are the conspicuous part of the flower the corolla itself is much smaller. They bloom from June through July. The flowers are loved by hummingbirds. The pea-shaped legume (pods), to 6 inches long, are flat, dry, and papery with 10 to 15 smooth brown seeds.

DISTRIBUTION

The silk tree is found from Iran to India, China, and Japan, and is naturalized in the United States. It is found on mountainsides, in mountain valleys, and along forest edges of central China. In China it is planted in most provinces, both north and south, occurring in Liaoning, Hebei, Shaanxi, Gansu, Ningxia, Xinjiang, Shandong, Jiangsu, Anhui, Jiangxi, Fujian, Henan, Hubei, Hunan, Guangxi, Guangdong, Sichuan, Guizhou and Yunnan. The provinces of Jiangxi, Anhui, Zhejiang, and Sichuan are the main production regions. It is said to be most common in eastern Sichuan and western Hubei. It is sometimes planted as an ornamental around temples.

In the United States it is naturalized, primarily in the Southeast, occurring in waste places, along roadsides, fence rows, borders of woods, and clearings, from Delaware west to Indiana and Missouri, and south to Florida and Texas.

CULTIVATION

The small, fast-growing silk tree likes warm moist surroundings and full sun, though it is quite adaptable, as evidenced by the fact that it is used in sidewalk plantings (along with ginkgo) in downtown Manhattan. The plant can tolerate cold conditions and poor dry soils. A temperature of -14°F in the winter of 1985 killed the tops of many "mimosa" trees in northern Arkansas, but new growth sprouted from the main trunks the following summer. In China, seedlings are started in early spring. The hard seeds are scarified (the seed coat is nicked with a file or sandpaper), and then soaked in water for 8 to 10 hours. Sometimes the seed is immersed in water at 160°F for five to six minutes to kill potentially harmful microorganisms. The seeds are planted out in rows spaced at two feet, and covered with about an inch of soil. The beds are kept moist until the seeds sprout, which takes about 10 days. Cultivars (cultivated varieties) are propagated vegetatively from cuttings. Young seedlings in nursery beds are kept well weeded. The following spring or autumn, seedlings are transplanted to permanent locations.

Albizia is sometimes attacked by a fungal blight that enters the roots and destroys the sap wood. Infected individuals die relatively quickly; however, only older, larger trees seem to be affected.

HARVESTING

In spring, summer, or autumn the lateral branches of the tree are lopped off. Bark harvested before April 5 (Qing Ming Festival) is considered to be the highest quality. The bark is removed, cut into pieces, and dried in the sun. The flower buds (the inflorescence with a small piece of the peduncle or flower stalk) are harvested from May to July on a sunny day, just before they begin to open. After harvest, the flowers are dried quickly in the sun, or more slowly under shade. Frequent stirring is required to retain the color of the flowers.

PROCESSING

In production areas in China, the bark is soaked in clean water for a short time, and then covered with a wet cloth until it is uniformly moist. It is then cut into long strips, which are again cut into square pieces that are dried in the sun.

ADDITIONAL SPECIES

Albizia kalkora (Roxb.) Prain is used in some parts of China as a substitute for *A. julibrissin*. The former is rare in cultivation in the United States. Another species considered closely related to *A. julibrissin*, *A. lebbeck* (L.) Benth., is from tropical Asia. Its uses in India are similar to Chinese uses for *A. julibrissin*.

OTHER USES

A decoction of silk tree leaves is considered insecticidal against maggots. The leaves have also been suggested as a fodder for farm animals.

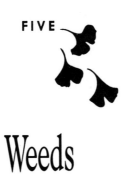

FIVE

Weeds

Achyranthes
Niu-xi

Botanical Name: *Achyranthes bidentata* Blume.
Chinese Names: Pinyin: *Niu-xi* (root). Wade-Giles: *Niu-hsi* (root).
English Name: Achyranthes.
Pharmaceutical Name: Radix Achyranthis.
Family: Amaranthaceae—amaranth family.

HISTORY

In 1958, Prof. Yue worked on farms in Wu-zhi in Henan province, where he participated in the harvest and processing of *Achyranthes bidentata*. The root is known in China as *niu-xi*. *Niu-xi* means "ox-knee," in reference to the somewhat swollen leaf nodes, which resemble the knee of an ox. Four famous traditional herbal medicines, known collectively as *huai* drugs, are produced in this area, including *niu-xi*, *Rehmannia glutinosa* (rehmannia root), *Dioscorea opposita* (wild yam root), and the flowers of the mum (*Chrysanthemum morifolium*). The plant is little known in the United States, although is a naturalized weed in the Gulf states.

The genus *Achyranthes* of the amaranth family contains at least ten species of variable tropical and subtropical weeds of the Old World. Another species, *Achyranthes aspera*, also found in China and common in India, was the first *Achyranthes* species named by Linnaeus in 1753. *Achyranthes bidentata* was the name given to the plant in an 1825 publication by Carl Ludwig von Blume. It has become a cosmopolitan weed in subtropical areas, including the southern United States. The exact date of its arrival in the New World is unclear.

Niu-xi is fist mentioned in *Shen Nong Ben Cao Jing* in the first class of herbal medicine. The most famous production area for this herb is in Wu-zhi county in Henan province.

TASTE AND CHARACTER

A little sweet, bitter, sour, neutral.

FUNCTIONS

Niu-xi expels blood stasis and reduces swelling. Processed *niu-xi* invigorates the liver and kidneys and strengthens bones and tendons.

USES

Niu-xi is used in prescriptions for turbid urine, difficult urination with blood, suppressed menstruation, difficulty in childbirth, difficulty in expelling the placenta, blood stasis after giving birth causing abdominal pains, sore throats, carbuncles with swelling, and traumatic injuries.

Processed *niu-xi* is used for waist, knee, and bone pains, and for stiffness, muscle spasms, pain, flaccidity, and high blood pressure.

Niu-xi, an official listing in the 1985 Chinese *Pharmacopeia*, is a famous traditional Chinese herb used to nourish the "kidney and liver," and to strengthen the bones and sinews for treating aches of the back and knees or debility or lack of strength in the lower limbs. It is also used in prescriptions for the treatment of hypertension. The root is considered to be diuretic as well. A traditional prescription for difficult urination, pain within the urethra, and blood stasis in women calls for one handful of *niu-xi*, including the leaves and stems. The herb is decocted and then taken with alcohol. It has also been used as a folk treatment for sores of the mouth and tongue. A tincture of *niu-xi* is used as a gargle for this purpose. Externally, a poultice of the root has been used as a folk remedy for knife injuries or wounds caused by metal objects.

A very interesting clinical report in the Chinese literature details how the root is used in some hospitals as an aid in performing dilation of the cervix and curettage of the uterus (commonly referred to as D & C). It is an excellent example of the combination of TCM and conventional medical techniques in modern Chinese health care. *Niu-xi* dry roots, 0.2 to 0.3 cm wide and 7 to 9 cm long, are chosen. The crown of the root must be round, not very sharp, and narrow. First the root is washed. A string is tied on the end of the root, or a hole drilled in the end, through which a string is tied. It is then placed in an autoclave to disinfect and completely sterilize the root. Surgical tongs are used to place the root inside the vagina (leaving the string outside for easy removal of the root). The root may be wrapped in sterile gauze. After twelve to twenty-four hours, the *niu-xi* root is removed and the D & C is performed. In 78 reported cases that used this technique, the root helped to engorge the cervix with blood, so that it was soft, and easily dilated. Using this method reportedly made the D & C easier and quicker to perform.

Experimentally, the root has been shown to have an analgesic effect, functions as an anti-inflammatory, has a gastrointestinal antispasmodic effect, is diuretic, and has the hypotensive effect of dilating blood vessels for a brief period of time. Water extracts have potential antiallergic action. The herb has a strong protein anabolism action—it increases the weight of laboratory animals and enhances protein anabolism of the kidneys and liver.

In Western terms, the root is considered an anodyne, analgesic, antirheumatic, diuretic, emmenagogue, stimulant, and tonic. The root is sometimes sold in herb combination products in health and natural food markets in the United States, although it is generally unfamiliar to the American herb consumer. In the United States, its use is primarily limited to prescriptions by TCM practitioners.

DOSE

4.5—15 g, in decoction, tincture, extract, pills, powders, and poultice.

WARNING

Contraindicated during pregnancy.

DESCRIPTION

Niu-xi is a squared-stemmed perennial herb growing from 15 to 38 inches in height. The branching stems are swollen at the nodes. The leaves are opposite and ovate-oblong, 2 to 4 inches long and about 1½ to 2 inches wide. There are dense velvety hairs on both surfaces. The flower stalks are terminal or axillary spikes with numerous inconspicuous greenish flowers.

DISTRIBUTION

The plant occurs wild in mountains and grassy areas in Shanxi, Shaanxi, Shandong, Anhui, Jiangsu, Zhejiang, Jiangxi, Taiwan, Hunan, Hubei, Sichuan, Guizhou, and Yunnan. The major cultivated production of the plant is in Wu-zhi county, Henan province, and other nearby counties. Some *niu-xi* is also produced in Hebei, Shanxi, Shandong, Jiangsu, and Liaoning. The cultivated roots from Henan are the highest quality. They are sold throughout China, and exported as well.

Achyranthes bidentata has become a cosmopolitan subtropical weed naturalized in the southern United States, the warmer parts of Asia, and other regions of the world.

CULTIVATION

Niu-xi grows best in warm areas in a rich, loose, sandy, well-drained soil. It does not do well in alkaline or clay soils, preferring a somewhat acid situation. The plant needs very deep soil to produce the highest quality roots. The soil should be liberally supplied with good-quality, well-rotted manure to ensure quick and vigorous growth. It is hardy to about 10°F.

Propagation is by seeds, planted in late spring. In China, it is planted out in rows spaced at about 1½ feet. They are covered lightly with soil. Seeds usually germinate in 5 to 7 days. When the seedlings are 3 to 4 inches high, they are thinned to a spacing of about six inches. Plantings are kept weeded during the growing season. To stimulate more root growth, the lower leaves and stems are removed from the first eight inches of the main stalk.

A benchmark of root quality is the length of the root, measured in "hands" (fist atop fist, basically the same measure used to determine the height of a horse). The highest-quality *niu-xi* root is 16 hands long, followed by roots that are 12 hands long. In the market, roots run from 2 to 6 hands (6 to 20 inches) in length. However, roots of exceptional quality may be more than 36 hands long—more than the height of an average person.

The root is harvested with a special tool called a *da-qian (ta-ch'ien)*, basically a long narrow shovel. Attached to a wooden handle about five feet long, the blade itself is about five inches wide and 15 inches long. The *da-qian* has an incurved blade with two teeth on either side. It is stabbed hard into the soil and then pressed in deep with the foot. The knee is used as a fulcrum to lift deep roots from the soil while keeping them intact.

HARVESTING

Cultivated roots are harvested after being grown for one or two years. Sometimes wild roots are dug from mountain fields or roadsides. It is collected in late fall, after the leaves have shriveled. After the roots have been dug up, thin lateral rootlets are removed and the roots are washed and tied into bundles. Roots are dried in the sun until the surface is wrinkled, but not 100 percent dry. They are then fumigated with sulphur fumes twice. Next, the crown of the root is cut off and the root is dried to

100 percent. Wild *niu-xi* is collected in autumn or winter, washed, and dried in the sun.

Another method is to simply clean the roots, cover them with a moist cloth until uniformly moist and soft, cut off the crown, and cut the root in slices. They are then dried in the sun.

PROCESSING

Rice (yellow) wine is used to produce processed *niu-xi*. The root is stir-fried until very hot. Then yellow wine is sprinkled on it, and it is fried again until a little dry, after which it is taken off the fire and cooled. For every 50 pounds of root, 5 pounds of yellow wine are used.

ADDITIONAL SPECIES

Achyranthes aspera, a wild species in Fujian, Guangdong, Guangxi, Sichuan, and Yunnan, is sometimes used as an herb or local medicine, not an official drug. It is called *ju-niu-xi* or *wei-niu-xi*. *Achyranthes longifolia* Mak. is also used as *niu-xi* in Jiangsu, Anhui, Zhejiang, Jiangxi, Fujien, Hubei, Hunan, Sichuan, Guizhou, and Yunnan. *Cyathula officinalis* is also used as a type of *niu-xi*. *Strobilanthes nemorosus* R. Ben, a member of the acanthus family (Acanthaceae) is used in some areas as a substitute for *niu-xi*. It, too, is called *wei-niu-xi*. This plant has the function to expel blood stasis, reduce swelling and pain, and strengthen the bones and muscles. *Cucubala baccifer* L., *bai-niu-xi*, a member of the pink family (Caryophyllaceae), is sometimes used as a low-quality, inferior substitute for *niu-xi* in some areas of Yunnan province.

Achyranthes rotundata is a rare shrub found only in arid and semiarid coastal lowlands of the island of Oahu in Hawaii. It is now known from only two populations, which include about 400 individual plants. It is on the federal list of endangered species.

OTHER USES

The root is the part of the drug most often used, but the leaves and the stem are also used as a folk medicine. The stems and leaves are collected in July and August. They are used for rheumatic pains due to cold and wetness, pains of the lower back, malaria, and turbid urine; 3 to 9 g of the dried leaves are used, or the fresh leaves are crushed for the juice or tinctured.

In India, the seed has been eaten as a grain in times of scarcity.

Japanese Honeysuckle
Jin-yin-hua and *Ren-dong-teng*

Botanical Name: *Lonicera japonica* Thunb.
Chinese Names: Pinyin: *Jin-yin-hua* (flowers); *Ren-dong-teng* (stems with leaves attached). Wade-Giles: *Chin-yin-hua* (flowers); *Jen-tong-teng* (stems).
English Name: Japanese honeysuckle.
Pharmaceutical Name: Caulis Lonicerae (dried stems with attached leaves); Flos Lonicerae (dried flowers).
Family: Caprifoliaceae—honeysuckle family.

HISTORY

An Englishman, William Kerr, who collected botanical specimens in Guangtong (Canton) for the Royal Botanical Garden at Kew, introduced Japanese honeysuckle into England by 1806. It came in the ship *Hope* captained by James Pendergrass. In the same year, Japanese honeysuckle arrived in the United States as a potential ornamental. Through the ensuing decades, the plant was considered a welcome ornamental among rare plant collectors. But in 1862, George Hall introduced a new vigorous variety to Parson's Nursery in Flushing, New York. This new introduction, *Lonicera japonica* "Halliana," (*L. Halleana* Hort. ex C. Koch) was touted in a 1912 nursery catalog as "Grand for trellises and ground cover. One of the best." The difference between this and other forms of Japanese honeysuckle is simply that Hall's honeysuckle is more vigorous in growth. This cultivated variety has become the most hated alien weed species of the eastern United States. First recorded as a garden escape in the 1890s, by 1919 it was considered a rank aggressive invader. Now it is recognized as one of the most ruthless weeds in America, especially the Southeast.

The genus *Lonicera* of the honeysuckle family includes about 180 species of shrubs and twining vines native to the northern hemisphere. Many species are cultivated as ornamentals. *Lonicera* is named after a German botanist, Adam Lonicer, who died in 1596.

The Chinese name *jin-yin-hua* means gold and silver flower. This refers to the fact that the white flowers turn golden yellow one or two days after blooming. Another Chinese name, *ren-dong*, referring to the stems with the leaves attached, means "stand winter" in reference to the fact that the leaves are evergreen.

The medicinal use of the flowers is mentioned in early Chinese herbals including *Ming Yi Bie Lu*, attributed to Tao Hong-jing (about 500 A.D.) and *Lu Chan Yan Ben Cao* (Materia Medica from Steep Mountainsides) attributed to Wang-jie, and dated about 1163–1224 A.D. Only one hand-written copy of the book survives from the Ming dynasty. The use of the stems is first mentioned in *Ben Cao Jing Ji Zhu*, attributed to Tao Hong-jing, published around the year 500 A.D.

TASTE AND CHARACTER

Flowers: a little sweet, cold. Stems: a little sweet, cold.

FUNCTIONS

Flowers: disperse heat and toxic matter. Stems: disperse heat and toxic materials, stimulate the menses, and allow energy to flow through the meridians.

USES

Flowers are used in prescriptions to treat infections of the upper respiratory tract, fever, colds, flu, acute conjunctivitis, acute mastitis, acute tonsillitis, pneumonia of the large lobes, lung abscesses, bacillus dysentery, leptospirosis, acute appendicitis, fever, headache, stuffy nose and sore throat, carbuncles, furuncles with pus and swelling, inflammatory diseases with redness of the skin, infections due to injuries, and ulcerations of the cervix. In short, it is considered to be a febrifugal (fever-reducing) agent and detoxicant for feverish conditions and acute infections.

Stems (branches) are used for rheumatism, urticaria, mumps, upper respiratory tract infections, pneumonia, flu, furuncles and swelling, appendicitis, and infectious hepatitis.

The flowers and the stems of Japanese honeysuckle comprise two separate herbal medicines in the 1985 Chinese *Pharmacopeia*. The flowers are used more often than the stems. An injectable form of the flowers is used in Chinese hospitals. For infected injuries with pus, the Japanese honeysuckle flower injection (in 4–6 ml dosage) is administered once every 4 to

6 hours. An injection of 2 percent procaine is used in conjunction with the treatment. A tincture of the flowers is also prescribed in Chinese hospitals for the treatment of cervical ulcers, utilizing 1000 g of the rough powder of the dried flowers, soaked in 1500 ml of 40 percent alcohol for 48 hours. The tincture is then filtered, decocted down to 400 ml, and poulticed on the affected area for 7 to 12 days. A decoction of the flowers along with the branches and leaves has long been used as a treatment for swellings with toxic matter (pus), both open and closed; or in the beginning stages of infection where the skin feels very hot, boils are present, or the patient has a sore throat. About one cup of juice of the fresh flowers, branches, and leaves is decocted to 80 percent of the original volume and then drunk. The spent herb material is used as a poultice on the affected area.

The action of the stems is considered similar to that of the flowers. It has primarily been used for dispersing heat and as an adjunct in the treatment of acute rheumatoid arthritis. The stems are also used for colds. A prescription for the common cold, characterized as "four seasons cold," with fever, accompanied by thirst and general aching, calls for 30 g of the dried stem with leaves (90 g fresh), which is decocted and drunk instead of tea. A thick decocted extract of the stem has been used as a traditional treatment for dysentery with bleeding. To treat chronic sores that have come to a head, the stem is made into an alcohol tincture, which is taken internally. A folk treatment for mushroom poisoning consisted of simply chewing the young branches and leaves very slowly, and swallowing the juice. One clinical study reports positive results using a strong decoction of the stem (with leaves) in the treatment of infectious hepatitis.

A clinical report to reduce the incidence of strep throat in 425 high school students used equal quantities (unspecified) of dried honeysuckle flowers and the root of *Belamcanda chinensis* (blackberry lily), with a small amount of borneol. The powder was blown on to the back of the patients' throats. Positive results were reported.

Another clinical study reports on the treatment of babies with pneumonia using a 20 percent intramuscular injection of the flowers (2 mls). Seriously ill patients received a 50 percent injection, with 10 to 30 percent of patients receiving the treatment intravenously. The treatment was used in 25 cases. Sixteen returned to good health, while 9 were much improved. After 2.5 days of treatment, the fever was reduced; 2.8 days later, labored breathing was allayed, and after 3.7 days, gurgling sounds in the chest were reduced.

For the treatment of acute bacillus dysentery, 300 g of honeysuckle flowers, 90 g of *Coptis chinensis* (Chinese goldthread), and 90 g of *Scutellaria baicalensis* (Baikal scullcap) are made into a 100 ml decoction. 30 ml of the decoction are taken 4 times per day. Out of 80 patients, 77 responded favorably to the prescription.

For wounds with pus infections, distilled water is used to make a 100 percent intramuscular injection of the flowers. The injection was administered every four to six hours, in 4–10 ml doses. For mild cases the injection was used only once. The same preparation (with procaine) was also reported to treat acute mastitis, carbuncles, and perforated appendix. A 90 percent success rate was reported.

Clinical reports have also been published on the use of honeysuckle flower preparations in the treatment of symptoms of cervical cancer, acute eye inflammations, urticaria, diarrhea in children, pneumonia, infectious hepatitis, hyperlipidemia, and leptospirosis.

Pharmacological research has shown that flower extracts have a strong antibacterial effect against *Salmonella tyhpi*, *Pseudomonas aeruginosa*, *Staphylococcus aureus*, *Staphylococcus pneumoniae*, and *Mycrobacterium tuberculosis*. In vitro studies have indicated antiviral activity. Studies with rats suggest that honeysuckle flower preparations may lower serum cholesterol levels. Components of the flowers have experimental antispasmodic, diuretic, and stomachic effects. Preparations of the flowers have been shown to promote leukocytic phagocytosis and phagocytic activity of inflammatory cells, suggesting immunostimulent activity.

In Western terms, febrifugal, astringent, depurative, corrective, antidiarrhetic, antiphlogistic, diuretic, and refrigerant qualities are attributed to the plant. Stuart states, "Prolonged use is said to increase vitality and strengthen life" (1911, p. 247). Japanese honeysuckle flowers and stems are used in some Chinese herb combination products available in health and natural food stores in the United States, though it is most likely to be used by TCM practitioners.

DOSE

Flowers 9–15 g in decoction, pills, powders, or poultice of the powder. Stems: 9–30 g in decoction, pills, powders, tincture, poultice, or dry extract.

DESCRIPTION

Japanese honeysuckle is a high-climbing or trailing woody vine. Young branches are pubescent. The evergreen opposite leaves are oval or elliptical-shaped, 1 to 3 inches long, with sparse hairs on the midribs above and below. The margins are entire (toothed in young growth), and pubescent. The sweetly fragrant white (fading to yellow) flowers are axillary, in pairs or solitary. The funnel-shaped corolla divides above and below. The top lobe is four-divided, the lower lip has one lobe. Flowers are 1¼ to 2 inches long, with strongly protruding stamens and style. It blooms from May to August. The fruit is a black, globe-shaped berry.

DISTRIBUTION

In China, Japanese honeysuckle grows in hillsides or valleys, forest margins, and is cultivated. It is found in most of China. Notably, the highest quality comes from Shandong, and Henan. The vine also grows in Japan and Korea.

In the United States, Japanese honeysuckle is widely naturalized in thickets, fields, and along roadsides and woodlands from southern New England west to Missouri and Kansas, and south to Florida and Texas. It is considered one of the most pernicious of introduced weeds that have become naturalized in the United States, more often than not completely dominating and eradicating native vegetation.

CULTIVATION

To suggest that Japanese honeysuckle be consciously planted by persons south of northern New England is simple blasphemy. After its introduction, Hall's honeysuckle (once called *Lonicera Halleana*) was considered one of the best of the climbing species and was valued because it was a free grower and bloomed throughout the summer. Within a few decades after its introduction to eastern North America, it became one of the most tenacious and hated weeds, spreading from birds eating the fruits and excreting the seeds in open areas, where it quickly took hold and choked out thousands of acres of native vegetation. The plant is extremely vigorous and aggressive. Unlike most native woody vines, Japanese honeysuckle is a twining vine that climbs and chokes vegetation, especially small trees and shrubs. It grows extremely fast—one plant can grow as much as 48 feet in a single year! Most efforts relative to the plant in the United States focus on eradicating it. Some even call for making the planting of Japanese honeysuckle illegal. But perhaps the best way to eradicate it is to find a way to use it, for medicinal or material purposes. The following is the Chinese experience in cultivating the plant. It is *not* recommended for planting in the United States.

Japanese honeysuckle is a pernicious perennial that will grow in average soil. In China it is grown in mountainside ditches near houses, in fields, backyards, or wherever idle land is available. Cuttings are used for propagation. In north China during July and August, when it is hot and humid, a rainy day is chosen to make cuttings of two- to three-year-old strong branches. They are cut into sections 1 to 1½ feet long, the lower leaves are removed, and the cuttings are placed obliquely in the soil, to a depth of two thirds the length of the cutting. Rows are spaced at 3 to 5 feet, with 2 to 3 feet between holes. Three to five cuttings are placed in each hole. With temperatures between 46 and 86°F, roots should develop in about 15 days. Japanese honeysuckle is also propagated by root divisions in spring or autumn; before the plant develops buds, or after it is hit by frost. Lateral young shoots are chosen for division.

HARVESTING

The stems are harvested in autumn and winter. The stems and leaves are cut off, tied into small bundles, and dried in the sun. The flowers are harvested in May through June. Before sunrise or in early morning after the dew has dried from the flowers, large flower buds that have not yet opened are picked. They are spread evenly on a stone slab or reed mat, and dried in the sun on the same day in which the flowers are harvested. Once spread out to dry, the flowers are not handled, turned, or allowed to become wet; otherwise they bruise and turn an undesirable black color, which affects the quality of the drug. If harvested on a rainy day, they must be dried indoors or baked over very low heat. If dried in this manner the flowers must be turned every few hours. However, if baked or dried in shade the color becomes darker, lessening the quality. The flowers should be stored in a dry place with good air circulation to prevent insect infestation and darkening of the dried flowers.

PROCESSING

The stems are sorted, soaked in water for a short time, and covered with a wet cloth until the stems are uniformly moist. They are then cut into small sections and dried in the sun.

To clean the dried flowers, they are sifted to remove dust and leaves. Some prescriptions call for fried *jin-yin-hua*, in which case the flowers are stir-fried for a short time. Another processing method is to stir-fry them over high heat for a short time until the exterior is black (charcoaled) while retaining the medicinal "character" of the flower interior. This is called "charcoaled" *jin-yin-hua*. Water is sometimes sprinkled on the cleaned flowers during the frying process to keep them from burning too quickly.

Another traditional method is to make a distilled fragrant water of the flowers. One pound of the cleaned fresh flowers are distilled in water. One pound of flowers can make 2.5 pounds of distilled honeysuckle water.

ADDITIONAL SPECIES

Many flowers in the same genus from different parts of China are used as substitutes for *L. japonica*. *Lonicera japonica* stems and flowers are official drugs of the 1985 Chinese *Pharmacopeia*. Interchangeable substitutes listed in the *Pharmacopeia* include *L. hypoglauca* Miq., *L. confusa* DC, and *L. dasystyla* Rehd.

A number of species are used locally as substitutes in various parts of China. The functions and uses are considered similar. These include *L. tragophylla* Hemsl., *L. similis* Hemsl., *L. macranthoides* Hand-Mazz., *L. hispida* (Steph.) Pall., *L. henryi* Hemsl., *L. longiflora* DC, *L. lanceolata* Wall., *L. reticulata* Champ., and *L. macrantha* Sprengel. Some of these species have also found their way into American horticulture.

OTHER USES

The fruit of Japanese honeysuckle is recorded as a relatively recent folk medicine of China. The fruits are collected during the last ten days of September or first ten days of October. They are then stir-fried for a short while until the fruits feel a little hot and are sticky to the touch. The taste and character is bitter, astringent, and cool. It is used to disperse blood heat and disperse wetness-heat in the treatment of uterine bleeding or dysentery with bleeding. 3 to 9 g of the fruits are used in decoction.

WARNING

Honeysuckle fruits are considered toxic.

The very fragrant flowers are sometimes harvested for use in potpourri mixes. The evergreen leaves could also be used as a bulk filler in potpourri. The stems are sometimes used as a basket-weaving material. The leaves have also been used as a tea subtitute.

Kudzu
Ge-gen

Botanical Name: *Pueraria lobata* (Willd.) Ohwi.
Botanical Synonyms: *P. thunbergiana* (Sieb. et Zucc.) Benth.,
   Dolichos lobatus Willd.
Chinese Names: Pinyin: *Ge-gen* (root). Wade-Giles: *Ko-gen* (root).
English Name: Kudzu.
Pharmaceutical Name: Radix Puerariae.
Family: Leguminosae (Fabaceae)—pea family.

HISTORY

Pueraria lobata, source of the Chinese herbal root *ge-gen*, is better known
to Americans, especially in the Southeast, as kudzu—perhaps the most
infamous of all alien weeds to take hold in the United States. Kudzu, or
kuzu, is an ancient Japanese name for the plant, perhaps derived from a
place name in Nare prefecture. The genus *Pueraria* of the pea family
contains about 20 species, mostly tropical vines.

Kudzu was introduced to the United States from Japan before 1876. It
was shown at the Centennial Exposition held in 1876 in Philadelphia, as
well as the 1883 New Orleans Exposition. The plant promised to be a
food, fodder, fiber, shade-producing economic bonanza. From 1910 to
1953, realizing its potential as a hay and fodder crop, USDA researchers
pushed its development as a new crop. The Soil Erosion Service, started
in 1933 during Frankin Roosevelt's New Deal, saw the plant as a means
of controlling soil erosion. That agency, which changed its name to the
Soil Conservation Service two years later, extensively planted kudzu for
erosion control. By 1945, an estimated 500,000 acres of the southeastern
United States was covered in kudzu. Today, the plant is the vegetative
plague of southern fields and forests. Like Japanese honeysuckle, perhaps
the best way to control kudzu is to find a way to utilize it. The irony, of
course, is that the plant was initially introduced for its many economic and
practical benefits, purposes now largely forgotten.

The German botanist Karl Ludwig Willdenow (1765–1812) published
a description of the plant in 1802, calling it *Dolichos lobatus*. The genus

name *Pueraria* was first published in 1825, named in honor of Prof. M. M. N. Puerari of Copenhagen. In 1867, George Bentham (1800–1884), a distinguished English botanist, named the plant *Pueraria thunbergiana* (Sieb. et Zucc.). Kudzu's Latin name went through several more phases of evolution. Finally, in 1947, the Japanese botanist, Jisaburo Owhi, published the currently accepted botanical name *Pueraria lobata.*

Ge-gen, the root of kudzu, is first mentioned in the middle class of herbs in *Shen Nong Ben Cao Jing* in the first century A.D. Since that time it has been mentioned in the *ben cao* of every dynasty. The source plant mentioned in the ancient *ben cao* is the same plant that is used today.

TASTE AND CHARACTER

A little sweet, hot, neutral.

FUNCTIONS

Promotes sweating, promotes the production of body fluids, helps quench thirst, stops diarrhea, and reduces fever.

USES

Ge-gen is used in the treatment of wei syndrome, or "superficial syndrome" (disease manifest just under the surface, mild, not yet severe, with fever), lack of sweat, thirst, headache, stiff neck with pain due to high blood pressure, allergies, headaches (including migraines), inadequate measles eruptions of children, diarrhea, dysentery, skin eruptions, acute gastroenteritis, diarrhea of children, intestinal obstructions, high blood pressure, angina pectoris, sudden deafness, drunkenness, and to improve cerebral blood circulation. To reduce fever, the crude root is used. To stop diarrhea, the roasted root is used.

Official in the 1985 Chinese *Pharmacopeia*, kudzu root, or *ge-gen*, is traditionally used as a diaphoretic for fevers accompanied by discomfort or pain in the neck and back. It is also used to relieve thirst caused by fevers, for hypertensive headaches, and for coronary heart disease. In cases of measles, it is given to help promote eruptions. It is used as a folk remedy to sober up an unconscious drunk. For this purpose the root is pulverized to obtain the fresh juice, enough to obtain 12 shot-glasses full. This treatment is said to help the drunk regain consciousness.

In modern China, 9–12 g of *ge-gen* may be prescribed for high blood pressure with stiff neck and pain if other medicines to reduce blood pressure are ineffective. It is taken in powdered form or as a water extract (1 g of extract equals 5 g of crude root). Two grams per day are taken, separated into two doses. Some patients reportedly develop dermatitis after taking the extract, in which case the treatment is discontinued.

Tablets made from the root are also used clinically in modern China. For the treatment of angina pectoris, a recent Chinese health guide calls for *ge-gen* tablets. Each 10 mg of weight per tablet equals 1.5 g of the crude root. The daily dose ranges from 30–120 mg, separated into 2 or 3 administrations per day.

In modern times, clinical reports were initiated to study the effect of *ge-gen* on high blood pressure, based on the traditional use of the root to cure headaches due to the common cold. A decoction of 10–15 g of the root was given every day, separated into two doses. The treatment was continued for two to eight weeks. In the treatment of 52 cases, 17 patients had significant improvement of symptoms. Thirty patients had marked improvements.

A clinical study of the treatment of angina pectoris used *ge-gen* tablets (tableted alcohol extract). The course of treatment was 4 to 22 weeks. Of 71 patients, 29 were much improved; 20 patients showed some improvement. Twenty-two patients showed little or no improvement.

In laboratory experiments intravenous injections of the active component of the root (flavonoids, including daidzin, daidzein, and puerarin) reduce blood pressure and venous obstruction. Oral administration of the crude root slightly reduces blood pressure. It has improved symptoms associated with high blood pressure, such as headache, vertigo, stiff neck, and tinnitus. It has also been shown experimentally useful in the treatment of angina pectoris. A cold infusion of the crude root in 2 g/kg of body weight dosages has reduced typhoid fever in animal subjects. The glycoside of the root is experimentally antispasmodic. The decoction is antibacterial. Oral administration of the decoction shows a rise in blood sugar in the first hour after administration, followed by a reduction to previous levels by the second hour. In the fourth to fifth hour, blood sugar seems to be significantly lower. Experiments with female mice have indicated a potential contraceptive effect.

Ge-gen has been studied for its effects on the treatment of headaches and sudden deafness that is believed to be of cochlear origin and spasms of the internal auditory artery, not traumatic injury or other common causes of acute deafness. For sudden deafness, *ge-gen* tablets, standardized to 10 mg equalling 5 g of crude root, are used. Two tablets are specified, 2 to 3 times per day.

In Western terms, *ge-gen* and its preparations are considered antipyretic, antidiarrheal, stomachic, secretory, and spasmolytic. In American herb markets kudzu root is sold primarily for use as a thickening starch, rather than as a traditional Chinese herb product.

DOSE

4.5–9 g; juice of roots is sometimes used. The dried root is poulticed. *Ge-gen* is considered nontoxic.

DESCRIPTION

Kudzu is a coarse, high-climbing, twining, trailing, fast-growing, weedy, perennial vine. The young stems are densely hairy and herbaceous; once old, and grown to 10 to 35 feet long, they become woody. Mature stems can be as much as 2 inches thick. Leaves are alternate, pinnately three-divided; leaflets are more less ovate, or rounded, without teeth, often two- or three-lobed, tapering to an abrupt, acuminate tip. The leaves, densely hairy on the lower surface, are up to 8 inches long. The leaf stalks are about ½ inch long. The flowers are in a raceme up to 8 inches long, borne in leaf axils. The showy flowers are purple or reddish-purple, about 1 inch long, and have a grapelike fragrance. Kudzu flowers in August and September. The hair-covered, flat seed pods are about 2 inches long.

DISTRIBUTION

Wild kudzu grows in moist shaded areas in mountains and fields, and along roadsides, thickets, and thin forests throughout most of China, except Xinjiang, Xizang, and Qinghai provinces.

Ge-gen is produced in most provinces for local use. Major commercial production of *ge-gen* is in Hunan, Henan, Guangdong, Zhejiang, and Sichuan. Their surpluses are sold to other Chinese provinces as well as exported.

In the United States, kudzu occurs from Pennsylvania south to Florida, west to Texas, and north to Kansas and southern Illinois. In the deep South it is a particularly pernicious weed, covering hundreds of acres of roadside embankments, fields borders, and woods, often completely engulfing native vegetation, including shrubs and trees, along with telephone poles and even buildings. In the northern part of its U.S. range, the plant winterkills and is only a localized weed problem. Perhaps the best way to control an established planting is to fence off the area and allow livestock to overgraze the area. Control and eradication of kudzu is extremely difficult. If just a small section of its enormous root is left in the ground, new plants can sprout from it.

Kudzu is also common in Korea, Japan, and adjacent Pacific islands.

CULTIVATION

In the United States, much more focus is now placed on eradicating the plant rather than attempting to grow it. In some parts of the South if you hinted at a desire to cultivate the plant, your sanity would certainly be questioned.

In China the plant is grown in warm moist soils, though it is tolerant of drought and cold temperatures as well. Kudzu is not particular about soils. A rich, sandy soil, however will produce the most vigorous growth. Kudzu is propagated by seeds, root division, or layering. Seeds are planted in spring after being soaked in water for one day and night. They are planted directly in the soil, covered with about an inch of earth, in rows spaced at about 2 feet apart. Individual seedlings are spaced at one foot. Trellising is provided in commercial plantings.

HARVESTING

The root is collected from October through the following April. After digging, the root is cleaned, the outer bark is shaved off, and the root is cut vertically into slices from ¼ to ⅜ inch thick, or cylindrical pieces 4 to 6 inches long. The root is dried in the sun or baked over light heat until dry. In Fujian and Guangdong provinces, to retain a desirable white color roots slices are soaked in salt, rice, or alum water to which sulphur is added and then dried in the sun.

The best quality is large pieces of firm, white, starchy roots, high in starch, with little fiber.

PROCESSING

To make roasted *ge-gen*, wheat bran is placed in a very hot pan. When it begins to smoke, slices of *ge-gen* are added, covered with another layer of wheat bran, and roasted until the bran turns dark yellowish-brown. At this point, the *ge-gen* slices are constantly turned until they are a deep yellow color. They are then cooled, and the wheat bran is sifted off. For every 100 pounds of the root, 25 pounds of wheat bran is used.

ADDITIONAL SPECIES

A number of other *Pueraria* species are used to produce *ge-gen*. *Pueraria thomsonii*, grown commercially and collected wild from mountains and shrub thickets in Guangdong, Guangxi, Yunnan, and Sichuan, is an official source plant of *ge-gen* in the 1985 edition of the Chinese *Pharmacopeia*. Most cultivated production is in Guangdong and Guangxi.

Pueraria edulis, distributed in Xizang, Yunnan, Guizhou, and Sichuan is used locally as *ge-gen*. Its quality is considered much poorer than that of *P. lobata*. *Pueraria omeiensis*, from Sichuan, Guizhou, and Yunnan, is used as *ge-gen* in some areas of Guizhou and Sichuan. *Pueraria phaseoloides*, occurring in Zhejiang, Fujian, Taiwan, Guangdong, and Guangxi, is used locally in Zhejiang province. *Pueraria peduncularis*, distributed in Sichuan, Yunnan, and Xizang, is called "bitter *gen*." It is used as a folk substitute for *ge-gen* in Xizang. A component of the root of this species is also used as an agricultural pesticide.

OTHER USES

The flowers, *ge-gen-hua*, are also used in TCM. The flowering raceme is collected in late summer or early autumn, when about half of the blooms are open. The stem is removed, and the flowers are dried in shade. Flowers are commercially produced in Hunan, Henan, Guangdong, Guangxi, Zhejiang, Sichuan, and Anhui.

The taste and character is a little bitter, cool, and neutral. The function is to expel drunkenness and awaken the spleen. The flowers are used to wake up a drunk the morning after having too much to drink, to quench thirst, for vomiting with blood, fresh bloody stool, acidic stomach, and lack of appetite. The dose is 3 to 9 g, in pills or powdered.

The starch of the root, *ge-fen*, is considered a little bitter and very cold in character. It is used to stop thirst, promote production of body fluids, and disperse heat in cases of gastrointestinal irritation, diarrhea, fevers, "hot" sores, and sore throat.

For the treatment of "vexation" in the chest with heat and thirst, 120 g of the starch and 250 g of millet are used. The millet is soaked in water overnight. The following morning the kudzu root starch is mixed with the millet and made into porridge.

The seeds of kudzu, *ge-gu*, are considered a little sweet and neutral. They have been used as a folk remedy for the treatment of dysentery and to disperse alcohol intoxication. A decoction of 9–16 g is used.

The stems, *ge-man*, are used for the treatment of boils, swelling and sore throat. A decoction of 6–9 g of the dried stems, or 30–60 g of the fresh stems, is used. For the treatment of boils, the dried stem is roasted until charcoaled, (retaining its character). The ash is powdered and applied directly on the boil. For mastitis, the charcoaled stem is taken in 6 g doses with alcohol.

The leaves, *ge-ye*, are traditionally used as a poultice to stop bleeding in the treatment of knife wounds.

The root starch is widely available in Asia as a colloidal thickener, used like cornstarch. It is used as a jelling agent in the production of various food goods, and for making noodles.

The vines have been used for the production of a resilient fiber. After being processed it is handwoven into textiles that are considered as soft as silk.

Perilla
Zi-su

Botanical Names: *Perilla frutescens* (L.) Britt., *P. frutescens* var. *crispa* (Benth.) Dcne.

Botanical Synonyms: *Perilla ocymoides* L., *P. ocymoides* var. *nankinensis* (Lour.) Voss; *P. nankinensis* (Lour.) Dcne.

Chinese Names: Pinyin: *Zi-su-zi* (seeds); *Zi-su-ye* (leaves); *Zi-su-geng* (stems). Wade-Giles: *Tsu-su-tsu* (seeds); *Tzu-su-yeh* (leaves); *Tzu-su-keng* (stems).

English Names: Perilla, beefsteak plant.

Pharmaceutical Names: Fructus Perillae, Folium Perillae, Caulis Perillae.

Family: Labiatae (Lamiaceae)—mint family

HISTORY

Perilla is widely grown in American herb gardens, primarily for the ornamental effect of the purple-leaved and crisped-leaved varieties. While seldom used in the United States, the seed, leaves, and stems are used as traditional Chinese herbal products. In Japan the young shoots, flowering stalks, and seeds are all used for culinary purposes. The leaves are pickled in Korea, and leaves packaged in sardine-type cans are available in Asian groceries throughout North America. Perilla is a common weed in the southern United States. In some places in the Ozarks, it blankets moist woods. The dried seed-encasing stalks rattle as one walks through a patch in autumn; hence, in the Ozarks perilla is called rattlesnake weed.

The genus *Perilla* includes six species native to Asia, from India to Japan. This Asian native came to the West by the 1750s. Pierre d'Incarville, a French Jesuit missionary who served in Beijing from 1740 until he died in 1757, collected dried plant specimens and seeds for his former botany professor in Paris, Bernard de Jussieu. Perilla was among the specimens. In 1764 Linnaeus applied the Latin name *Perilla*, which also serves as a common English name for the plant. The exact derivation of the name is unclear, but it may have originated in India.

Perilla seems to have arrived in the United States sometime in the midnineteenth century. When the sixth edition of *Gray's Manual of Botany* (1889) was published, perilla had escaped from gardens, growing in southern Illinois "about dwellings and roadsides." By the turn of the century it had become a widespread weed, occurring from Illinois to New York south to Georgia.

As a medicinal herb, the use of the seeds and the leaves were first mentioned in *Ming Yi Bie Lu* by the great physician Tao Hong-jing (452–536 A.D.). Like *Shen Nong Ben Cao Jing*, this herbal contains 365 herbs which had been praised by other physicians during the previous thousand years. The seeds were placed in Tao Hong-jing's middle class of drugs.

TASTE AND CHARACTER

Hot and warm.

FUNCTIONS

The seeds lower adverse rising energy (making *qi* move in a downward direction), stop asthma, expel phlegm, relieve coughs, strengthen the diaphragm, and widen the intestines. The leaves expel cold, lower adverse rising energy, regulate vital energy (*qi/ch'i*), and expand the chest. The stem of the plant regulates vital energy, expands the chest, disperses depressed vital energy, and is soothing to a fetus.

USES

The seeds are used in prescriptions for cough, excessive phlegm, asthma, constipation and an oppressed or full feeling in the chest, hiccups, and blockages of vital energy.

The leaves are used for cold due to wind and coldness, aversion to coldness with fever, headache, coughs, asthma, stuffy nose, fullness of the chest and abdomen, excessive fetal movement, mastitis with pain and swelling, wounds, snakebite, and poisoning from eating too many crabs or fish. The fresh leaves are mashed and then poulticed for wounds, mastitis, or snakebites.

The seeds, leaves, and stems of perilla are all official medicines in the 1985 Chinese *Pharmacopeia*. The seeds are primarily valued as an anti-asthmatic and expectorant for chronic bronchitis characterized by a stuffy chest, with thin white phlegm. A strong tea of two ounces of dried leaves combined with three large slices of fresh ginger, drunk frequently, is given as an antidote from eating too much crabmeat or fish. In conjunction with poulticing, the juice of the fresh leaves is sipped to treat snakebites. The tea of the leaves is given for mastitis, and a leaf poultice is applied at the same time. A traditional prescription for the common cold consists of a decoction including 6 g each of perilla leaves, mint leaves (*Mentha*), and licorice root (*Glycyrrhiza uralensis*); 4.5 g of *ma-huang* (*Ephedra sinica*), 9 g of kudzu root (*Pueraria lobata*), and two slices of fresh ginger. This prescription is sipped in wine-glassful doses four times a day. Mint leaves, *ma-huang*, and fresh ginger are commonly used as cold remedies in Western herbal traditions.

One clinical study in China reported on using the fresh leaves to treat warts. The leaves were rubbed on the warts for ten to fifteen minutes, then the leaves were poulticed on the wart (tied with a cloth) for the rest of the day. The treatment was repeated for two to six days. The warts shortly disappeared in all of the 20 patients involved in the study.

In a clinical report for the treatment of chronic bronchitis, the dried leaves, in a 10:1 ratio with dried ginger root, were made into a 25 percent infusion. A dose of 100 ml of the infusion was taken morning and evening. The course of treatment was for ten days, with a three-day resting period between courses of treatment. In 554 cases, 27.2 percent showed marked improvement, 38.6 percent showed some improvement, and it was of no use in 23 percent. Sixty-two patients (11.2 percent) served as controls in this clinical study. A few individuals experienced an increase in urination and reduction of edema. One or two of the patients developed dry mouth. These side effects were reported as light, lasting only for a short time.

Extracts of the leaves have been found to prolong the duration of sleep, have a mild fever-reducing effect and be antibacterial against *Staphylococcus aureus*.

The stems are used for an oppressed feeling in the chest, abdominal fullness and distention, stagnation of vital energy, difficulty in digesting food, stomach and abdominal pains, morning sickness, and excessive fetal movement.

In Western terms, the leaves and flower tops are considered slightly sedative, antispasmodic, and diaphoretic. They have been used in prescriptions for coughs and lung ailments as well as uterine troubles and cephalic disease. Perilla leaves, stems, and seeds are used in some herbal combination products sold in American health and natural food markets. The plant is very commonly grown as an herb garden specimen, and the leaves are used sparingly for flavoring purposes.

DOSE

Seeds, 3–10 g powdered, decocted, or in powder. Dried leaves, 3–9 g. Stems, 4.5–9 g.

WARNING

While the plant is widely used in food and medicine in Asia, a 1974 study showed that an isolated ketone-substituted furan from perilla causes severe lung lesions in mice, rats and sheep. Cattle who eat the plant may contract acute pulmonary emphysema. Its use in human foods and medicine has, therefore, been questioned.

DESCRIPTION

Perilla is an annual growing from 1½ to 3 feet in height. The much-branched stems have opposite, oval-shaped leaves of up to five inches long. Leaves have a peculiar varnishlike fragrance, are strongly toothed and often wrinkle-edged, with a purple or bronze tint or all purple in *Perilla frutescens* 'Atropurpurea,' a cultivated form. Plants with strongly wrinkled leaves have been described as a separate species (*P. crispa*), but it is now considered a cultivated variety of the regular form. The white or purplish flowers are in dense or loose racemes, encased by a ⅛ inch long calyx, which remains once the plant goes to seed.

DISTRIBUTION

The plant occurs throughout much of China, including Hebei, Shanxi, Jiangsu, Zhejiang, Hubei, Sichuan, Jiangxi, Fujian, Guangdong, Guangxi, Guizhou, and Yunnan. Perilla is an escaped weed in eastern China but occurs naturally south of the Yangtze River valley, and grows in Taiwan and Japan. It is cultivated throughout China and is common near villages and along roadsides. While most areas of China produce perilla for local consumption, Hubei province produces it commercially.

In the United States it grows throughout most of the eastern half of the country, from Massachusetts to Florida west to Texas and Iowa, occurring in damp woods, along fence rows, old gardens, roadsides, and old logging roads. While considered a common weed, it is also widely cultivated in herb gardens.

CULTIVATION

Perilla is an annual that can be easily grown from seed. Seeds germinate prolifically in the garden if plants from the previous autumn are allowed to go to seed. Once plants self-sow, you will probably spend more time weeding seedlings out of the garden than you do actually planting seed. In the Yangtze River region of China, seeds are planted around April 5. Two-inch-tall seedlings are thinned to spacings of about two feet. It does well in full sun or partial shade. It becomes most luxuriant in a moist, rich, well-drained soil, but will grow in just about any garden soil.

HARVESTING

The seeds are collected in autumn as they ripen. The whole plant is cut, dried, and threshed to remove the seeds. The leaves are harvested as they become most luxuriant, from June to the first two weeks of September, when the flowers fully open. The whole plant is cut and hung to dry, and then the leaves are removed by rubbing or threshing. If the stems are used they may be harvested from June to August, or after the plant has gone to seed. Stem harvested early in the season is called "young stem" of perilla. If harvested after going to seed it is called "old stem" of perilla. Some Chinese herbalists consider the "young stem" to be of better quality. The stems are cut into sections, then dried. Or, after the leaves are removed, they may be soaked in water for a short time and covered with a moist cloth until the middle part of the stem is whitish in color. They are then cut into slices and dried in the sun.

Processing

After the seeds are cleaned by winnowing away dust and other debris, they may be processed into "fried *su zi*," preferred in some prescriptions. When clean, they are stir-fried (without oil) under a light fire, stirring frequently for a few moments until the seeds become fragrant and begin to crackle or hiss. Before use, they are bruised in a mortar and pestle.

Other Uses

In a fifth-century work by Chia Ssu-hsieh, *Ch'i Min Yao Shu*, it is stated that perilla is an important crop for the production of the leaves as a vegetable as well as for the oil from the seed.

While underutilized as a culinary herb in American herb gardens, it is widely used as a condiment in Japan and China. In Japan the leaves are considered edible, though not necessarily eaten, much as Americans use parsley. The fresh flower spikes and dried seed stalks are also used as a garnish. In Japan if you let the plant go to seed in your garden and seedlings become a weed problem the next year, the small 2- to 3-inch-tall plants can be used as a spice to flavor *sashimi* (raw fish), or be fried in a tempura batter. The mature leaves are used to flavor bean curds and pickles, as well as being used as a garnish. Pickled apricots, plums, and ginger are colored with the purple-leaved forms of perilla. The fading leaf stalks are sometimes used in soups. The seeds are also harvested, salted, and used as a condiment.

The edible seeds have an antioxidant function and produce a valuable drying oil, similar to linseed oil, that comprises up to 51 percent of the seed's weight. The oil is very high in linolenic acid. The seeds have been produced in China, Japan, Korea, and northern India for oil production. After harvest the seeds are roasted, and the oil is obtained by expression or solvent extraction. The oil is glossier, tougher, harder, has greater durability, and is more water resistant than linseed oil and dries about three times as fast. However, the oil has a tendency to yellow, shrivel, and crack when exposed to heat. It has been used in Asia for paints, varnishes, printing inks, Japanese oil papers, and cheap lacquers. The seed cake remaining after oil production has been used as a fertilizer in Japan for mulberry trees and rice.

The dried leaves have an essential oil containing a component that is converted to a sweetener 2,000 times sweeter than sugar. Its commercial applications include use as a substitute for maple sugar or licorice to flavor tobacco products in Japan. The substance, an antioxime of perilla-alde-hyde, is considered too toxic for food use. In minute amounts it has also been used as a flavoring in sauces, dentifrices, and confections.

Sicklepod
Jue-ming-zi

Botanical Names: *Cassia obtusifolia* L., *C. tora* L.
Botanical Synonyms: *Senna obtusifolia* (L.) H. Irwin and Barneby, *Senna tora* (L.) H. Irwin and Barneby.
Chinese Names: Pinyin: *Jue-ming-zi* (seeds). Wade-Giles: *Chueh Ming-tzu* (seeds).
English Names: Sicklepod, cassia seed.
Pharmaceutical Name: Semen Cassiae.
Family: Leguminosae (Fabaceae)—pea family.

HISTORY

You are more likely to see sicklepod listed on the label of an herbicide container than in an herb garden in the United States. Sicklepod, includ-ing both *Cassia tora* and *Cassia obtusifolia*, is considered a nuisance weed rather than a useful plant in America. In Asia, it is thought of in a different light. The seeds are the traditional Chinese herbal product *jue-ming-zi*. In Africa, nomadic groups in the Sudan plant sicklepod and use it in the manufacture of a high-protein fermented food. Perhaps this plant has more value than is appreciated by Americans.

The genus *Cassia*, of the pea family, contains more than 535 species. Both *Cassia tora* and *C. obtusifolia* were named by Linnaeus in 1753. The generic name, *Cassia*, derives from the Greek, *kassia*, the name of a woody plant with fragrant bark. *Tora* is from the Latin *torus*, denoting a soft object to lie or sit on. It may refer to the shape of the gland between the lowermost pair of leaflets. These plants occur in many parts of the world. Western cultures regard them as weeds, yet many traditional cultures have used these two species as food and medicine.

Cassia tora and *C. obtusifolia* are very closely related. The source plant of *jue-ming-zi* was long thought to be *C. tora*, but when Chinese researchers were working on the 1977 edition of the Chinese *Pharmacopeia*, it was discovered that the source plant for most of the supply was actually *C. obtusifolia* rather than *C. tora*, although the latter was found to be used in tropical and subtropical regions of China. *Cassia obtusifolia* is called big *jue-ming-zi* because of its larger seeds. *Cassia tora*, which produces smaller seeds, is known as little *jue-ming-zi*. The Chinese name derives from the use of the seeds to clear vision. The seeds look something like horses hooves, so the seeds are called "horse" *jue-ming* in Chinese folk traditions. The first mention of the plant comes in the superior class of herbs in *Shen Nong Ben Cao Jing*.

TASTE AND CHARACTER

A little sweet, bitter, salty.

FUNCTIONS

The seeds function to disperse liver fire to treat eye diseases; they improve eyesight and relax the bowels.

USES

Jue-ming-zi is used in prescriptions for headaches due to high blood pressure, ulcerated cornea, vertigo, red eyes with swelling and pain, conjunctivitis, glaucoma, liver heat, cataracts, ocular swelling and pain, blurred vision, and constipation.

The seeds are used to improve eyesight by improving the liver. In TCM the eyes and liver are related to one another. To strengthen eyesight, for example, the livers of goats or ewes are eaten. If the liver is strong, the eyes become stronger as well. The Zaghawa tribe of the northern Darfur region of Sudan in Africa, like the Chinese, also use *Cassia obtusifolia* seeds for the treatment of headaches, as well as for stomachache and fatigue.

The seeds of both *C. obtusifolia* and *C. tora* are official in the 1985 Chinese *Pharmacopeia*. They are frequently used for the treatment of eye diseases, especially those involving acute inflammation.

A traditional treatment for acute blindness calls for two "bowls" of *jue-ming-zi* coarsely ground, to be taken with rice porridge. To achieve efficacy, the remedy must be continued for a long time. The patient is directed not to eat pork, fish, garlic, or hot-tasting vegetables during the course of treatment. For conjunctivitis with swelling and pain, the roasted seeds are made into an extract that is then rubbed on to the temples. Once the poultice begins to dry, it is replaced. To improve eyesight by improving the liver, one bowl of *jue-ming-zi* and one bowl of *Vitex negundo* fruits are decocted in 5 bowls of good wine. The herbs are extracted until they completely absorb the liquid and then are dried in the sun, pulverized, and sifted. After supper, before going to bed, 6 g of the powdered extract is taken in warm water.

In addition, *jue-ming-zi* is widely used in prescriptions for helping to reduce blood pressure and blood cholesterol levels. A traditional treatment for high blood pressure calls for the seeds to be stir-fried until they turn a yellowish color; they are then pulverized into a coarse powder. Sugar is added, and the seed powder is soaked in hot water. A dose of 3 g of the powder is given 3 times per day. Another treatment for high blood pressure calls for 15 g of *jue-ming-zi* stir-fired until yellow. It is then decocted and drunk instead of tea.

A study by Anthony Koo, W. S. Chan and K. M. Li (1976) showed that an extract of *C. tora* seeds consistently reduced arterial blood pressure in anesthetized rats. The hypotensive response occurred without significant heart rate changes, indicating that it was not the result of a direct action of the extract on the heart. Instead, the immediate hypotensive action involves a blocking effect on the vagus nerves and sympathetic nervous systems.

Chinese clinical studies have reported that *jue-ming-zi* seed extracts produce a reduction in serum cholesterol levels. In the treatment of 100 patients with high serum cholesterol, levels returned to normal in 98 percent of the patients after one month. Eighty-five percent of the patients also reported subjective improvement in symptoms including dizziness, headaches, and lethargy.

Water and alcohol extracts of the seeds have a hypotensive (blood pressure-lowering) effect in animal trials. They are experimentally diuretic, may reduce fat levels in the blood, and are antibacterial; water extracts have antifungal activity.

While thirty years ago *C. tora* was listed as the source plant in Chinese materia medica, it is now known that much of the supply is actually from the closely related *C. obtusifolia*, as previously mentioned. The latter species has some differences in chemical components and varying pharmacological action. Some Chinese researchers think they should be separated into two different drugs. The plant is little known in American herb markets.

DOSE

6–15 (20–25) g.

DESCRIPTION

Cassia tora is an erect, much-branched, ill-scented annual herb, 10 to 12 inches in height. The obovate leaflets are in three pairs; they are 1 to 2 inches long, and about a third as wide. The leaf stalk (petiole) is ¼ to 2½ inches long. The leaf rachis has a cylindrical gland between the lowest two pairs of leaflets. The yellow to orange flowers are in short axillary clusters with one to two flowers per cluster. The somewhat flattened or four-angled pods are 4 to 6 inches long and sickle-shaped, hence the common name sicklepod. The individual angular ripe seeds (about 20 to 30 per pod) are used as *jue-ming-zi*. The plant flowers from June to August.

Historically, *Cassia obtusifolia* has been considered both distinct from and synonymous with *C. tora*. In *Flora of Okinawa and the Southern Ryukyu Islands*, E. H. Walker notes that they have been previously separated on the presence of one or two foliar glands, and short or long flower stalks. *Cassia tora* is considered by some to have a strong fetid odor, not common to *C. obtusifolia*. However, Walker notes that these differences do not hold up in the material he observed and that the two should be recognized as one variable species until a large number of specimens from its entire range can be critically studied on a purely morphological basis. Microscopic evaluation of *C. obtusifolia* seed powder, however, show only a few cluster crystals, whereas *C. tora* has a greater number of larger crystals.

DISTRIBUTION

Cassia obtusifolia grows in the countryside along roads, mountains, and riverbanks in Jiangsu, Anhui, and Sichuan. In recent decades it has been cultivated in most of China. Supplies of wild-harvested or cultivated material are abundant. *Cassia tora* grows along roadsides and in waste places, especially rich soils high in organic matter, in subtropical or tropical areas such as Taiwan, Guangxi, and Yunnan. The supply of *C. tora* is smaller than that of *C. obtusifolia*. It is mainly produced in Guangxi.

Both species are found throughout warm temperate and tropical regions, including much of East Asia, India, Africa, South America, and North America. In the midwestern United States, where it is known as sicklepod, it is targeted in television herbicides commercials as a plant that should be eradicated. In the United States, *C. obtusifolia* grows on arable land, waste places, garbage dumps, gravel of railroads, highway shoulders, and gravel bars of intermittent creeks. In Sudan, Africa, it it is one of the few plants to grow where soil erosion and desertification occur.

CULTIVATION

Cassia tora and *Cassia obtusifolia* are not particular about soils. They will grow virtually anywhere, preferring full sun and good drainage. They are easily propagated by seeds and will self-sow in the garden. Germination seems to be hastened by soaking the seeds in water overnight. The plants produce an abundance of seeds as well. Foster has collected twelve ounces of seed from just four plants. In North China it is planted in the first two weeks of April. In South China it is planted in March. Individual plants are spaced at about 2 feet. Seeds are covered with about ¼ inch of soil. Young seedlings appear after about 10 days. The seedlings are thinned when they are 2 to 3 inches high. They are side-dressed with a nitrogen fertilizer during the middle of the growing season. Toward the time seeds develop, they are side-dressed with a phosphorus source. Rock phosphate may be added the previous season to supply phosphorus.

HARVESTING

In September to November, after the fruit has ripened, the whole plant is cut, dried in the sun, and threshed once the pods have dried.

PROCESSING

The seeds are stir-fried until they are a little swollen, and have a pleasant but not strong fragrance, then cooled. The whole seed is stored until needed; then it is pulverized into coarse or fine powder.

ADDITIONAL SPECIES

Several substitutes or adulterants are found in Chinese markets including the seeds of *Cassia occidentalis* (known as "rounded *jue-ming-zi*"), as well as the coarse ground seeds of *Celosia argentea*.

Most *Cassia* species were placed in the genus *Senna* by H. Irwin and R. C. Barneby in a 1982 publication, including *Cassia obtusifolia* and *Cassia tora*. The subjects of this chapter are now called *Senna obtusifolia* (L.) H. Irwin and Barneby and *Senna tora* (L.) H. Irwin and Barneby. We have chosen to use the older Linnean names used in the vast majority of works on Chinese medicinal plants in order to avoid further confusion. Various sennas are source plants for senna leaf and senna pods, widely used throughout the world in stimulant laxative products.

OTHER USES

The whole herb and leaves of *C. tora*, *ye-hua-sheng*, is mentioned in a relatively new book on medicinal plants produced in Ssu-mao, a small city in southwestern Yunnan. It is considered bitter, a little sweet, and cool. The leaves expel wind, disperse heat, and improve eyesight. It is used for the treatment of eye disease, the common cold, and flu. A decoction of 15 to 30 g of the herb is used. For the common cold or flu, 15 to 30 g of the whole plant of *Cassia tora* has been decocted with a suitable amount of *Glycyrrhiza uralensis*. In China a decoction is used as a wash for vaginitis. It is reported to improve or eliminate the symptoms of vaginitis in clinical trials.

In a 1984 publication, Hamid A. Dirar, reported on the potential of the plant as a protein source especially for drought-stricken regions of Africa. Certain tribes of Sudan use the green leaves of *C. obtusifolia* to produce a fermented food product known as "kawal." The product is sun-dried then eaten as needed. It contains about 20 percent protein on a dry weight basis. The food use of the plant is looked down upon by the cultural elite in Sudan because of its strong, characteristic odor. However, the use of kawal has spread across most of the Sudan in recent years.

The seeds of *C. tora* have also been used as a coffee substitute. The ripe seeds have been used as a high-protein feed for livestock. In India, seeds dried in the sun for 15 to 20 days were gradually added to livestock feed over a two-week period to introduce them to the diet. In the subcontinent, the seeds have also been used as a laxative.

In India and Burma, *C. obtusifolia* is used as a folk medicine for the treatment of skin diseases. The leaves have been used as a poultice to draw out pus and are applied as a warm poultice for gout, sciatica, and joint pains. Chakramardha, an oil containing *C. obtusifolia* and *Eclipta alba*, has been used externally for the treatment of ringworm. The leaves of *C. obtusifolia*, fried with castor oil, have been poulticed on foul ulcers. In India, the root has also been used to treat ringworm. The root is rubbed on a stone, and then mixed with the juice of a lime. The ground seeds mixed with soured buttermilk were once applied to itchy skin eruptions.

Summer Cypress
Di-fu-zi

Botanical names: *Kochia scoparia* (L.) Schrad., *Kochia scoparia* f. *trichophylla* (Schmeiss) Schinz. & Thell.
Botanical Synonyms: *Bassia scoparia* (L.) A. J. Scott, *Chenopodium scoparia* L.
Chinese Names: Pinyin: *Di-fu-zi* (fruits). Wade-Giles: *Ti-fu-tzu* (fruits).
English Names: Summer cypress, belvedere, kochia.
Pharmaceutical Name: Fructus Kochiae.
Family: Chenopodiaceae—goosefoot family.

HISTORY

A farmer in the midwestern United States may consider summer cypress, or kochia, to be a noxious weed. Gardeners grow cultivars of the large shrublike, annual herb for its brilliant red autumn foliage. The Chinese grow it for production of its seeds, producing the Chinese traditional herbal product *di-fu-zi*.

The genus *Kochia* of the goosefoot family contains about 40 species of herbs and subshrubs. Recently the genus *Kochia* has been transferred to *Bassia*. In some recent botanical works the plant is known as *Bassia scoparia*

(L.) A. J. Scott. Considering that virtually all botanical works on the plant published since 1809 place it under the genus *Kochia*, a modern name change is utterly annoying. The first botanical name, bestowed by Linnaeus, was *Chenopodium scoparia*. The German botanist Heinrich Adolph Schrader (1767–1836) transferred the plant to the genus *Kochia*, which is named in honor of the German botanist, W. D. J. Koch (1771–1849). The specific name *scoparia* is derived from a Latin word root, meaning "a sweeper," referring to the use of the plant as a broom. It is grown as an ornamental in the United States, and as a medicinal plant and an ornamental in China. In other parts of Asia it is grown as a food and broom-producing plant.

In a letter written in 1736, a French missionary, Francis Xavier d'Entrecolles (1662–1741), noted that summer cypress seeds were used as a famine food in times of scarcity. The plant, now occurring throughout much of East and Central Asia, with a range extending into Central Europe, is mentioned by Pliny, who noted its strong-scented leaves, and by authors of medieval European herbals. It is believed to have been introduced into China from the Mediterranean region at least 2000 years ago.

Kochia was first mentioned in the superior class of herbs in *Shen Nong Ben Cao Jing*. The plant is found in many ancient *ben cao*. Li Shi-zhen noted that the plant is soft, not very strong, and that old dry plants were used as brooms. The plant mentioned in the old *ben cao* is the same source plant that is used today. The seeds are used today in TCM, and the young leaves and stem are also used as a folk medicine.

TASTE AND CHARACTER

A little sweet, bitter, cold.

FUNCTIONS

Disperses wetness and heat, stops itching, promotes diuresis.

USES

Kochia seeds are used in prescriptions for painful or difficult urination, sudden need to urinate, turbid urine, vaginal discharges, hernia, eczema due to wind, jock itch, skin itch, urticaria, eczema, sores, scabies, and as a diuretic.

While not one of the most famous medicinal plants of Chinese traditions, the seed, *di-fu-zi*, is an official listing in the 1985 Chinese *Pharmacopeia*. The seed is primarily used for its effect on various urinary disturbances, as well as in prescriptions for impotence. Cardiotonic properties have also been ascribed to the fruits. A wash of the seeds has been used for the treatment of skin conditions and abscesses. The juice, squeezed from the fruits, is recorded for use as eye drops for heat and pain in the eyes (perhaps conjunctivitis). Combined with warmed alcohol, the powdered seeds have been used in the treatment of mastitis. The mixture apparently produces sweating, which is said to improve the condition. Also in combination with alcohol, the seeds, fried until fragrant, were used for the treatment of hernias. As a folk treatment for warts, the seeds were mixed with alum and applied as a wash. Combined with equal amounts of radish seeds and decocted, kochia seeds have been used as a wash to relieve the pain and swelling of carbuncles. Antifungal and diuretic activity have been confirmed in laboratory studies.

In Western terms, the seeds are considered diuretic, astringent, antiphlogistic, and antiscorbutic. It is rarely seen on American herb markets.

DOSE

3–15 g of dried fruits, poultice, or wash.

DESCRIPTION

Kochia is a much-branched, silky-haired, close-leafed annual, with a rounded, pyramidal, or columnar habit, growing from 3 to 6 feet in height. The alternate leaves are lance shaped or linear, and up to 3 inches long. The flowers, born in axillary clusters, are small and inconspicuous. The fruit is bladderlike, one-seeded, and develops five transverse wings when mature. Basically, the flower calyx grows to envelop the seed, producing the urticle or bladderlike winged enclosure.

Kochia scoparia f. *trichophylla*, sold as burning bush, firebush, and red summer cypress in American horticulture, is a dense, globe-shaped cultivated form with threadlike leaves that turn bright reddish-purple in autumn. The fruits of this cultivar, which occurs in northeast China, are used as a substitute for typical *di-fu-zi*.

Swollen fruit of a grayish-green color is considered the best quality.

DISTRIBUTION

The plant occurs as a wild weed in mountains, waste ground, fields, roadsides, or in gardens near villages or homes. It is grown throughout China. It occurs wild in Heilongjiang, Jilin, Liaoning, Hebei, Shandong, Shanxi, Shaanxi, Henan, Anhui, Jiangsu, and Gansu. Major production is in the north part of Jiangsu, Shandong, Henan, and Hubei. Material from these provinces is sold throughout China.

The plant also occurs in Japan and Korea west to Central Europe, north to Siberia and far eastern parts of Russia, and is naturalized in North America. In the United States it occurs from Maine south to the Carolinas, west through to the rangelands of Nevada, and north to Montana. Here it is considered a weed. At least 10 different herbicides are approved and labeled for use to eradicate the plant.

CULTIVATION

Kochia is a rank annual very adaptable to its surroundings, and is grown in both North and South China. It is not particular about soils, doing well in any average garden soil, though it thrives best in warm, moist, rich, friable, well-drained soils. In China, it is grown in front yards or on idle land in corners of fields. Seeds are used for propagation. In the first ten days of April, the seeds are planted. If started in flats, seedlings are transplanted once they develop two true leaves. In April one can direct-seed the plant in rows, spaced at 1½ to 2 feet, and covered with about ½ inch of soil. If the soil is quite moist, seedlings will appear in about ten days. Seedlings are thinned one or two times in order to space plants on two-foot centers. Plantings are cultivated and weeded every two weeks. They are watered during periods of drought and side-dressed with manure two or three times during the growing season. Night soil is considered the best fertilizer.

HARVESTING

The whole plant is harvested in autumn when the fruit is ripe. The plant is dried and then threshed to remove the fruits. The chaff is sifted off. If the stems and leaves are saved for use as well, they are cut into sections and dried in the sun.

Processing

None noted.

Additional Species

In some parts of China, *Chenopodium album* L. is used as a substitute for the herb. In Liaoning, Jiangsu, Anhui, Fujian, Hubei, Hunan, Jiangxi, Guangdong, and Guizhou, *Chenopodium album* is used as a substitute. In other parts of China, including some areas of Sichuan and Yunnan, *Melilotus suaveolens* is used as *di-fu-zi*. *Baeckea frutescens* L. has also been used as a substitute, especially in Guangxi.

Besides the typical species, *K. scoparia* f. *trichophylla* Schinz. et Thell. is used in Heilongjiang, Jilin, and Liaoning. *Kochia sieversiana* (Pall.) C. A. Mey. is used as a substitute in Heilongjiang, Jilin, Liaoning, and Shaanxi.

Kochia indica has been relished as a camel, cattle, and mule feed in India. It has also been used as a cardiac stimulant. The dried plant has been burned as a fuel.

Other Uses

The young stem and leaves of kochia, *di-fu-miao*, are considered bitter and cold. They dispel heat, detoxify, and have diuretic qualities. This herb is used for turbid urine, "red and white" dysentery, diarrhea, hot urine, red eyes, skin reddened and swollen due to wind and heat. The leaves have also been used for digestive disorders in a decoction of 30–60 g. The fresh juice of the plant is used as a wash or poultice.

The plant is widely grown as an ornamental, has been used as an emergency food in times of famine, and is grown for making brooms. In Japan the young tips of the plant are eaten as a potherb. The seeds have also been used for making breads. In northwest India, the plant is eaten by cattle. Canadian and American researchers have studied the plant as a potential livestock feed. Young plantings yield hay and silage high in crude protein. Experimental plantings produced three to five tons of young dried herb per acre. Older plants tend to become woody and are less palatable.

Sweet Annie
Qing-hao

Botanical Name: *Artemisia annua* L.

Chinese Names: Pinyin: *Qing-hao* (herb). Wade-Giles: *Ching-hao* (herb).

English Names: Sweet Annie, sweet sagewort, annual wormwood, annual sweet wormwood, sweet wormwood.

Pharmaceutical Name: Herba Artemisiae Annuae.

Family: Compositae (Asteraceae)—aster family.

HISTORY

This relatively nondescript, green-leaved herb with inconspicuous flowers has gained popularity in the last ten years as an herb garden specimen in American horticulture, where the plant is most commonly known as sweet Annie. It has also become a common weed of waste places in North America. The dried leaves are widely used in herbal decorative arts in America, primarily for wreaths and dried arrangements. The whole plant is the Chinese traditional herbal medicine *qing-hao*. *Qing-hao* has emerged as the most promising new treatment for malaria in over 300 years.

The genus *Artemisia* contains about 300 species of annual, biennial, and perennial aromatic herbs and shrubs, primarily indigenous to dry regions of the northern hemisphere. A few species are represented in South America, and one species hails from South Africa. Linnaeus named the plant *Artemisia annua* in 1753. The generic name, *Artemisia*, is an ancient name believed to honor Artemisia the younger, wife of Mausolus (Maussollus), satrap of Caria (350–353 B.C.). Artemisia, a botanist and medical researcher, was undoubtedly named after Artemis, (Diana in Roman tradition), Greek goddess of wild nature (wild animals, vegetation, chastity, childbirth, and the hunt), the twin sister of Apollo. The specific name *annua*, of course, denotes that the plant is an annual. *Artemisia annua* probably arrived as a vagrant in the United States from ships trading with Asia.

The use of the extract of *qing-hao* is mentioned in a work known as "Prescriptions for 52 Kinds of Diseases." This document was found in the Mawangui Han dynasty tombs. Dated to 168 B.C., it recommends the use of the herb extract for the treatment of hemorrhoids. A 340 A.D. work by

Ge-hong, *Zhou Hou Bei Ji Fang* (Handbook of Prescriptions for Emergency Treatments) is the earliest record suggesting the use of the herb for the treatment of malarial fevers. It was also mentioned in Li Shi-zhen's *Ben Cao Gang Mu.*

TASTE AND CHARACTER

Bitter, cold.

FUNCTIONS

Qing-hao dispels heat, cools the blood, removes fever, and reduces summer heat syndrome (characterized by headache, dry mouth, fever, profuse sweating, irritability, and other symptoms).

USES

The whole herb is used for the intermittent fever of tuberculosis and malaria and for low fever from sunstroke (without sweating).

Qing-hao, the whole herb of *Artemisia annua*, is an official listing in the 1985 Chinese *Pharmacopeia*, and has attracted attention from research groups around the world as a treatment for malaria. A traditional prescription for the treatment of malaria calls for a decoction of 30 g of *qing-hao*. One dose per day is taken. Another malaria prescription calls for 3 g of the dried leaves, ground into powder. It is taken one time per day, 4 hours before the return of the fever, and continued for 5 days. The juice of the fresh plant has also been used to treat malaria. The fresh herb is pulverized. A 3 g dose of the juice is taken one time per day.

In the 1970s and 1980s, Chinese researchers devoted tremendous amounts of time and energy to the study of *qing-hao* and its antimalarial component, known as *qinghaosu*. In the international literature the name artemisinin has been adopted for this component. A number of scientific institutions from several provinces in China have taken part in the research. At the Institute of Chinese *Materia Medica*, in the Academy of Traditional Chinese Medicine, for example, about 60 workers have taken part in the work.

A study published in 1979 by the Coordinating Research Group on *qinghaosu* reported on a nearly 100 percent success rate in treating 2,099 patients infected with the malarial organisms *Plasmodium vivax* (1511) and

Plasmodium falciparum (588). The study was carried out from 1973–1978 in Yunnan and Henan provinces and on Hainan Island. The work excited widespread international interest.

Artemisinin was first isolated by a Chinese research group in 1972. *Artemisia annua* is the only *Artemisia* species that is known to contain appreciable levels of artemisinin. Dozens of species have been studied by Chinese, Japanese, and American scientists in an attempt to find other source plants for the compound. Artemisinin has been synthesized by research groups in Switzerland, China, and the United States, but it is still much less expensive to produce the component from the plant itself.

Since the early 1970s Chinese scientists have intensively studied the pharmacology, pharmacokinetics, and toxicology of artemisinin. In addition to Chinese studies, research groups working on artemisinin include the Walter Reed Army Institute of Research and the UNDP/World Bank/WHO Special Programme for Research and Training in Tropical Diseases.

While malaria was once widespread in the United States from New England to California, and caused widespread epidemics in the United States during the early nineteenth century, it was generally eradicated in the United States by the end of the Second World War. Still, a thousand cases of malaria are reported in the United States each year, mainly from travelers and immigrants. The disease had a strong impact on the United States military during the Vietnam War. In 1965, the number of troops sent home from contracting malaria equaled the number of troops wounded. To most Americans, malaria is considered a disease of the past, but it is still a major world health concern.

Malaria is the most common infectious disease on earth affecting between 200 and 300 million people per year and causing as many as 3 million deaths. While malaria has been controlled in many countries by the use of DDT (eradicating the mosquitos that carry malaria-causing parasitic protozoans) and by the use of chloroquine drugs, it remains a major health problem worldwide. What's more, malarial parasites have developed resistance to chloroquine drugs used to treat the disease. Chloroquine is a derivative of quinine, which itself comes from South American cinchona (Jesuit's bark) trees. Cinchona first became known to Europeans as a potential malarial treatment in the 1630s.

As the result of the extensive Chinese research on *artemisinin* over the past twenty years, this chemical extract of *Artemisia annua* has emerged as the most important new antimalarial drug in over 300 years. It is a major

Chinese achievement in blending traditional medicine with Western ("modern") medicine to develop solutions to world healthcare problems.

While the use of the herb and isolation of the active components are from China, Western research groups have attempted to patent the use of the plant to treat malaria, raising the question of who should benefit from the commercial development of the plant. Ethically, the benefits of commercial development should rest with the original discoverers, Chinese scientists, not Westerners with a better understanding of world patent laws.

In Western terms *Artemisia annua* is considered antimalarial and antipyretic. Water extracts of the plant have an antibacterial effect. An acid isolated from the plant, known as qinghaoic acid, is antibacterial against *Staphylococcus aureus*, *Escherichia coli*, *Salmonella typhosa*, and other bacteria.

DOSE

4.5–9 g in decoction.

DESCRIPTION

Sweet Annie is a smooth, sweetly pungent, bushy annual from 1½ to 9 feet tall. The leaves are broadly oval to lance-shaped in general outline, and up to 4 inches long. The lower and middle leaves are three-pinnatisect (three-divided into fernlike segments) and without stalks. Uppers leaves are one- to two-pinnatisect. Individual leaf segments are linear-lanceolate, entire or with a few teeth. The flowers are in a loose, broad panicle or are racemose. The individual tiny, inconspicuous, greenish-yellow flowerheads, about ¹⁄₁₆ inch in diameter, are round and somewhat nodding.

DISTRIBUTION

Sweet Annie is native to Eurasia, from southeast Europe to China, Japan, Siberia, Korea, India, and West Asia. It has become widely naturalized in central and southern Europe. It is a weed found throughout much of China on mountainsides, disturbed soil, fallow ground, and along roadsides. In the past decade, commercial cultivation of the plant has commenced in China as well as the United States.

In North America it is a weed of waste places, fallow ground, roadsides, barnyards, and neglected gardens from Prince Edward Island south to

Alabama, and from Tennessee west to Arkansas, Missouri, and Kansas. In recent years it is met with more frequently, as it has been widely planted in herb gardens and then escaped from cultivation. Given its recent proliferation in cultivation, it will, no doubt, spread across the continent within the next ten years.

CULTIVATION

Sweet Annie is not particular about soil conditions and grows in a wide variety of soils, including sand, sandy loam, and clay. An average sandy-loam with good drainage would seem to suit the plant. It prefers full sun. An annual easily grown from seed, it can be direct-sown in the garden in early spring before the last spring frost. Young seedlings are frost tolerant. The seeds, however, are very tiny, and a more uniform stand can be established by planting the seeds indoors in flats. Emergence occurs in about a week. Plants can be transplanted outdoors about six weeks after they are sown.

According to a study conducted by researchers at Purdue University's Department of Horticulture, if the plant is grown on a large scale for production of artemisinin, the greatest amount of biomass is achieved with plants spaced on a 12 inch center (Simon and Cebert 1988). If plants are grown as decorative material, plants spaced on 3 feet centers are more manageable. As much as 35 metric tons of fresh material per hectare have been obtained. The plant is highly variable in its growth habit, morphological characteristics, and chemical composition. Varieties are being selected that will produce the highest amounts of artemisinin. While malaria is primarily a disease of tropical regions, *Artemisia annua* is most easily grown in temperate climates.

HARVESTING

Chinese works suggest harvesting the entire above ground portion of the plant in August to October, before flowering (depending upon planting date). Dr. Daniel Klayman, the leading American researcher on *Artemisia annua* at the Walter Reed Army Institute of Research, determined that artemisinin content of the leaves is at a maximum in late July or August (in naturalized plants harvested in Virginia). After harvest, the plant is cleaned and used fresh or dried. Chinese works suggest drying in the sun. However, if the plant is to be used for decorative purposes, dry in a well-ventilated, shaded area. Avoid drying under direct sun, which will discolor the leaves.

PROCESSING

Some buyers may require that the leaves be removed from the stem. Artemisinin itself is extracted using one of a number of solvents.

ADDITIONAL SPECIES

In southwest China, *Artemisia annua* form *macrocephala* is used. *Artemisia apiacea* Hance is used as *qing-hao* in some parts of China. The flowers are about twice as large, and the leaves twice-pinnate. *Artemisa capillaris* Thunb. and *A. scoparia* Waldst. et Kitab have also been used as substitutes in Chinese tradition. At least one quarter of all *Artemisia* species have been screened in a search for new sources of artemisinin. The results were negative. Well-known European species include common wormwood *Artemisia absinthium*, and the common culinary herb, tarragon *Artemisia dracunculus*.

OTHER USES

In addition to being produced in the United States for experimental development of the active constituents, the plant is widely planted in herb gardens for use in dried arrangements, potpourri, and wreaths. The plant also produces an essential oil.

In China the leaves are burned as a fumigant insecticide to kill mosquitos.

The seeds are also used as a folk medicine in China. The fruits (seeds) are considered slightly hot, cool, without poison. The seeds are used for lack of appetite, flatulence, dyspepsia, and night sweats of tuberculosis patients. Three to nine grams are used in decoction.

Glossary

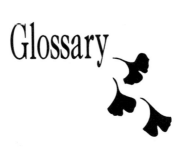

Absolute: a preparation in perfumery in which the fragrance principles of flowers are concentrated through alcohol extraction.

Achene: small, hard one-seeded fruit.

Adaptogen: a substance that has a "tonic" effect irrespective of the disease condition (see *Ginseng*).

Adulterant: an unacceptable additive or replacement of a specified herb (see also: **substitute**).

Analgesic: a substance that relieves pain.

Anodyne: a pain-relieving agent that locally numbs terminal sensory nerves.

Anti-inflammatory: a substance that reduces inflammation.

Antianemic: a substance that allays anemia.

Antipyretic: a substance that reduces fever.

Antiscorbutic: a substance that treats scurvy, such as vitamin C.

Antispasmodic: an agent that relieves spasms or cramps.

Antitussive: a cough-relieving agent.

Astringent: an agent causing the contraction of tissues.

Bechic: tending to relieve a cough.

Calyx: external floral envelope; the sepals collectively.

Cardiotonic: an agent that increases tonicity or heart muscles.

Carminative: an agent that expels gas from the digestive tract.

Cultigen: a plant arising in cultivation and not known from the wild, such as garlic.

Cultivar: a plant variety produced in cultivation, retaining its characteristics when propagated.

Cytotoxic: a substance toxic to cells.

Decoction: a preparation made by simmering plant parts in water for a specified period of time.

Demulcent: a substance that soothes and protects surfaces to which it is applied.

Deobstruent: a substance that removes obstructions.

Depurative: a cleansing agent such as a "blood purifier."

Detoxicant: a substance tending to remove toxins.

Discutient: an agent that disperses or dissipates lesions or tumors.

Diuretic: a substance that increases urinary flow.

Emmenogogue: a substance that aids in menstrual function.

Expectorant: an agent inducing bronchial secretion.

Extract: a preparation in which the properties of an herb are drawn out by solvents, heat, or other processes.

Hemostatic: an agent that stops bleeding.

Hyperglycemic: an agent increasing blood sugar as in diabetes.

Hypoglycemic: an agent that reduces blood sugar.

Hypotensive: an agent that lowers blood pressure.

Immunostimulant: an agent that stimulates the immune system in a non-specific manner.

Larvacidal: an agent that kills insect larvae.

Meridians: in Chinese medicine, the specific pathways of energy flow in the body.

Molluscicidal: an agent that kills mollusks, such as snails and slugs.

Moxabustion: the use of burning substances placed on an acupuncture point for therapeutic benefits.

Palmate: in a leaf, where three or more leaflets or lobes radiate from a central point of origin.

Poultice: external application of dried or fresh herb.

Qi/ch'i: in Chinese, the concept of life force; vital energy.

Raceme: unbranched flower stalk, with individual flowers on distinct stalks.

Resolvant: an agent that promotes the dispersion of inflammation.

Rhizome: an underground stem, often creeping.

Scion: a shoot or twig (usually of a woody plant) used for grafting or propagation.

Spasmolytic: tending to check spasms.

Stipule: leaflike appendages found at the base of true leaves.

Substitute: a plant that is an acceptable replacement for another herb (see also: **adulterant**).

Tincture: a preparation made by soaking (macerating) an herb in a specified amount of ethanol (alcohol) to extract its properties.

Bibliography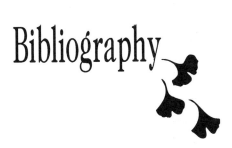

Abdullah, T. H., D. V. Kirkpatrick, and J. Carter. 1989. Enhancement of Natural Killer Cell Activity in AIDS with Garlic. *Deutsch Zeishrift für Onkologie* 21:52–53.

Bailey, L. H. 1953. *The Garden of Bellflowers in North America.* New York: Macmillan.

_____. 1939. *The Standard Cyclopedia of Horticulture.* 3 vols. New York: Macmillan.

Bailey, L. H., and E. Z. Bailey. Expanded by the Staff of the Liberty Hyde Bailey Hortorium. 1976. *Hortus Third.* New York: Macmillan.

Baranov, A. I. 1979. On a Technical English Name for *Eleutherococcus. Taxon* 28:586–587.

Barkley, T. M., ed. 1986. *Flora of the Great Plains.* Lawrence: University Press of Kansas.

Barneby, R. C. 1964. Atlas of North American Astragalus. Special issue of the *Mem. New York Botanical Garden* 13:1–1188.

Beijing Medical College, eds. 1984. *Dictionary of Traditional Chinese Medicine.* Hong Kong: The Commercial Press.

Beijing Traditional Chinese Medical College, eds. 1971. *The Prescriptions of Traditional Chinese Drugs (Zhong Yao Fang Ji Xue).* Beijing: Beijing Traditional Chinese Medical College (in Chinese).

Bensky, D., and A. Gamble. 1986. *Chinese Herbal Medicine: Materia Medica.* Seattle, WA: Eastland Press.

Bingel, A. S., and H. H. S. Fong. 1988. Potential Fertility-regulating Agents from Plants. *In* H. Wagner, H. Hikino and N. R. Farnsworth, eds., *Economic and Medicinal Plant Research*, vol. 2. Orlando, FL: Academic Press, 73–18.

Block, E. 1986. Antithrombic Agent of Garlic: A Lesson from 5000 Years of Folk Medicine. *In* R. P. Steiner, ed., *Folk Medicine: The Art and the Science.* Washington, DC: American Chemical Society, 125–138.

Braly, B. 1987. *Supplement to the Ginseng Research Institute's Indexed Bibliography.* Wausau, WI: Ginseng Research Institute.

Braquet, P., ed. 1988. *Ginkgolides—Chemistry, Biology, Pharmacology and Clinical Perspectives.* Barcelona, Spain: J. R. Prous.

Brekhman, I. I. *et al.*, eds. 1986. *New Data on Eleutherococcus: Proceedings of the Second International Symposium on Eleutherococcus (Moscow, 1984).* Vladivostok: Academy of Sciences of the USSR Far East Science Center.

Bretschneider, E. 1898. *History of European Botanical Discoveries in China.* 2 vols. Reprint. Leipzig: Zentral-Antiquariat der Deutschen Demokratischen Republik, 1981.

Burkill, I. H. 1966. *A Dictionary of the Economic Products of the Malay Peninsula.* 2 vols. Kuala Lumpur: Ministry of Agriculture and Cooperatives.

But, P. P. H., S. Y. Hu, and C. Y. King. 1980. Vascular Plants Used in Chinese Medicine. *Fitoterapia* 51(5):245—264.

Chang, H. M., and P. P. H. But, eds. 1986–1987. *Pharmacology and Applications of Chinese Materia Medica.* Vol. 1: 1986, Vol. 2: 1987. Singapore: World Scientific Publishing Co.

Chang, H. M, H. W. Yeung, W. W. Tso, and A. Koo. 1985. *Advances in Chinese Medicinal Materials Research.* Singapore: World Scientific Publishing Co.

Chen, W. B., T. Q. Li, L. Q. Yan, Z. Y. Li, and M. Y. Liu. 1983. Boosting Effects of Drugs Benefiting Vital Energy and Activating Blood and Transfer Factor on the Immunity of Patients with Chronic Cor Pulmonale. *Jour. Trad. Chin. Med.* 3(1):63–68.

Cheung, S. C. and N. H. Li, eds. 1978–1986. *Chinese Medicinal Herbs of Hong Kong.* 5 vols. Hong Kong: Commercial Press.

Chow, H. Y., J. C. C. Wang, and K. K. Cheng. 1976. Cardiovascular Effects of *Gardenia Florida* (*Gardeniae Fructus*). *Am. Jour. Chin. Med.* 4 (1):47–51.

Chun, W. Y. 1921. *Chinese Economic Trees.* Shanghai: Commercial Press.

Council of Scientific and Industrial Research. 1948–1985. *The Wealth of India.* 11 vols. New Delhi: Publications & Information Directorate, Council of Scientific & Industrial Research.

Cullen, W. 1808. *A Treatise of the Materia Medica.* 2 vols. Philadelphia: Mathew Carey.

Cunningham, I. S. 1984. *Frank N. Meyer: Plant Hunter in Asia.* Ames: Iowa State University Press.

Del Tredici, P. 1991. Ginkgos and People: A Thousand Years of Interaction. *Arnoldia.* 51(2):2–15.

DeWolf, G. P. Jr. 1968. *Albizia julibrissin* and its Cultivar 'Ernest Wilson.' *Arnoldia* 28 (4–5):29–35.

Dirar, H. A. 1984. Kawal, Meat Substitute from Fermented *Cassia obtusifolia* Leaves. *Economic Botany* 38(3):342–349.

Dirr, M. A., and C. W. Heuser, Jr. 1987. *The Reference Manual of Woody Plant Propagation.* Athens, GA: Varsity Press, Inc.

Duke, J. A., 1984. Parallels in Amerindian and Chinese Phytotherapy. *Botanical Grower* 2(2):4–5.

_____. 1985. *CRC Handbook of Medicinal Herbs.* Boca Raton, FL: CRC Press.

_____. 1989. *Ginseng: A Concise Handbook.* Algonac, MI: Reference Publications, Inc.

Duke, J. A., and E. A. Ayensu. 1985. *Medicinal Plants of China.* 2 vols. Algonac, MI: Reference Publications, Inc.

Duke, J. A., and S. Foster. 1989. *Trichosanthes kirilowii:* A New Hope in the AIDS-Relief Search? *HerbalGram* 20(Spring):20–21, 25, 46–47.

Duncan, A. 1789. *The New Edinburgh Dispensatory.* Edinburgh: Charles Elliot.

Dymock, W. n.d. *The Vegetable Materia Medica of Western India.* Bombay: Education Society's Press, Byculla.

_____. 1890, 1891, 1893. *Pharmacographia Indica: A History of the Principal Drugs of Vegetable Origin Met with in British India.* 3 vols. Bombay: Education Society's Press, Byculla.

Eastman, L. M. 1976. Ginseng *Panax quinquefolius* L. in Maine and its relevance to the Critical Areas Program. Augusta, ME: State Planning Office.

Eddison, S. 1988. Daylilies. *Fine Gardening* No. 3, pp. 22–26.

Farnsworth, N. R. 1975. The Validation of Claims for Traditional Medicines. *In Herbal Pharmacology in the People's Republic of China; A Trip Report of the American Herbal Pharmacology Delegation.* Washington, DC: National Academy of Sciences, pp. 67–70.

Farnsworth, N. R., A. D. Kinghorn, D. D. Soejarto, and D. P. Waller. 1985. Siberian Ginseng (*Eleutherococcus senticosus*): Current Status as an Adaptogen. *In* H. Wagner, H. Hikino, and N.R. Farnsworth, eds., *Economic and Medicinal Plant Research.* Vol. 1. Orlando, FL: Academic Press, pp. 155–215.

Felter, H. W. and J. U. Lloyd. 1898. *King's American Dispensatory.* Reprint. Portland, OR: Eclectic Medical Publications, 1983.

Fernald, M. L. 1950. *Gray's Manual of Botany.* 8th ed. New York: D. Van Nostrand.

Flückiger, F. A. and D. Hanbury. 1879. *Pharmacographia. A History of the Principal Drugs of Vegetable Origin met with in Great Britain and British India.* 2d ed. London: Macmillan and Co.

Foster, S. 1984. *Herbal Bounty: The Gentle Art of Herb Culture.* Layton, UT: Gibbs M. Smith, Inc.

_____. 1984. Embracing Traditional Chinese Medicine. *East West Journal.* 14(11):64–67.

_____. 1986. *East West Botanicals: Comparisons of Medicinal Plants Disjunct Between Eastern Asia and Eastern North America.* Brixey, MO: Ozark Beneficial Plant Project.

_____. 1987. Prof. Yue Chongxi—An Interview. *Business of Herbs* 5(4):1–4.

_____. 1988. Motherwort—An Ancient Link to the Future. *Business of Herbs*. 6(4):12–14.

_____. 1988. Medicinal Ornamentals. *Fine Gardening* No. 3, pp. 28–30.

_____. 1989. Phytogeographic and Botanical Considerations of Medicinal Plants Disjunct in Eastern Asia and Eastern North America. *In* L.E. Craker and J.E. Simon, eds., *Herbs, Spices, and Medicinal Plants: Recent Advances in Botany, Horticulture, and Pharmacology*. Vol. 4. Phoenix, AZ: Oryx Press., pp. 115–140.

_____. 1990. Chinese Medicinal Herbs. *The Herb Companion*. 2(3):28–33.

_____. 1990. The China Prescription. *Harrowsmith/CountryLife*. 5(30):78–83

_____. 1991. Siberian Ginseng, *Eleutherococcus senticosus*. *Botanical Series*, No. 302. Austin, TX: American Botanical Council.

_____. 1991. Asian Ginseng, *Panax ginseng*. *Botanical Series*, No. 303. Austin, TX: American Botanical Council.

_____. 1991. Ginkgo, *Ginkgo biloba*. *Botanical Series*, No. 304. Austin, TX: American Botanical Council.

_____. 1991. American Ginseng, *Panax quinquefolius*. *Botanical Series*, No. 308. Austin, TX: American Botanical Council.

_____. 1991. Garlic, *Allium sativum*. *Botanical Series*, No. 302. Austin, TX: American Botanical Council.

Foster, S., and J. A. Duke. 1990. *A Field Guide to Medicinal Plants: Eastern and Central North America*. (Peterson Field Guide Series #40). Boston: Houghton Mifflin.

Foster, S., and C. H. Yueh. 1991. Disjunct Occurrence and Folk Uses of Medicinal Plants in the Ozarks and in China. *Missouri Folklore Society Journal*. 10(1988):27–36.

Fulder, S. 1980. The Drug that Builds Russians. *New Scientist*. 21:576–579.

_____. 1980. *The Root of Being: Ginseng and the Pharmacology of Harmony*. London: Hutchinson.

_____. 1990. *The Tao of Medicine: Ginseng and Other Chinese Herbs for Inner Equilibrium and Immune Power*. Rochester, VT: Healing Arts Press.

Fulder, S., and J. Blackwood. 1991. *Garlic: Nature's Original Remedy*. Rochester, VT: Healing Arts Press.

Gerarde, John. 1633. *The Herball or Generall Historie of Plantes*. Revised and enlarged by Thomas Johnson. New York: Dover Publications. Reprinted, 1975.

Gleason, H. A., and A. Cronquist. 1963. *Manual of Vascular Plants of the Northeastern United States and Adjacent Canada*. New York: D. Van Nostrand.

Goldstein, B. 1975. Ginseng: Its History, Dispersion, and Folk Tradition. *Am. Jour. Chin. Med*. 3(3):223–234.

Gray, A. 1889. *Manual of Botany of the Northern United States*. 6th ed. New York: American Book Company.

Guan, K. J. and C. Y. Cheng. 1974. *Latin-Chinese Names of Seed Plants*, 2d ed. Beijing: Scientific Publishing House.

Halstead, B. W., and L. L. Hood. 1984. *Eleutherococcus senticosus, Siberian Ginseng: An Introduction to the Concept of Adaptogenic Medicine*. Long Beach, CA: Oriental Healing Arts Institute.

Hardt, R. A. 1986. Japanese Honeysuckle: From "One of the Best" to Ruthless Pest. *Arnoldia* 46(2):27–35.

Hartwell, J. L. 1982. *Plants Used Against Cancer*. Lawrence, MA: Quarterman Publications. Previously published as Plants Used Against Cancer: A Survey. *Lloydia*, 1967–71.

Hedrick, U. P., ed. 1919. *Sturtevant's Notes on Edible Plants*. State of New York, Dept. of Agriculture, Twenty–seventh Annual Report, vol. 2, part II.

———. 1950. *A History of Horticulture in America to 1860*. Reprint. Portland, Oregon: Timber Press, 1988.

Henderson, P. 1889. *Henderson's Handbook of Plants and General Horticulture*. New York: Peter Henderson & Co.

Hill, M., and G. Barclay. 1987. *Southern Herb Growing*. Fredericksburg, TX: Shearer Publishing.

Hoo, G., and C. J. Tseng. 1978. Araliaceae. *Flora Reipublicae Popularis Sinicae*. 54: 1–210.

How, F. C. 1982. *A Dictionary of the Families and Genera of Chinese Seed Plants (Zhong Guo Zhong Zi Zhi We Ke Shu Ci Dian)*. Beijing: Scientific Publishing House.

Hsu, H. Y. 1980. *How to Treat Yourself with Chinese Herbs*. Long Beach, CA: Oriental Healing Arts Institute.

Hsu, H. Y., Y. P. Chen, S. J. Shen, C. S. Hsu, C. C. Chen, and H. C. Chang. 1986. *Oriental Materia Medica—A Concise Guide*. Long Beach, CA: Oriental Healing Arts Institute.

Hsu, H. Y. and W. G. Preacher, eds. 1981. *Sang Han Lun: The Great Classic of Chinese Medicine*. Long Beach, CA: Oriental Healing Arts Institute.

Hsu, H. Y. and S. Y. Wang, trans. 1983. *Chin Kuei Yao Leuh: Prescriptions from the Golden Chest*. Long Beach, CA: Oriental Healing Arts Institute.

Hu, S. L., ed. 1990. *Abstracts of the First International Symposium on Rhubarb*. Beijing: State Administration of Traditional Chinese Medicine.

Hu, S. Y. 1957. An Enumeration of the Food Plants of China with Their Vernacular Names in Chinese. *Flora of China* Project of Arnold Arboretum, pp. 1–33.

———. 1968. An Early History of Daylily. *American Horticultural Magazine* 47 (2): 51–85, Spring. (Readers are referred to this article and other's by Dr. Hu, (The Species of *Hemerocallis, Ibid*, pp. 86–120; Uses of Daylily in Food and Medicine, *Ibid*, pp. 214–218) for a fascinating and complete account of the history, botany, and uses of daylilies, including recipes for food use of the flowers.

———. 1976. The Genus *Panax* (Ginseng) in Chinese Medicine. *Economic Botany* 30:11–28.

_____. 1976. A Contribution to Our Knowledge of *Leonurus* L., *I-mu-ts'ao*, the Chinese Motherwort. *Am. Jour. Chin. Med.* 4(3):219–237.

_____. 1977a. Knowledge of Ginseng from Chinese Records. *Journ. of the Chinese University of Hong Kong* 4(2):283–305.

_____. 1977b. A Contribution to Our Knowledge of Ginseng. *Am. Jour. Chin. Med.* 5:1–23.

_____. 1977c. The Origin and Meaning of the Generic Names of Chinese Orchids. *Quart. Journ. Taiwan Museum* 30(1&2):123–186.

_____. 1979a. Letter to S. Foster, March 20, 1979, p. 44 *In*. S. Foster "Ginseng: Are You Confused?" *Well-Being* No. 46:43–50.

_____. 1979b. A Contribution to Our Knowledge of Tu-chung—*Eucommia ulmoides. Am. Journ. Chin. Med.* 7(1):5–37.

_____. 1980a. *An Enumeration of Chinese Materia Medica.* Hong Kong: The Chinese University Press.

_____. 1980b. *Eleutherococcus* vs. *Acanthopanax. Jour. Arnold Arboretum* 61:107–111.

_____. 1990. History of the Introduction of Exotic Elements into Traditional Chinese Medicine. *Jour. Arnold Arboretum* 71: 487–526.

Hunan Province Revolutionary Health Committee. 1977. *A Barefoot Doctor's Manual* (reprinted ed.). Seattle: Cloudburst Press.

Ibragimov, F. I. and V. S. Ibragimova. 1964. *Principal Remedies of Chinese Medicine.* English translation from the Russian by Foreign Technology Division of United States Air Force Systems Command. Ohio: Wright-Patterson Air Force Base.

Institute of Chinese Materia Medica, Academy of Traditional Chinese Medicine. 1975–1978. *All China Traditional and Herbal Drugs* (*Quan Guo Zhong Cao Yao Hui Bian*). Beijing: People's Health Publishing House. 2 vols (in Chinese).

Jartoux, P. 1714. The Description of a Tartarian Plant Called Ginseng. *Phil. Trans. Roy. Soc. London* 28:237–247

Jiangsu New Medical College, eds. 1977–1979. *Encyclopedia of Traditional Chinese Medicine.* (*Zhong Yao Da Ci Dian*). Shanghai: Shanghai Science and Technology Publishing Co., 3 vols (in Chinese).

Kariyone, T. and R. Koiso. 1971. *Atlas of Medicinal Plants.* Osaka, Japan: Takeda Chemical Industries, Ltd.

Keys, J. D. 1976. *Chinese Herbs: Their Botany, Chemistry, and Pharmacodynamics.* Rutland, VT: Charles E. Tuttle Company.

Kitagawa, M. 1979. *Neo-Lineamenta Florae Manshuricae or Enumeration of the Spontaneous Vascular Plants Hitherto Known from Manchuria (North-Eastern China) Together with Their Synonymy and Distribution.* Vaduz: J. Cramer.

Klayman, D. L. 1985. *Qinghaosu* (Artemisinin): An Antimalarial Drug from China. *Science* 228:1049–1055.

_____. 1989. Weeding Out Malaria: American Scientists Pursue a Cure from a Chinese Plant. *Natural History* 10:18.

Kong, Y. C., H. W. Yeung, Y. M. Cheung, and J. C. Hwang. 1976. Isolation of the Uterotonic Principle from *Leonurus artemisia*, the Chinese Motherwort. *Am. Journ. Chin. Med.* 4(4):373–382.

Kong, Y. C., C. T. Che, T. T. Yip, and H. M. Chang. 1977. Effects of Fructus Gardeniae Extract on Hepatic Function. *Comparative Medicine East and West* 5 (3–4):241–255.

Koo, A., and K. M. Li. 1977. Phytochemical Properties and Hypotensive Mechanism of Extracts from *Gardenia jasminoides* Seeds. *Am. Journ. Chin. Med.* 5 (1):31–37.

Koo, A., W. S. Chan, and K. M. Li. 1976. A Possible Reflex Mechanism of Hypotensive Action of Extract from *Cassia tora* Seeds. *Am. Journ. Chin. Med.* 4(3):249–255.

Kuang, P. G., X. F. Zhou, F. Y. Zhang, and S. Y. Lang. 1988. Motherwort and Cerebral Ischemia. *Journ. of Trad. Chin. Med.* 8(1):37–40.

Kunming Institute of Botany, Academy of Sciences, eds. 1984. *Index Florae Yunnanensis*. 2 vols. Kunming, Yunnan: The People's Publishing House.

Lafitau, J. F. 1718. *Mémoire Présenté à son Altesse Royale monsigneur le Duc d'Orléans*, p. 8–18. Paris: Joseph Monge.

Laufer, B. 1919. *Sino-Iranica: Chinese Contributions to the History of Civilization in Ancient Iran*. Chicago: Field Museum of Natural History Publication 201.

Leung, A.Y. 1980. *Encyclopedia of Common Natural Ingredients Used in Food, Drugs, and Cosmetics*. New York: John Wiley & Sons.

_____. 1984. *Chinese Herbal Remedies*. New York: Universe Books.

_____. 1990. Chinese Medicinals: A Review of Chinese Materia Medica. *HerbalGram*. 23(Summer):21–31.

Lewis, W. H. 1986. Ginseng: A Medical Enigma. *In* N. L. Etkin, ed., *Plants in Indigenous Medicine and Diet: Biobehavioral Approaches*. Bedford Hills, NY: Redgrave, pp. 290–305.

Li, C. P. 1974. *Chinese Herbal Medicine*. Washington, DC: HEW Publ. No. 75-732. National Institutes of Health.

Li, H. L. 1942. The Araliaceae of China. *Sargentia* 2:1–134.

_____. 1952. Floristic Relationships Between Eastern Asia and Eastern North America. *Trans. Amer. Philos. Soc.* 42:371–429. (Reprinted, with foreword, as Morris Arboretum monograph, 1971).

_____. 1956. A Horticultural and Botanical History of Ginkgo. *Morris Arb. Bull.*, 7: 3–12.

_____. 1963. *Woody Flora of Taiwan*. Philadelphia: Morris Arboretum.

_____. 1969. The Vegetables of Ancient China. *Economic Botany* 23:253–260.

Li, H. L. 1982. *Contributions to Botany: Studies in Plant Geography, Phylogeny and Evolution, Ethnobotany and Dendrological and Horticultural Botany*. Taipei: Epoch Publishing.

Li, H. L., T. S. Liu, T. C. Huang, T. Koyama, and C. E. DeVol, eds. 1975–1979. *Flora of Taiwan*. 6 vols. Taipei: Epoch Publishing.

Liao, J. Z., Z. N. Chai, W. S. Li, X. F. Liu, S. R. Wang, L. M. Qin, and W. Q. Guo. 1988. Pharmacological Effects of Codonopsis Pilosula-Astragalus Injection in the Treatment of CHD Patients. *Jour. Trad. Chin. Med.* 8(1):1–8.

Liberti, L., ed. 1988. Ginkgo. *The Lawrence Review of Natural Products* (Feb.).

Lien, E. J., and W. Y. Li. 1985. *Structure Activity Relationship Analysis of Anticancer Chinese Drugs and Related Plants.* Long Beach, CA: Oriental Healing Arts Institute.

Linnaeus, C. 1753. *Species Plantarum.* 2 vols. Reprint. London: The Ray Society, vol. 1, 1957; vol 2, 1959.

Liu, Y. C. 1988. *The Essential Book of Traditional Chinese Medicine.* Vol. 1: Theory. Volume 2: Clinical Practice. New York: Columbia University Press.

Liu, G. Z., D G. Cai, and S. Shao. 1988. Studies on the Chemical Constituents and Pharmacological Actions of Dangshen *Codonopsis pilosula* (Franch). Nannf. *Jour. Trad. Chin. Med* 8(1):41–47.

Lloyd, J. U. 1921. *Origin and History of All the Pharmacopeial Vegetable Drugs.* Cincinnati, OH: Caxton Press.

Lorenzi, H. J., and L. S. Jeffery. 1987. *Weeds of the United States and Their Control.* New York: Van Nostrand Reinhold.

Lou, Z. C., P. G. Xiao, and G. J. Xu, eds. 1980–1987. *Chinese Materia Medica (Zhong Yao Zhi).* Beijing: People's Publishing House. 4 vols (in Chinese).

Lowe, D. W., ed. 1990. *The Official World Wildlife Fund Guide to Endangered Species of North America.* Vol. 1. Washington, DC: Beacham Publishing.

Lucas, R. 1973. *Eleuthero (Siberian Ginseng): Health Herb of Russia.* Spokane, WA: R&M Books.

Mabberly, D. J. 1987. *The Plant Book: A Portable Dictionary of the Higher Plants.* New York: Cambridge University Press.

McGrath, M. S., *et al.* 1989. GLQ 223: An Inhibitor of Human Immunodeficiency Virus Replication in Acutely and Chronically Infected Cells of Lymphocyte and Mononuclear Phagocyte Lineage. *Proc. Natl. Acad. Sci.* 86:2844–2848.

Marshall, D. E. 1988. *A Bibliography of Rhubarb and Rheum Species.* USDA, NAL, ARS, Bibliographies and Literature of Agriculture. No. 62.

Merrill, E. D. and E. H. Walker. 1938. *A Bibliography of Eastern Asiatic Botany.* Jamaica Plain, MA: Arnold Arboretum.

Miao, W. W. 1981. *Stories of Drugs and Herbs (Zhong Cao Yao De Gu Shi).* Beijing: Chinese Folk Literature Publishing House (in Chinese).

Moerman, D. E. 1986. *Medicinal Plants of Native America.* 2 vols. Technical Reports, No. 19, Research Reports in Ethnobotany, Contribution 2. Ann Arbor: University of Michigan Museum of Anthropology.

Morton, J. F. 1977. *Major Medicinal Plants: Botany, Culture, and Uses.* Springfield, IL: Charles C. Thomas.

Moule, A. C. 1937. The Name *Ginkgo biloba* and Other Names of the Tree. *T'oung Pao* 33:193–219.

Nanjing Medical College, eds. 1975. *A Microscopic Identification of Drug Powders.* (*Fen Mo Yao Cai Xian Wei Jian Ding*). Nanjing: Nanjing Medical College (in Chinese).

National Academy of Sciences. 1975. *Herbal Pharmacology in the People's Republic of China: A Trip Report of the American Herbal Pharmacology Delegation.* Washington, DC: National Academy of Sciences.

_____. 1980. *Proceedings U.S.–China Pharmacology Symposium.* Washington, DC: National Academy of Sciences.

National Institute for the Control of Pharmaceutical and Biological Products, eds. 1987. *Colour Atlas of Chinese Traditional Drugs.* Vol. 1. Beijing: Science Press.

Needham, J., G. D. Lu, and H. T. Huang. 1986. *Science and Civilization in China* Vol. 6. *Biology and Biological Technology.* Part 1: Botany. Cambridge: Cambridge University Press.

Ng, T. B. and H. W. Yeung. 1986. Scientific Basis of the Therapeutic Effects of Ginseng. *In* R. P. Steiner, ed., *Folk Medicine: the Art and the Science.* Washington, DC: American Chemical Society, pp. 139–151.

Nicholson, G. 1886–1905. *Dictionary of Gardening.* 8 vols. London: L. Upcott Gill.

Ohwi, J. 1965. *Flora of Japan.* Washington, DC: Smithsonian Institution.

Ou, M., C. Lu, *et al.* 1982. *Chinese-English Glossary of Common Terms in Traditional Chinese Medicine* (*Han Ying Chang Yong Zhong Yi Ci Hui*). Guangzhou: Guangdong Scientific and Technological Publishing House (in Chinese).

Perry, L. M. 1980. *Medicinal Plants of East and Southeast Asia.* Cambridge, MA: MIT Press.

Pharmacopeia Committee of the Ministry of Health. 1985. *Pharmacopeia of the People's Republic of China* (*Zhong Hua Ren Min Gong He Guo Yao Dian, Yi Bu*). Vol. 1. Beijing: People's Health Publishing House and Chemical Industry Publishing House (in Chinese).

_____. 1988. *Pharmacopeia of the People's Republic of China.* Hong Kong: China Pharmaceutical Books Company. (English edition of 1985 Chinese Pharmacopeia).

Pickering, C. 1879. *Chronological History of Plants.* 2 vols. Boston: Little, Brown.

Poyarkova, A. I. 1973. *Eleutherococcus. In* B. K. Shishkin ed., *Flora of the U.S.S.R.* (1950). Translated from the Russian. Jerusalem: Israel Program for Scientific Translations. pp. 16–23.

Radford, A. E., H. E. Ahles, and C. R. Bell. 1968. *Manual of the Vascular Flora of the Carolinas.* Chapel Hill: University of North Carolina Press.

Read, B. E. 1936. *Chinese Medicinal Plants from the Pen Ts'ao Kang Mu.* A.D. *1596.* Peking: Peking Natural History Bulletin.

Reid, D. P. 1987. *Chinese Herbal Medicine.* Boston: Shambhala.

Saito, H. 1980. Ginsenoside R$_{b1}$ and Nerve Growth Factor. *In Proceedings of the 3rd. International Ginseng Symposium.* Seoul, Korea: Korean Ginseng Research Institute, pp. 181–85.

Saito, H., Tsuchiya, H. and K. Takagi. 1974b. Effect of *Panax ginseng* Root on Spontaneous Movement and Exercise in Mice. *Journal of Japanese Pharmacology* 24:41–48.

Saito, H, Y. Yoshida, and K. Takagi. 1974a. Effect of *Panax ginseng* Root on Exhaustive Exercise in Mice. *Journal of Japanese Pharmacology* 24:119–27.

Sargent, C. S. 1905. *Manual of the Trees of North America.* Boston: Houghton Mifflin.

Shibata, S., O. Tanaka, J. Shoji, and H. Saito. 1985. Chemistry and Pharmacology of *Panax. In* H. Wagner, H. Hikino, and N. R. Farnsworth, eds., *Economic and Medicinal Plant Research.* Vol. 1. Orlando, FL: Academic Press. pp. 218–84.

Simon, J. E. and E. Cebert. 1988. *Artemisia annua:* A Production Guide. *In* J. E. Simon and L. Z. Clavio, eds., *Proceedings of the Third National Herb Growing and Marketing Conference.* West Lafayette, IN: Purdue Research Foundation. pp. 78–83.

Smith, H. H. 1928. Ethnobotany of the Meskwaki Indians. *Bulletin of the Public Museum of Milwaukee,* 4(2):175–326.

———. 1932. Ethnobotany of the Menominee Indians. *Bulletin of the Public Museum of Milwaukee,* 4(1):1–174.

———. 1932. Ethnobotany of the Ojibwe Indians. *Bulletin of the Public Museum of Milwaukee,* 4(3):327–525.

———. 1933. Ethnobotany of the Forest Potawatomi Indians. *Bulletin of the Public Museum of Milwaukee,* 7(1):1–230.

Soejarto, D. D. and N. R. Farnsworth. 1970. The Correct Name for Siberian Ginseng. *Botanical Museum Leaflets* 26:(9–10)

Song, W. Z., and P. G. Xiao 1982. Medicinal Plants of Chinese Schisandraceae and Their Lignan Components. *Chinese Traditional and Herbal Drugs* 13(1):40–48.

Spongberg, S. A. 1990. *A Reunion of Tress: The Discovery of Exotic Plants and Their Introduction into North American and European Landscapes.* Cambridge, MA: Harvard University Press.

Stearn, S. 1801. *The American Herbal.* Walpole, NH: Thomas and Thomas.

Steward, A. N. 1958. *Manual of Vascular Plants of the Lower Yangtze Valley, China.* Corvallis, OR: Oregon State College.

Stuart, G. A. 1911. *Chinese Materia Medica. Vegetable Kingdom,* extensively revised from F. Porter Smith (1871). Reprinted as *Chinese Medicinal Herbs.* San Francisco, CA: Georgetown Press, 1973.

Sun, Y., E. M. Hersh, M. Talpaz, S. L. Lee, W. Wong, T. L. Loo, and G. M. Mavligit. 1983. Immune Restoration and/or Augmentation of Local Graft Versus Host Reaction by Traditional Chinese Medicinal Herbs. *Cancer* 52(1):70–73.

Sun, Y., E. M. Hersh, S. L. Lee, M. McLaughlin, T. L. Loo and G. M. Mavligit. 1983. Preliminary Observations on the Effects of the Chinese Medicinal Herbs *Astragalus membranaceus* and *Ligustrum lucidum* on Lymphocyte Blastogenic Responses. *Journal of Biological Response Modifiers.* 2(3):227–237.

Thorton, R. J. 1814. *A Family Herbal.* London: R.and R. Crosby and Co., Stationers.

Thunberg, C. P. 1784. *Flora Japonica.* Lipsiae: Bibliopolio I. G. Mülleriano.

Torrey, J., and A. Gray. 1838–43. *A Flora of North America.* Reprint. New York: Hafner Publishing Company, 1969.

Trigg, P. I. 1989. Qinghaosu (Artemisinin) as an Antimalarial Drug. *In* H. Wagner, H. Hikino, and N. R. Farnsworth, eds., *Economic and Medicinal Plant Research.* Vol. 3. Orlando, FL: Academic Press, pp. 20–6.

Tucker, A. O., J. A. Duke and S. Foster. 1989. Botanical Nomenclature of Medicinal Plants. *In* L. E. Craker and J. E. Simon, eds., *Herbs, Spices, and Medicinal Plants: Recent Advances in Botany, Horticulture, and Pharmacology.* Vol. 4. Phoenix, AZ: Oryx Press, pp. 169–242.

Tyler, V. E. 1986. Plant Drugs in the Twenty-First Century. *Economic Botany* 40(3):279–288.

_____. 1987. *The New Honest Herbal.* 2d ed. Philadelphia: George F. Stickley.

Tyler, V. E., L. R. Brady, and J. E. Robbers. 1988. *Pharmacognosy.* 9th ed. Philadelphia: Lea & Febiger.

United States Consular Reports. 1885. *The Licorice Plant.* Washington, DC: Government Printing Office.

Unschuld, P. U. 1986. *Medicine in China: A History of Pharmaceutics.* Berkeley and Los Angeles: University of California Press.

Uphof, J. C. Th. 1968. *Dictionary of Economic Plants.* Lehre, Germany: J. Cramer.

Van Rensselaer, M. 1969. The Remarkable Ginkgo. *Plants & Gardens* 25(2):50–53.

Wagner, H. and A. Proksch. 1985. Immunostimulatory Drugs of Fungi and Higher Plants. *In* H. Wagner, H. Hikino, and N. R. Farnsworth, eds., *Economic and Medicinal Plant Research*, vol. 1. Orlando, FL: Academic Press, pp. 111–153.

Walker, E. H. 1943. The Plants of China and Their Usefulness to Man. *In Annual Report of the Smithsonian Institution*, pp. 352–61.

_____. 1960. *A Bibliography of Eastern Asiatic Botany; Supplement 1.* Washington, DC: American Institute of Biological Sciences.

_____. 1976. *Flora of Okinawa and the Southern Ryukyu Islands.* Washington, DC: Smithsonian Institution Press.

Wallnöfer, H., and A. von Rottauscher. 1965. *Chinese Folk Medicine.* New York: Crown Publishers.

Wang, X. T., ed. 1978. *The Process of Preparing and Uses of the Small Pieces of Chinese Materia Medica (Zhong Yao Yin Pian Pao Zhi Yu Ying Yong).* Beijing: Institute of Chinese Materia Medica, Academy of Traditional Chinese Medicine, (in Chinese).

Wang, Z. S., D. W. Li, W. J. Xia, H. Q. Qui, and L. Y. Zhu. 1988. The Therapeutic Effect of Herba Leonuri in the Treatment of Coronary Myocardial Ischemia. *Journ. Trad. Chin. Med.* 8(2):103–106.

Weng, P. 1983. Traditional Chinese Medicine. *In* R. H. Bannerman, J. Burton, and W. C. Ch'en, eds., *Traditional Medicine and Health Care Coverage*. Geneva: World Health Organization, pp.68–75.

Wilson, E. H. 1913. *A Naturalist in Western China*. 2 vols. London: Methuen & Co.

———. 1917. *Aristocrats of the Garden*. New York: Doubleday, Page & Co.

———. 1928. *More Aristocrats of the Garden*. Boston: The Stratford Co.

Wyman, D. 1950. The Forsythias. *Arnoldia* 10(2):9–16.

Xiao P. G., and S. L. Fu. 1987. Pharmacologically Active Substances of Chinese Traditional and Herbal Medicines. *In* L. E. Craker and J. E. Simon, eds., *Herbs, Spices, and Medicinal Plants: Recent Advances in Botany, Horticulture, and Pharmacology*, vol 2. Phoenix: AZ: Oryx Press, pp. 1–56.

Xu, G. J., ed. 1986. *A Glossary of Chinese–Latin–English Names of Chinese Traditional and Herbal Drugs*. Nanjing: Nanjing College of Pharmacy.

Yueh, C. H. 1985. Trichosanthes: Identification and Uses. *Update on Herbs* 2(4):23–24.

Yueh, C. H., and C. Y. Cheng. 1974. A Preliminary Study on the Chinese Medicinal Species of the Genus *Trichosanthes* L. *Acta Phytotaxonomica Sinica* 12(4):415–457 (in Chinese).

———. 1980. The Chinese Medicinal Species of the Genus *Trichosanthes* L. *Acta Phytotaxonomica Sinica* 18(3):333–354 (in Chinese).

———. 1982. Second Report of *Tian-hua-fen*. *Acta Pharmaceutica Sinica* 17(10) :766–782 (in Chinese).

Yueh, C. H., and L. T. Ching. 1980. Morphological and Histological Studies on the Chinese Drug *Tian-hua-fen*, its Adulterants and Substitutes. *Acta Pharmaceutica Sinica* 17(10):766–782 (in Chinese).

Yueh, C. H, and Y. L. Zhang. 1986. Studies on the Pollen Morphology of Chinese *Trichosanthes*. *Bulletin of Botanical Research*. 6(2):21–35 (in Chinese).

Yueng, H. C. 1983. *Handbook of Chinese Herbs and Formulas*. 2 vols. Los Angeles: Institute of Chinese Medicine.

Zhang, Q. C. 1990. *Compound Q: Trichosanthin and Its Clinical Applications*. Long Beach, CA: Oriental Healing Arts Institute.

Useful Addresses

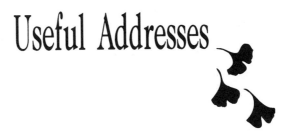

Please note: Most of these businesses charge for their catalogs. Send a self-addressed stamped envelope to inquire on catalog price.

Edible Landscaping
Rt. 2, Box 77
Afton, VA 22920
Good source for unusual fruit trees, including jujube.

Elixir Farm Botanicals
General Delivery
Brixey, MO 65618
Specializing in seed of Chinese herbs, notably astragalus and Baikal scullcap.

Forest Farm
990 Tetherow Rd.
Williams, OR 97544
Excellent source for unusual woody plants and perennials. Includes several species discussed in this book.

J. L. Hudson, Seedsman
P.O. Box 1058
Redwood City, CA 94064
Probably the most comprehensive seed catalog of the rare and unusual.

Logee's Greenhouses
545 North St.
Danielson, CT 06239
Famous source for unusual plants.

Otto Richter & Sons
Goodwood
Ontario LOC 1A0
Canada
Comprehensive herb seed source, including eleuthro.

Thompson & Morgan
P.O. Box 1308
Jackson, NJ 08527
Good general seed source for garden flowers.

We-Du Nurseries
Rt. 5, Box 724
Marion, NC 28752
Excellent source for rare and unusual perennials; many unique Asian offerings.

Woodlanders
1128 Colleton Ave.
Aiken, SC 29801
Excellent source for unusual woody plants, including many trees and shrubs mentioned in this book.

If you can't find specific plants or seeds in the above sources, the following directories are excellent guides to finding plant and seed sources:

Andersen Horticultural Library's Source List of Plants and Seeds (1989), compiled by Richard T. Isaacson. Available for $29.95 postpaid from:
>   The Andersen Horticultural Library
>   Minnesota Landscape Arboretum
>   3675 Arboretum Drive, Box 39
>   Chanhassen, MN 55317

Cornucopia: A Source Book of Edible Plants (1990), by Stephen Facciola. Available for $37.75 postpaid from:
>   Kampong Publications
>   1870 Sunrise Drive
>   Vista, CA 92084

Serious institutionally affiliated researchers can obtain germplasm for research purposes through the U.S. National Plant Germplasm System. See "Chinese Medicinal Plants in the U.S. National Plant Germplasm System," by Mark P. Widrlechner and Steven Foster. *The Herb, Spice, and Medicinal Plant Digest*, Vol. 9, No. 4 (Winter 1991), pp: 1–5. Subscriptions: $10 per year; back issues of the digest available for $3 postpaid from:
>   Dr. Lyle E Craker
>   Department of Plant and Soil Sciences
>   University of Massachussetts
>   Amherst, MA 01003

A new book with germination information on 2000 species of temperate zone plants and revolutionary seed germination concepts is: *Seed Germination: Theory and Practice* by Dr. Norman C. Deno; available for $15.50 postpaid from:
>   Dr. Norman Deno
>   139 Lenor Drive
>   State College, PA 16801

Plant Index

Subject Index

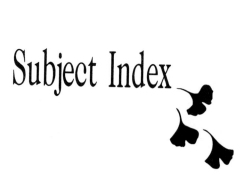